HEPATITIS C: STATE OF THE ART AT THE MILLENNIUM

Editors

Andrea D. Branch, Ph.D.
Associate Professor of Medicine
Division of Liver Diseases
Recanati/Miller Transplantation Institute
Mount Sinai School of Medicine
New York, New York

Leonard B. Seeff, M.D.
Senior Scientist for Hepatitis Research
National Institute of Diabetes and Digestive and Kidney Diseases
National Institutes of Health
Bethesda, Maryland

Project Editor

Paul D. Berk, M.D.
Lillian and Henry M. Stratton Professor of Molecular Medicine
Chief, Division of Liver Diseases
Mount Sinai School of Medicine
New York, New York

Thieme New York
333 Seventh Avenue
New York, NY 10001

Compositor: Compset, Inc.
Printer: The Sheridan Press

The material in this volume has been previously published in *Seminars in Liver Disease*, volume 20, numbers 1 and 2, 2000.

Library of Congress Cataloging-in-Publication Data are available from the publisher.

Printed in the United States of America

5 4 3 2 1

TNY ISBN 0-86577-998-8
GTV ISBN 3 13 127251 1

Contents

i   **Introduction — Hepatitis C: The Virus that Created Hepatology**
Paul D. Berk, M.D.

iii   **Foreword**
Andrea D. Branch, Ph.D. and Leonard B. Seeff, M.D.

1   **Epidemiology of Hepatitis C: Geographic Differences and Temporal Trends**
Annemarie Wasley, Sc.D. and Miriam J. Alter, Ph.D.

17   **Recovery, Persistance, and Sequelae in Hepatitis C Virus Infection:
A Perspective on Long-Term Outcome**
Harvey J. Alter, M.D. and Leonard B. Seeff, M.D.

37   **Transmission, Natural History, and Treatment of Hepatitis C Virus Infection in
the Pediatric Population**
Jeffrey B. Schwimmer, M.D. and William F. Balistreri, M.D.

47   **Fibrosis in Patients with Chronic Hepatitis C: Detection and Significance**
*Thierry Poynard, M.D., Ph.D., Vlad Ratziu, M.D., Yves Benmanov, M.D., Vincent Di
Martino, M.D., Pierre Bedossa, M.D., Ph.D., and Pierre Opolon, M.D.*

57   **Hepatitis C Virus RNA Codes for Proteins and Replicates: Does It Also Trigger
the Interferon Response?**
Andrea D. Branch, Ph.D.

69   **Biochemical and Immunologic Properties of the Nonstructural Proteins of the
Hepatitis C Virus: Implications for Development of Antiviral Agents and
Vaccines**
*Raffaele De Francesco, Ph.D., Petra Neddermann, Ph.D., Licia Tomei, Ph.D.,
Christian Steinkühler, Paola Gallinari, Ph.D., and Antonella Folgori, Ph.D.*

85   **Distribution of Markers of HCV Infection Throughout the Body**
Eric J. Gowans, M.D.

103   **Clinical Significance of Hepatitis C Virus Genotypes and Quasispecies**
Patrizia Farci, M.D. and Robert H. Purcell, M.D.

CONTENTS

127   Interaction between the Hepatitis C Virus and the Immune System
      Barbara Rehermann, M.D.

143   The Lymphoid System in Hepatitis C Virus Infection: Autoimmunity, Mixed
      Cryoglobulinemia, and Overt B-Cell Malignancy
      Franco Dammacco, M.D., Domenico Sansonno, M.D., Claudia Piccoli, B.Sc.,
      Vito Racanelli, M.D., Francesca Paola D'Amore, B.Sc.,
      and Gianfranco Lauletta, M.D.

159   Diagnostic Testing for Hepatitis C
      Robert L. Carithers, Jr., M.D., Anthony Marquardt, and
      David R. Gretch, M.D., Ph.D.

173   Hepatitis C Kinetics: Mathematical Modeling of Viral Response to Therapy
      Thomas J. Layden, M.D., Brian Mika, B.S., and Thelma E. Wiley, M.D.

185   Antiviral Therapy of Patients with Chronic Hepatitis C
      Jenny Heathcote, M.B., B.S., M.D., FRCP, FRCP(C)

201   Hepatitis C after Liver Transplantation
      Patricia A. Sheiner, M.D.

211   Vaccine Development for Hepatitis C
      Martin Lechmann, Ph.D. and T. Jake Liang, M.D.

DIAGNOSTIC PROBLEMS IN HEPATOLOGY

227   A 67-Year-Old Man with Hepatitis C Virus Infection and a Liver Tumor
      Arief Suriawinata, M.D., Katya Ivanov, M.D., Menahem Ben Haim, M.D., and Myron E. Schwartz, M.D.

233   Afterword
      Andrea D. Branch, Ph.D. and Leonard B. Seeff, M.D.

239   Index

This volume is a compilation of the articles published in *Seminars in Liver Disease*, volume 20, numbers 1
and 2, 2000.

Introduction
Hepatitis C: The Virus that Created Hepatology

This first issue of *Seminars in Liver Disease* of the 21st century is also the first of two issues of volume 20 devoted to the hepatitis C virus (HCV). Since its discovery by a team at Chiron Corporation in 1989,[1,2] this virus and the disease(s) it causes has dominated both the literature and the practice of clinical hepatology. Following on the heels of the dramatic clinical impact of liver transplantation (to be reviewed in November 2000, with Dr. Michael F. Sorrell as Guest Editor), hepatitis C has been one of the major factors contributing to the emergence of hepatology as a widely recognized and respected independent discipline. HCV is the subject of hundreds of abstracts submitted to the annual meetings of each of the major national and international associations devoted to the study of the liver, the subject of the numerous drug company-sponsored satellite symposia that have become the standard appendages to these meetings, and the sole focus of a growing number of hepatitis C-specific conferences each year around the world. Hepatitis C has become not only big science, but also big business, making hepatology and hepatologists, for better or worse, the recipients of a degree of industry-sponsored attention and generosity not previously known in our field.

As these first sixteen articles of the year 2000 will clearly document, hepatitis C is, in fact, a puzzling and fascinating pathogen. Its quasispecies nature, its confusing and uncertain natural history, its involvement in the pathogenesis of a variety of disorders of the immune system including cryoglobulinemia and B-cell lymphomas, and its stimulation of a hepatic fibrotic process that evolves to cirrhosis at a rate largely independent of the degree of inflammatory activity, are among the interesting characteristics described in these issues, but requiring still further study. Even the genomic organization of the virus is not yet fully defined, as illustrated by the recent discovery of an alternative (+1) reading frame encoding previously unrecognized viral protein(s).[3] One of the most unusual features of HCV is the extent to which what we know about it has been so largely defined by elements of the pharmaceutical industry.

The Guest Editors for these two issues of *Seminars* are Andrea Branch, Ph.D. and Leonard Seeff, M.D. Dr. Branch refers to herself as an RNA biochemist. Many consider her a molecular virologist. In either case, after a distinguished career defining the nature and life cycles of plant viroids and the hepatitis delta agent (HDV), she now focuses her remarkable analytical skill on hepatitis C. Indeed, it was her laboratory that deduced, on purely theoretical grounds, the likely existence of an alternate reading frame in the HCV genome, and then documented its existence by demonstrating that patients with chronic HCV infection have antibodies against peptides encoded in such a reading frame. Dr. Seeff, in contrast, is the consummate creative clinical investigator. He has long been at the forefront of studies aimed at determining the natural history of hepatitis C and is responsible for some of the most compelling data that indicate that, overall, the majority of chronically infected patients do not develop symptomatic liver disease from HCV for three or more decades after infection, if ever. Together, their expertise covers the broadest possible spectrum of HCV virology, pathology, and disease. They and the colleagues they have selected to contribute to these issues tell a remarkable and challenging story.

However, even two full issues of *Seminars* do not cover all aspects of this fascinating subject in detail. The pathogenetic role of hepatitis C in hepatocellular carcinoma was examined just two issues ago, in August 1999,[4,5] and articles one issue earlier examined the role of cytokines in HCV etiopathogenesis and in fibrogenesis.[6,7] The February 1995 issue, devoted entirely to hepatitis C and again guest edited by Dr. Seeff (clearly a glutton for punishment), contains many still highly important articles, of which I will cite only two.[8,9]

Hepatitis C did not make it into *Seminars'* first issue (February 1981), edited by Dr. Harvey Alter, and devoted to hepatitis B. However, when we returned to the subject in the second Alter-edited issue on viral hepatitis five years later (February 1986), two seminal articles anticipated the subsequent discovery of HCV.[10,11] And our tenth anniversary issue on viral hepatitis (May 1991), edited by Dr. Jules Dienstag, devoted all or at

0272–8087,p;2000,20,01,000i,00ii,ftx,en;sld00050b

least a portion of five of its eight articles to the recently discovered hepatitis C virus. There is little doubt that further issues of *Seminars* will be devoted to this virus in the future.

For illness resulting from hepatitis C, as with many other hepatic disorders of both infectious and noninfectious etiologies, the obvious goal of hepatologists is disease eradication. In the short run, this means effective treatment of existing cases and in the longer run, disease prevention. Although articles in these two issues document that progress is being made on both fronts, treatment of established infection, while clearly improving, is far from optimal and a proven hepatitis C vaccine does not appear to be around the corner. Neither the clinicians who treat HCV-infected patients nor the scientists who work on the fundamental problems of the biology of the virus and the body's responses to infection are threatened with impending unemployment. HCV is providing plenty of work for all.

In the battle against hepatitis C, therefore, these issues of *Seminars* describe a work in progress. While progress there is, there are also many obvious and important, yet incompletely answered questions. A critical function of these issues is not only to convey what is known, but to focus attention on the many things that are not.

Paul D. Berk, M.D.
Editor in Chief

REFERENCES

1. Choo QL, Kuo G, Weiner AJ, et al. Isolation of a cDNA clone derived from a blood-borne non-A, non-B viral hepatitis genome. Science 1989;244:359–362
2. Kuo G, Choo QL, Alter HJ, et al. An assay for circulating antibodies to a major etiologic virus of human non-A, non-B hepatitis. Science 1989;244:362–364
3. Walewski JL, Stump DD, Keller TR, Branch AD. HCV patients have antibodies against a novel protein encoded in a second reading frame. Hepatol 1998;28:279A (Abstr)
4. Colombo M. Hepatitis C virus and hepatocellular carcinoma. Semin Liver Dis 1999;19:263–269
5. Bosch FX, Ribes J, Borras J. Epidemiology of primary liver cancer. Semin Liver Dis 1999;19:271–285
6. Koziel MJ. The role of cytokines in viral hepatitis. Semin Liver Dis 1999;19:157–169
7. Friedman SL. Cytokines and fibrogenesis. Semin Liver Dis 1999;19:129–140
8. Goodman ZD, Ishak KG. Histopathology of hepatitis C viral infection. Semin Liver Dis 1999;15:70–81
9. Koff RS, Dienstag JL. Extrahepatic manifestation of hepatitis C and the association with alcoholic liver disease. Semin Liver Dis 1999;15:101–109
10. Bradley DW, Maynard JE. Etiology and natural history of posttransfusion and enterically-transmitted non-A, non-B hepatitis. Semin Liver Dis 1999;6:56–66
11. Dienstag JL, Alter HJ. Non-A, non-B hepatitis: Evolving epidemiologic and clinical perspectives. Semin Liver Dis 1999;6:67–81

Foreword

Guest Editors: Andrea D. Branch, Ph.D. and Leonard B. Seeff, M.D.

Five years ago, the winter issue of *Seminars in Liver Disease* was devoted to hepatitis C virus (HCV). Articles described the epidemiology of HCV, diagnostic assays, genetic diversity (quasispecies and genotypes), hepatocellular carcinoma, histopathology, therapies, transplantation, and extrahepatic manifestations. The studies reviewed in that issue established a foundation for much of the subsequent research in the field. Many of these advances will be presented in this year's winter and spring issues of *Seminars*.

The winter issue begins with a series of four articles providing an updated view of HCV's impact on human populations. HCV epidemiology, natural history in adults and children, and risk factors for disease progression (fibrosis) are reviewed. Attention then shifts to the virus itself with four articles describing HCV RNA, nonstructural proteins, genetic diversity, and distribution throughout the body. HCV molecular virology is presented with an emphasis on the clinical implications of basic research findings. Potential pharmaceutical targets and vaccine components are identified, genotypes and interferon sensitivity are analyzed, and measurements of HCV products in the liver are related to pathogenesis. The clinical consequences of HCV infection will be the focus of the spring issue, with articles on immune responses to HCV, B-cell abnormalities (including cryoglobulinemia), diagnostic tests, kinetic studies of HCV clearance during therapy, factors influencing responses to interferon–ribavirin combination therapy, liver transplantation, and vaccine development.

To provide a backdrop for the next two issues of *Seminars*, HCV's indolent lifestyle and unusual biologic niche are discussed below. HCV survives because it is able to hide in plain sight, using a variety of adaptations to elude the immune system and maintain chronic viremia. Understanding these adaptations will help us to prevent their pathogenic consequences and to break the chain of HCV transmission.

GETTING BY WITH A LITTLE HELP

HCV is a subtle pathogen with a unique *modus operandi*. It lingers in the blood for years waiting for human activities—needlesticks, ceremonial cutting, medicinal exchanges of human blood, perhaps even hand-to-hand combat—to move from one person to another. Sexual and perinatal transmission may occur, but only at a low rate. New infections are usually established in immunocompetent adults (see Wasley and Alter), although children are also at risk (see Schwimmer and Balistreri). HCV has used its unusual mode of transmission to establish a global presence. Other pathogens use more familiar routes, such as oral/fecal (used by hepatitis A virus [HAV] and many bacteria), arthropod vectors (used by the agents of yellow fever and lyme disease), airborne respiratory secretions (which spread tuberculosis and rhinoviruses), and sexual contact (responsible for gonorrhea and human immunodeficiency virus).

By providing transportation out of the bloodstream and into new hosts, humans unwittingly provide an important service to the virus. Unlike most other microbes, HCV does not need to breach epithelial barriers on its own (Fig 1). Thus, HCV does not need to pass out of the body in excretions or secretions nor does it need strategies for gaining access to these substances. Furthermore, HCV does not need protection against extremes of heat, cold, high acidity, or any other harsh environmental conditions. It is exempt from selection pressures that constrain most other infectious agents. This exemption may confer an extra degree of freedom and account for the plasticity of the HCV genome, which is manifested by the variability of HCV genotypes and quasispecies (see Farci and Purcell). Its ability to accommodate genetic change may be one of several characteristics that benefits HCV in an ongoing war with the immune system.

0272–8087,p;2000,20,01,0iii,00iv,ftx,en;sld00048c

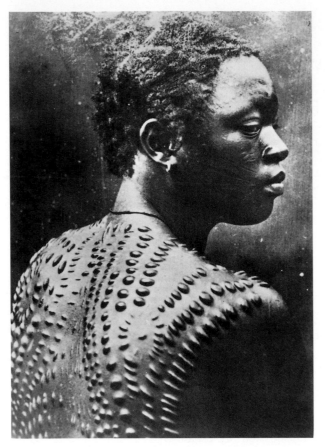

FIG. 1. Cultural practices may have contributed to HCV transmission: Tabwa woman with scars on face and back, circa 1900. Beginning in childhood, razors made by local blacksmiths were used to slit skin plucked up with an acacia thorn, fishhook, or arrowhead. Elaborate scar patterns were created on their faces, chests, abdomens, and backs of women to prove their ability to endure pain; men bore simpler patterns. The original photograph, part of the White Fathers' Central Archives, Rome, was reproduced by A.F. Roberts in *Marks of Civilization*, University of California, L.A., and is shown here with the kind permission of the author.

SURVIVAL STRATEGIES

Frustrating the immune system has been one of HCV's central accomplishments. The others are infecting liver cells and persisting in the bloodstream. Its unusual mode of transmission frees HCV to focus its genetic capital on these three objectives. HCV has evolved a series of adaptations that serve it well. HCV routinely establishes a chronic liver infection and often remains in the blood at levels exceeding one million genomes per milliliter for decades.

Because HCV has no need to rupture cells or to cause lesions in the body, it has little to gain, and much to lose, by causing liver pathology. Accordingly, many patients have little evidence of liver injury (see Alter and Seeff). This suggests that HCV has adaptations to minimize both direct and indirect (immune-mediated) cell damage. Unfortunately, the relationship between

HCV and the liver is not entirely harmonious. The immune system makes a relentless effort to eradicate the virus, which takes a toll on the liver, especially in older men who drink alcohol (see Poynard et al.). HCV infection has a number of immunologic consequences, including stimulation of specific T-cell and B-cell responses, development of cryoglobulinemia, and elevations of certain cytokines. HCV is reported to replicate in lymphocytes and may alter their functioning. Other viruses, such as dengue fever virus, turn human immune responses to their advantage. It is possible that HCV does this as well, although not necessarily through the same mechanism as dengue fever virus. Unlike liver pathology, which appears to have no up side for HCV, some of the immune responses it provokes may be advantageous.

BLESSINGS OF HEPATOTROPISM

The liver is the body's largest internal organ and has a tremendous potential for self-renewal. Adaptations that allow HCV to reach the liver and to replicate within the hepatic environment are essential for viral survival. The liver's regenerative capacity allows it to endure years of cell damage and death. Lesser organs would shrivel if forced to produce over one trillion virions per day, but the liver can sustain this rate of viral production, and the consequent immune responses, for decades.

The liver's vast size means that a substantial viremia can result even if each cell produces only a few virions a day. This low yield per cell may be essential for a virus that needs to elude the adult immune system. During chronic infection, HCV RNA and proteins are present in such low amounts that they are difficult to detect in biopsy specimens (see Gowans).

LIVING TO FIGHT ANOTHER DAY

The low rate of production may benefit HCV by ensuring that infected cells are difficult for the immune system to recognize. Minimal production occurs even in cell culture systems, suggesting that HCV has built-in mechanisms for downregulating production (see Branch).

In addition, several lines of evidence suggest that signals from the immune system diminish the rate of viral production. For example, serum levels of HCV are higher during acute infection than during chronic infection, and this decline is usually accomplished without clinical evidence of hepatitis. It is likely that the reduction in viremia testifies to a partial victory by the immune system. Similarly, interferon treatment causes a rapid reduction in the serum levels of HCV RNA without causing a rise in serum levels of liver enzymes. Finally, in a related system, hepatitis B virus (HBV) gene expression in transgenic mice can be abolished by treatment with cytokines in the *absence* of cell lysis. HCV proteins may mediate viral responses to interferon: If viral proteins, such as NS5a, have affinity for interferon-inducible proteins, high levels of interferon (whether produced naturally or administered pharmaceutically) will cause these viral proteins to be sequestered, attenuating HCV production. Interactions between viral and cellular proteins may also contribute to persistence by blocking the interferon response and other immune defenses (see De Francesco et al.). As a final adaptation, HCV may respond to interferon treatment by shifting genetically toward a more benign population of sequences. Such a shift is in accord with the observation that interferon treatment confers long-term benefit even in the absence of viral clearance (see Poynard et al.).

HEPATIC CLOAKING DEVICE

The liver not only provides HCV with a vast and durable production site, its unusual relationship with the immune system may contribute to persistence. The liver is associated with dramatic displays of tolerance. For example, liver grafts can protect transplanted kidneys that would otherwise be rejected. Moreover, a high percentage of infants born to HBV-infected mothers develop a chronic infection even though they are capable of mounting protective immune responses if inoculated with the HBV vaccine in the early postnatal period. Thus, the HBV surface antigen is tolerated when produced by the liver but confers protective immunity when presented from an extrahepatic site as part of a vaccine. This latter example is especially noteworthy because it suggests that once immune responses have been stimulated elsewhere in the body, they are capable of clearing an infection that has already been estab-

lished in the liver. The immune system is clearly capable of responding to HBV antigens, and it may be capable of responding to HCV proteins if they are presented in the proper context. Chronic infection may occur, in part, because parenteral transmission allows HCV to enter the human body without activating the immune system.

In contrast to HCV and HBV, HAV and hepatitis E virus (HEV) are transmitted by the oral/fecal route and generally do not establish chronic infections. To gain access to the bloodstream, lymph, and eventually the liver, HAV and HEV must cross the gut. During this passage, these viruses are likely to trigger immune responses. This initial activation may set the stage for clearance from the liver. The body's major portals—the gastrointestinal, the respiratory, and the urogenital tracts—are all monitored by the immune system. Parenteral transmission cuts across the immune defenses at these ports of entry. Of course, parenteral transmission has a downside: When there is no way out, home can turn into prison.

The success of the HBV vaccine bodes well for the development of an HCV vaccine. However, development of an HCV vaccine may be considerably more difficult. HBV depends more heavily on vertical transmission than HCV, and the immune system of neonates may be easier to thwart than that of adults. Perhaps as a reflection of its reliance on infection of neonates, HBV strains from around the world share a conserved surface feature, the "a" determinant, which has no known counterpart in HCV. The preservation of this conserved feature suggests that HBV has not been under as intense pressure to evolve escape variants as HCV. Nonetheless, by understanding the interplay between HCV and the immune system, it may be possible to lift the hepatic cloaking device, paving the way for vaccines and immunotherapies that are more effective and less toxic than the current regimens.

Epidemiology of Hepatitis C: Geographic Differences and Temporal Trends

ANNEMARIE WASLEY, Sc.D. and MIRIAM J. ALTER, Ph.D.

ABSTRACT: *Hepatitis C Virus (HCV) infection appears to be endemic in most parts of the world, with an estimated overall prevalence of 3%. However, there is considerable geographic and temporal variation in the incidence and prevalence of HCV infection. Using age-specific prevalence data, at least three distinct transmission patterns can be identified. In countries with the first pattern (e.g., United States, Australia), most infections are found among persons 30–49 years old, indicating that the risk for HCV infection was greatest in the relatively recent past (10–30 years ago) and primarily affected young adults. In countries with the second pattern (e.g., Japan, Italy), most infections are found among older persons, consistent with the risk for HCV infection having been greatest in the distant past. In countries with the third pattern (e.g., Egypt), high rates of infection are observed in all age groups, indicating an ongoing high risk for acquiring HCV infection. In countries with the first pattern, injection drug use has been the predominant risk factor for HCV infection, whereas in those with the second or third patterns, unsafe injections and contaminated equipment used in healthcare-related procedures appear to have played a predominant role in transmission. Much of the variability between regions can be explained by the frequency and extent to which different risk factors have contributed to the transmission of HCV. Because different strategies are required to interrupt different patterns of HCV transmission, determining the epidemiology of HCV infection in areas where that information has not yet been assessed is critical for developing appropriate prevention programs.*

KEY WORDS: hepatitis C, epidemiology

Hepatitis C virus (HCV) is a bloodborne pathogen that appears to be endemic in most parts of the world. HCV is the most common cause of posttransfusion hepatitis worldwide and a leading cause of end-stage liver disease requiring liver transplantation. There is, however, considerable geographic and temporal variation in the incidence and prevalence of HCV infection. Much of this variability can be explained by differences in the frequency and extent to which different risk factors have contributed to the transmission of community-acquired HCV infection.

Objectives

Upon completion of this article the reader should be able to: 1) list five known risk factors for HCV infection, and 2) describe how the relative contribution of those risk factors as sources of infection has varied geographically and temporally.

Accreditation

The Indiana University School of Medicine is accredited by the Accreditation Council for Continuing Medical Education to sponsor continuing medical education for physicians. The Indiana University School of Medicine takes responsibility for the contents, quality, and scientific integrity of this activity.

Credit

The Indiana University School of Medicine designates this educational activity for a maximum of 1.0 hours credit toward the AMA Physicians Recognition Award in category one. Each physician should claim only those hours of credit that he/she actually spent in the educational activity.

Disclosure

Statements have been obtained regarding the authors' relationships with financial supporters of this activity. There is no apparent conflict of interest related to the context of participation of the author of this article.

From the Hepatitis Branch, Centers for Disease Control and Prevention, Atlanta, Georgia.
Reprint requests: Annemarie Wasley, Sc.D., Hepatitis Branch, Mailstop G37, Centers for Disease Control and Prevention, Atlanta, GA 30333.
Copyright © 2000 by Thieme Medical Publishers, Inc., 333 Seventh Avenue, New York, NY 10001, USA. Tel.: +1(212) 584-4663.
0272–8087,p;2000,20,01,0001,0016,ftx;en;sld00049x

GEOGRAPHIC PATTERNS OF HCV INFECTION

It is estimated by the World Health Organization that the global prevalence of HCV infection averages 3%, representing approximately 170 million HCV-infected persons worldwide.[1] Although the most valid estimates of the prevalence of HCV infection are provided by data from population-based surveys, such information is not available from most parts of the world. Consequently, prevalence estimates from selected populations, such as blood donors, are frequently used to assess the burden of HCV infection. Many published studies reporting the prevalence of antibody to HCV (anti-HCV) among blood donors have been based on repeatedly reactive results by enzyme immunoassays (EIA) without supplemental testing, which may have resulted in their overestimating the prevalence of infection in this population group.

On the basis of studies among blood donors that used both EIA and supplemental testing (Fig. 1), the lowest anti-HCV prevalence rates (0.01–0.1%) have been reported from the United Kingdom [2–4] and Scandanavia.[5,6] Low but slightly higher rates (0.2–0.0.5%) have been reported from Western Europe,[7–10] North America,[11–13] most areas of Central and South America,[14–18] Australia,[19] and limited regions of Africa, including South Africa.[20–22] Intermediate rates of anti-HCV prevalence (1–5%) have been reported from Brazil,[23,24] Eastern Europe, the Mediterranean,[25–30] the Mideast, the Indian subcontinent,[31–35] parts of Africa,[36–41] and Asia.[42–56] A single study from Libya re-

ported a rate of 7%,[57] but by far the highest HCV prevalence rates (17–26%) have been reported from Egypt.[58–60] Although estimates of prevalence derived from studies of blood donors provide information about the relative magnitude of regional differences in the prevalence of HCV infection, they underestimate the absolute burden of infection, because even first-time blood donors are highly selected populations and are not representative of the infection rates in the general population. For example, in the United States, the prevalence of HCV infection among volunteer blood donors in 1990 was 0.6%, threefold lower than the 1.8% prevalence in the general population.[61] Furthermore, even among studies of similar populations, such as blood donors, comparisons may not be valid because of differences in testing methodologies, as well as in the degree to which individuals with risk factors for HCV infection may have been excluded.

There are a limited number of population-based studies on the age-specific prevalence of HCV infection. These studies demonstrate at least three distinct epidemiologic profiles of HCV transmission that can be identified worldwide (Fig. 2). These profiles reflect not only regional variations in the prevalence of HCV infection but also variations in the time period(s) during which there was an increased risk for acquiring HCV infection.

In the first pattern, age-specific prevalence is low among persons less than 20 years old; rises steadily through middle age, with most infections occurring among adults 30–49 years old; and declines sharply among persons greater than 50 years old. This pattern,

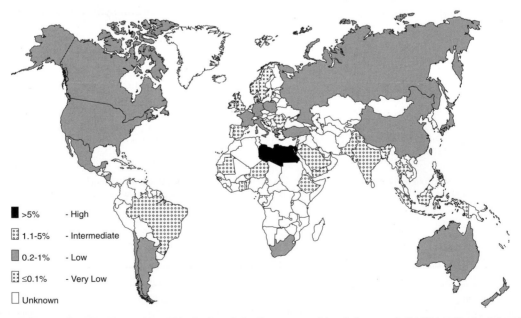

FIG. 1.   Global prevalence of antibodies to hepatitis C virus infection among blood donors. Anti-HCV antibody determined by EIA with supplemental testing. The figure is based on the data available in January 2000.

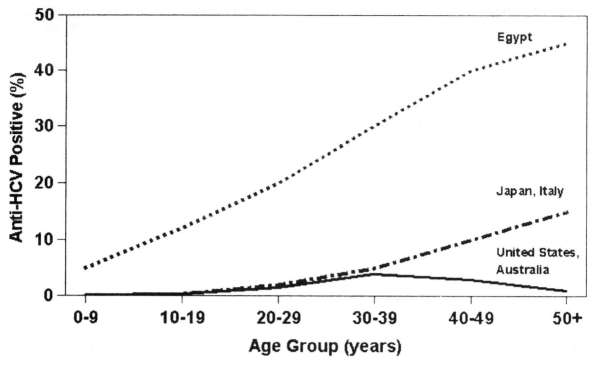

FIG. 2. Patterns of HCV infection: geographic differences in the age-specific prevalence of anti-HCV antibodies.

found in the United States[61] and Australia,[62,63] suggests that most HCV transmission occurred in the relatively recent past (10–30 years ago) and primarily among young adults. In the United States, estimates derived from catalytic modeling of these age-specific prevalence data indicate that the incidence of newly acquired HCV infection was low (18/100,000) before 1965, increased steadily through 1980, and remained high (130/100,000, corresponding to an average of 240,000 infections per year) through 1989.[64] Since 1989, the incidence of HCV infection has declined more than 80% based on trends in reported cases.[65]

In the second pattern, age-specific prevalence is low in children and younger adults but increases sharply among older persons, who account for most infections. This type of pattern is seen in Japan[66,67] and Italy[68,69] and is consistent with the risk for HCV infection having been greatest in the distant past (30–50 years ago).

In the third pattern, the prevalence of HCV infection increases steadily with age, and high rates of infection are observed among persons in all age groups. This pattern, seen in Egypt,[70,71] indicates an increased risk in the distant past followed by an ongoing high risk for acquiring HCV infection.

These age-specific prevalence patterns provide information to assess how the burden of disease due to HCV infection may change during the coming years. In the United States and other countries where the emergence of HCV infection is a relatively recent event, the magnitude of the burden of HCV-related chronic liver

disease has yet to be realized. In contrast, in countries where the emergence of HCV infection occurred in the distant past, the burden of disease might have already peaked, although changes in disease transmission patterns that result in increased infection rates among younger persons could result in future increases in chronic disease as this cohort ages. In countries where there have been ongoing high levels of HCV transmission, the magnitude of both the current and future burden of disease are of concern.

DISEASE TRANSMISSION PATTERNS

Many geographic and temporal differences in prevalence of HCV infection can be related to the relative importance of different risk factors over time. Globally, the most frequently cited risk factors for HCV infection are blood transfusion from unscreened donors and injection drug use. However, in some parts of the world, exposures to infectious blood from other health-care-related procedures and cultural practices are being increasingly recognized as playing an important role in HCV transmission.

Injection Drug Use

Injection drug use is one of the most efficient routes for HCV transmission. In the United States and Australia (pattern 1), where most infections have been acquired in young adults, illegal use of injection drugs has been the dominant mode of HCV transmission during the past 30 years, accounting for 60%[61] and 80%,[62,63] respectively, of prevalent infections. HCV infection is acquired more rapidly after initiation of injection drug use than other viral infections, and after 5 years of injection, 50–90% of users are infected with HCV.[72–74]

In the United States, drug-use-related risk factors for acquiring HCV infection include frequent use, sharing of drug paraphenalia, injecting cocaine, and first injecting with an older user.[72,73] Thus, the rapid acquisition of HCV infection among injection drug users is likely explained by their high prevalence of chronic infection and their particular drug-using behaviors, both of which facilitate the likelihood of exposure among new users to an HCV-infected person. A high proportion of new HCV infections continues to be associated with injection drug use, but for reasons that are unclear, the dramatic decline in the incidence of acute hepatitis C since 1989 in the United States correlates with a decrease in cases among injection drug users.[65,72,75]

In countries where the increased incidence of HCV infection occurred in the distant past (patterns 2 and 3), injection drug use appears to have played a minor role, although its contribution to more recent transmission may be increasing. In both Japan and Italy, the highest incidence of infection is now among young adults.[76,77] In Italy, a history of injection drug use is reported by half of persons with newly acquired hepatitis C and by 40% of persons less than 40 years old with chronic hepatitis C.[77,78] In contrast, none of those with chronic infection over 40 years old reported injection drug use.[78] In one study from Egypt, a history of injection drug use was reported by two thirds of HCV-positive paid professional blood donors.[58]

Intranasal cocaine use as a route for HCV transmission remains to be established. Although it is biologically plausible that such transmission could occur through the shared use of blood-contaminated straws, to date only one study has reported an association between intranasal cocaine use and HCV infection that was independent of injection drug use.[79] Not only was this study performed in a highly selected population (i.e., volunteer blood donors), but cross-sectional seroprevalence surveys have serious limitations for making causal inferences, particularly when the studies do not use random (probability) sampling.[80] Furthermore, cocaine use (by injection or noninjection) has been reported by a high proportion (13% overall; 22% among 25–39 year olds) of the general population in the United States,[61] and intranasal cocaine use specifically has been reported by >10% of HCV-negative blood donors.[79,81] In contrast, such a history is uncommon (<5%) in the absence of injection drug use among patients with recently

acquired hepatitis C.[65] Thus, we cannot conclude that intranasal cocaine use places persons at risk for HCV infection until more data are available, including whether persons with a history of intranasal cocaine use alone are likely to be infected with HCV.

Transfusions and Transplants

Transfusion of blood or plasma-derived products and transplantation of solid organs from HCV-infected donors to their recipients are highly effective routes for transmitting HCV.[82] In areas of the world where HCV testing of blood and organ donations has not been feasible, these exposures remain important sources for infection. However, in most developed countries, infectious disease screening and testing practices have eliminated most transfusion- and transplant-related transmission of HCV and other bloodborne pathogens. In such countries, incidence rates of posttransfusion hepatitis C ranged from 5% to 13% before 1986,[83–90] declined to between 1.5% and 9% from 1986 to 1990,[85,87,89] and then to between 0.6% and 3% after the introduction of first-generation anti-HCV testing.[88,90–92] The implementation of more sensitive multiantigen testing has further reduced the risk of transfusion-associated HCV infection to an estimated 0.01%–0.9% per recipient transfused.[90,93] It can be assumed that the use of anti-HCV-negative organ and tissue donors also has reduced the risk of HCV transmission from transplantation.

Hemophilia patients who were heavily transfused with nontreated factor concentrates have prevalence rates of anti-HCV exceeding 90%, which along with those for injection drug users are the highest of any group studied.[82] However, in countries that have implemented effective viral inactivation of clotting factor concentrates, these blood products as a source for HCV infection have been virtually eliminated.

Unsafe Injections and Other Healthcare-Related Procedures

In developed countries, appropriate use of disposable equipment and effective disinfection and sterilization procedures have reduced the transmission of bloodborne pathogens, including HCV. Transmission of HCV from healthcare-related procedures is rarely reported (except in the chronic hemodialysis setting) , and in the United States, case control studies have not found an association between standard medical care procedures and transmission of HCV.[94,95] However, because most individuals acutely infected with HCV have no or mild symptoms, detecting cases of nosocomial transmission of HCV is difficult, and those episodes that are detected may represent a relatively small proportion of health-care-related cases of HCV infection. Consequently, although it is still unlikely that such infections occur frequently, it is possible that they may occur more often than is currently recognized.

In the healthcare setting, patients may serve as a reservoir for transmission, and the prevalence among patients in hospital-related (inpatient and outpatient) settings has been reported to range from 2 to 18%[96–99] and in chronic hemodialysis settings to average 20%.[82] The few reported episodes of HCV transmission from patient to patient in hospital-related settings have mostly involved unsafe injection practices resulting in contamination of equipment used for phlebotomy or flushing intravenous lines or of multiple dose medication vials.[100–103] Contaminated equipment that was not adequately cleaned or disinfected and was shared among patients has been implicated in one report of HCV transmission to two patients during colonoscopy[104] and is the likely source for transmission among chronic hemodialysis patients.

Among hemodialysis patients, the prevalence of HCV infection varies widely across different geographic regions,[25,105–125] which may reflect differences not only in background rates of infection but also in practices related to infection control. The lowest rates have been reported in the United Kingdom and South Africa (1–5%) and the highest in Eastern Europe (20–91%). Intermediate anti-HCV prevalence rates of 10–50% have been reported among hemodialysis patients in North America, Scandanavia, Western and Southern Europe, and Asia. Among anti-HCV-negative hemodialysis patients with no other identified risk factors for infection, the incidence of HCV infection has been estimated at approximately 2–2.6%/year.[105,125–127] A correlation between increasing years on dialysis and anti-HCV positivity that was independent of blood transfusion has been demonstrated in both incidence and prevalence studies.[105,112,122,128–130]

These studies, as well as investigations of dialysis-associated outbreaks of hepatitis C, indicate that HCV might be transmitted among these patients because of incorrect implementation of infection-control procedures. In a recent investigation of an outbreak of HCV infection among chronic hemodialysis patients in the United States, 17% of the susceptible patients acquired HCV infection during a 16-month period, and infection was associated with chronically infected patients at the same station (and same machine) on the same day (Centers for Disease Control and Prevention [CDC], unpublished data, 1999). Multiple opportunities for cross-contamination between patients were observed, including shared equipment and supplies that were not disinfected between patient use, shared multiple-dose medication vials that were placed at patients' stations on top of machines; and contaminated priming buckets that were not routinely changed or cleaned and disinfected between patients.

In countries where the period of increased risk for HCV infection occurred in the distant past, healthcare-related procedures performed both by professionals and nonprofessionals appear to have been a major mode of HCV transmission. In Japan and Italy, geographic clustering of infections among older persons has been reported that is associated not only with transfusions from unscreened donors but also with unsafe injection practices (including reuse of contaminated glass syringes and at-home administration by nonprofessionals using shared syringes among family, friends, and neighbors), surgical procedures, and folk medicine practices (e.g., in Japan, acupuncture performed by unlicensed therapists and traditional remedies performed by family members using nonsterile instruments).[68,78,131–133] The lower prevalence in younger age groups in these populations suggest that these exposures may no longer play a role in transmission.

In countries where the increased risk for HCV infection has been ongoing for many decades, there is evidence that healthcare-related procedures have been the major source for transmission. In Egypt, transmission of HCV has been attributed to unsafe injection practices associated with reuse of glass syringes during mass campaigns to treat schistosomiasis with injection therapy during 1960–1987.[59,70–71,134] Although those campaigns no longer exist, use of common syringes and a history of medical care procedures involving injections or hospitalization continue to be associated with HCV infection, suggesting that unsafe injection practices are playing an ongoing role in transmission.[59]

The role of unsafe injections in the transmission of bloodborne pathogens is being increasingly recognized and has been documented in several other countries, including Romania, Moldova, and Pakistan.[135–137] Injection-associated bloodborne pathogen transmission occurs when infection control practices are inadequate, and overuse of injections to administer medications might increase opportunities for transmission. In many developing countries, supplies of sterile syringes may be inadequate or nonexistent, injections are often administered outside the medical setting by nonprofessionals, and injections are often given to deliver medication that could be otherwise delivered by the oral route. In addition to unsafe injection practices, inadequate cleaning and disinfection of equipment used in medical and dental settings may also be a major source of HCV transmission in developing countries.

The risk of HCV transmission from infected healthcare workers to patients during the performance of invasive procedures appears to be very low. There have been two reports of HCV transmission attributed to healthcare workers performing such procedures, both involving HCV-infected cardiothoracic surgeons. In the one from Spain, the surgeon transmitted infection to five of his patients during a 6-year period, although the factors responsible for transmission were not identified.[138] In the second report from the United Kingdom, only a single episode of transmission was identified from among 277 patients of the surgeon (who was in training) during a 13-month period.[139]

In the United States, a retrospective investigation was performed of an HCV-infected plastic surgeon whose infection was diagnosed during a routine physical examination (CDC, unpublished data, 1999). HCV testing of 268 (85%) of the surgeon's patients was performed more than 6 months after their surgery, and no provider-to-patient transmission was detected. One other report of an HCV-infected healthcare worker from the United States involved a chronically infected outpatient surgical technician who did not perform exposure prone invasive procedures but who was addicted to narcotics and injected himself with patients' analgesic medications (L Sehulster, personal communication, 2000). Contamination of the medications resulted in HCV transmission to multiple patients.

Occupational Exposures

The proportion of all HCV infections attributed to occupational exposure is small and has shown little temporal or geographic variation. Although healthcare workers with exposure to blood are at risk for being infected with HCV and other bloodborne pathogens, the prevalence of HCV infection among healthcare workers appears to be no greater than that found in the general population of their native regions.[22,140–148] Studies done in the United States indicate that this is true even for specialties with a high likelihood of percutaneous exposures to blood, including orthopedic, general, and oral surgeons.[150–153]

Risk factors for HCV transmission in the occupational setting have not been well defined but appear to be primarily related to a history of accidental needlesticks.[142] Seroconversion after needlestick or sharps exposures averages 1.8% (range, 0–7%),[147,149,154,155] and one study found that such transmission occurred only from hollow-bore needles.[147] Transmission of HCV from blood splashes to the conjunctiva have been described,[156,157] but transmission via nonintact skin exposures has not been reported.

Perinatal Transmission

Perinatal exposures account for a small proportion of HCV infections, and there appears to be no geo-

graphic or temporal differences in the frequency of perinatal transmission. Data from the relatively large number of studies done to date indicate that perinatal transmission occurs exclusively from mothers who are HCV RNA positive at the time of delivery (Table 1).[158–189] Of the 25 studies that followed infants for at least 12 months and included testing for HCV RNA, only one episode of transmission was reported from an anti-HCV-positive HCV RNA-negative mother,[162] and the detection method used in this study might not have had sufficient sensitivity to detect lower levels of virus. Thus, it would seem appropriate to evaluate the risk of perinatal transmission only among infants born to HCV RNA-positive mothers (Table 1). A summary of such studies demonstrates an average risk for transmission of 6% (range, 0–42%) for infants born to HCV-positive mothers who are not infected with human immunodeficiency virus (HIV),[158–172,174,175,178–182,184,186–189] and 17% (range, 8.5–44%) for infants born to mothers co-infected with HCV and HIV.[159,162,164,167,168,173,175–177,185,188,189] Data on the relationship between risk of perinatal transmission and titer of HCV RNA are inconsistent. Studies of HCV/HIV-co-infected mothers more consistently have shown an association between virus titer and transmission. Only two studies of infants born to HCV-positive HIV-negative women reported an association with virus titer, and each reported a different level of HCV RNA related to transmission.[166,174]

Available data are limited on the relationship between the risk for perinatal transmission of HCV and mode of delivery or type of feeding. Nevertheless, such data indicate no increased risk for transmission related to either vaginal delivery or breast-feeding (Table 1). The average rate of HCV infection among infants born by vaginal delivery is 10% compared with 8.4% among infants born by cesarean section.[162,175,177,184,185] Similarly, the average infection rate is 5% among breast-fed infants compared with 8% among bottle-fed infants.[166,168,175,180,184,188,190]

Sexual Activity

The relative importance of sexual activity in the transmission of HCV remains controversial. Associations between sexual activity and infection with HCV have been reported from case-control studies of persons with acute hepatitis C, cross-sectional studies of groups with different types of sexual behaviors (heterosexuals and men who have sex with men [MSM] attending sexually transmitted disease [STD] clinics, female prostitutes), and a cross-sectional study of a representative sample of the general population.[61,94,95,191–199] Although compared with other groups at risk for HCV infection, the prevalence of HCV infection among male and fe-

TABLE 1. Perinatal Transmission of HCV Infection

Potential Risk Factor	Infants Born to Anti-HCV-Positive Mothers			Infants Born to HCV RNA-Positive Mothers		
	No. Studies	Total Tested (Range)	Percent (Range) HCV Infected	No. Studies	Total Tested (Range)	Percent (Range) HCV Infected
Maternal HIV status						
Negative	27	1,070 (10–252)	4 (0–23)	21	646 (7–174)	6 (0–42)
Positive	12	620 (8–155)	13 (5–40)	6	261 (8–140)	17 (9–44)
Type of delivery				Data not available		
Vaginal	5	336 (34–116)	10 (6–32)			
Cesarean	5	107 (7–33)	8 (0–14)			
Type of feeding*				Data not available		
Breast-fed	6	157 (11–71)	5 (0–25)			
Bottle-fed	6	74 (3–30)	8 (0–20)			

*Includes only infants born to HIV-negative mothers.

male heterosexuals and MSM attending STD clinics who denied injection drug use is relatively low (Table 2). Factors associated with HCV infection in these populations include early age at first intercourse, greater numbers of sex partners, a history of other STDs, and failure to use a condom.[24,25,191–197,199–210] Among female prostitutes, sexual activities involving trauma have also been found to be associated with HCV infection.[211] In addition, evidence from one study indicates that male-to-female transmission of HCV may be more efficient than female-to-male,[191] a pattern characteristic of a sexual route of transmission.

Unlike STD populations, there is a striking variation between different geographic regions in the prevalence of infection reported among spouses (i.e., long term steady sex partners) of persons with chronic hepatitis C (Table 3). In studies done in Western Europe and North America, the average anti-HCV positivity rate among spouses who report no other risk factor for infection is 1.3%.[79,192,212–222] In contrast, higher anti-HCV positivity rates among spouses have been reported from studies done in southern Europe (11%)[203,223–235] and

Asia (27%).[236–240] Some of these studies have reported a direct relationship between anti-HCV positivity and increasing years of marriage.[228,229,231,239] However, it is likely that this relationship, as well as the high infection rates, is mostly the result of percutaneous exposures commonly experienced by both spouses in the past, because these studies were done in countries where it appears that contaminated equipment used in traditional and nontraditional medical procedures was the major source for HCV infection.

Similar differences by region in HCV prevalence rates have been found among nonsexual household contacts (Table 3). In Western Europe and North America, the average anti-HCV prevalence rate among nonsexual household contacts is 0.7%[79,213,215,217,241] compared with about 4% among such contacts in southern Europe and Asia.[224,226,228–243] Thus, it is likely that transmission of HCV within households is uncommon in the absence of shared percutaneous exposures.

Only one study has found an association between HCV infection and MSM activity,[196] and at least in STD clinic settings, the prevalence rate of HCV infection

TABLE 2. Prevalence of HCV Infection in Populations with Different Sexual Behaviors and No History of Injection Drug Use by Geographic Region

Geographic Region*	MSM Attending STD Clinics		Heterosexuals Attending STD Clinics			Female Prostitutes		
	No. Studies	No. Tested (Range)	Anti-HCV Positive† (Range)	No. Studies	No. Tested (Range)	Anti-HCV Positive† (Range)	No. Studies	No. Tested (Range)	Anti-HCV Positive† (Range
North America	4	1,896 (38–926)	2.5% (1.5–18%)	5	4,124 (95–1257)	6% (3.4–10%)	1	535	12%
South America	3	533 (103–228)	8.6% (1–13%)	1	1147	11.5%	2	1,505 (539–966)	4.3% (0.7–11%)
Europe	8	1,534 (48–270)	3.5% (0–9%)	5	2,539 (82–1130)	1.9% (0.4–18%)	3	740 (203–310)	6.5% (4–9%)

*Sufficient data were available only from these three regions.
†Includes only studies that determined anti-HCV positivity by EIA and supplemental testing.

TABLE 3. Prevalence of HCV Infection in Contacts of HCV-infected Persons by Geographic Region

Geographic Region*	*Long-Term Spouses/Sex Partners*			*Nonsexual Household*		
	No. Studies	N (Range)	Anti-HCV Positive (Range)†	No. Studies	N (Range)	Anti-HCV Positive (Range)†
Western Europe, North America	12	636 (7–104)	1.3% (0–4.4%)	5	734 (47–231)	0.7% (0–1.3%)
Southern Europe	14	1,651 (18–455)	11% (0–34%)	12	2,644 (52–924)	4.3% (1.3–32%)
Asia	4	301 (48–95)	27% (21–36%)	3	580 (144–250)	4.5% (3.3–5.5%)

*Sufficient data were available for only these three regions.
†Limited to studies that determined anti-HCV positivity by EIA and supplemental testing and occurring in contacts with no reported percutaneous risk factors (i.e., injection drug use, transfusion).

among MSM generally has been similar to that of heterosexuals. Because sexual transmission of bloodborne viruses is recognized to be more efficient among MSM compared with heterosexual men and women, why HCV infection rates are not substantially higher among MSM compared with heterosexuals is unclear. This observation and the low prevalence of HCV infection observed among the long-term steady sex partners of persons with chronic HCV infection have raised doubts about the importance of sexual activity in the transmission of HCV. Unacknowledged percutaneous risk factors (i.e., illegal injection drug use) might contribute to increased risk for HCV infection among persons with high-risk sexual practices.

Nevertheless, the findings of existing studies support the conclusion that sexual transmission of HCV occurs but that the virus is inefficiently spread through this manner. Furthermore, in the United States, the low risk of transmitting HCV infection through sexual intercourse is not inconsistent with the results of both incidence and prevalence studies showing that high-risk sexual behavior accounts for 15–20% of HCV infections.[61,65] Among acute hepatitis C cases reported during 1991–1997, 17% were attributed to sexual exposure in the absence of other risk factors; two thirds of these had an anti-HCV-positive sex partner and one third reported more than two partners in the 6 months before illness (CDC, unpublished data, 1999).[65] In the general population, 15% of prevalent infections could be attributed to sexual exposures in the absence of injection drug use.[61] Sex is a common behavior in the general population, a substantial proportion of the adult population in the United States has had multiple partners, and there are a large number of HCV chronically infected persons in the population. Although there are other types of exposures (e.g., transfusion from an HCV-infected donor) more likely to transmit HCV, they account for a much smaller proportion of infections because of the relatively small proportion of the current population in whom these exposures have occurred.

Other Potential Risk Factors

In the United States, a commonly recognized risk factor can be identified among most (90%) patients with acute or chronic hepatitis C. During 1991–1997, 60% of newly acquired infections were associated with injection drug use, 21% with high-risk sexual exposures (HCV-positive partner, multiple partners, history of STD), 4% with occupational exposures to blood, 3% with household exposure to an infected contact, and 3% to blood transfusion (all of which occurred before 1995) (CDC, unpublished data, 1999).

There are a variety of other percutaneous exposures for which a biologically plausible link with transmission of HCV can be postulated but about which there are insufficient data to assess their role as sources for HCV infection in either developed or developing countries. Reused contaminated instruments and objects during the performance of rituals or cosmetic services, such as tattooing, body piercing, commercial barbering, circumcision, and scarification, have the potential to transmit HCV and other bloodborne pathogens. However, the few studies conducted to date have either used inappropriate control groups or have been done in highly selected groups, resulting in conclusions that cannot be extrapolated to other populations.[77,244–248] Thus, there are no studies demonstrating a causal link between these types of practices and HCV infection, and there are no data showing that persons with a history of exposures such as tattooing, body piercing, or being attended by a commercial barber are at increased risk for HCV infection based on these exposures alone.

In the United States, these types of exposures are rarely reported by persons with acute hepatitis C. Among patients reported with acute hepatitis C during the past 15 years who denied a history of injection drug use, only 1% reported tattooing or ear piercing and none reported a history of acupuncture.[75] However, the importance of some of these types of exposures as routes of transmission may differ according to the setting in which they occur. For example, although receiving a tattoo in a licensed commercial establishment may not be associated with an increased risk for HCV infection, when received in the setting of a correctional facility or in an unregulated commercial establishment, the risk associated with this type of exposure might be considerably greater. Similarly, although these types of exposures may not be significant sources for transmission in the United States or where the prevalence of infection is low and/or appropriate infection control standards are practiced, their role in other places or settings needs to be assessed.

PREVENTION AND CONTROL OF HCV INFECTION AND HCV-RELATED LIVER DISEASE

A comprehensive strategy for the prevention and control of HCV infection and HCV-related liver disease requires implementation of primary and secondary prevention activities,[1,75] although the degree to which the components of such a program can be implemented in individual countries will depend on the capacity and resources available.

Primary Prevention

Because there is currently no vaccine and no effective postexposure prophylaxis for hepatitis C, the major emphasis of activities aimed at the primary prevention of HCV is on the counseling of uninfected persons at increased risk for HCV infection about ways to protect themselves from becoming infected and the counseling of infected persons so that they can reduce their risk of transmitting to others. Primary prevention efforts should also include education to reduce the risk for transmission of HCV in healthcare and other settings by modifying such practices as unsafe injections, emphasizing the importance of infection control, and reducing the risk of percutaneous exposures to blood in these settings. Finally, the implementation of donor screening and testing is needed to prevent transmission of HCV via blood transfusions, blood components, or plasma derivatives.

All countries should develop and implement programs for the primary prevention of new infections. To develop effective approaches to primary prevention, it is necessary to know the relative contribution of various sources of HCV infection. In countries where this information is not available, studies should be performed to facilitate prioritization of possible preventive measures and to allow the most appropriate use of available resources.[1]

In developing countries, where donor screening and testing policies for HCV and inactivation procedures for plasma-derived products have not been implemented and transfusions and organ transplants continue to be major sources for HCV infection, improving the safety of the blood supply should be the highest priority.[1] However, programs should also be initiated to reduce the extent to which HCV is transmitted as a result of inadequate sterilization or disinfection of medical, surgical and dental equipment, reuse of contaminated equipment, and unsafe injection practices. Such programs should include training regarding appropriate infection control practices and use of devices or products that prevent reuse or contamination of equipment. In addition, efforts should be made to modify injection practices of professionals and nonprofessionals and to educate practitioners of folk medicine, rituals, and cosmetic procedures about the risk for transmission of bloodborne pathogens from nonsterile instruments or objects used in these procedures.

In developed countries, primary prevention of illegal drug injecting, which remains the single most important mode for transmission of HCV in these countries, should be a high priority. In addition, although the relative importance of sexual activity as a route for HCV transmission is still unclear, it is known that persons with multiple sex partners are at risk for a variety of STDs and should be counseled regarding behavioral modification to reduce risk for all STDs, which may include HCV. Healthcare professionals should routinely obtain a history that inquires about use of illegal drugs and evidence of high-risk sexual practices to identify individuals for appropriate testing and counseling. Counseling and education, especially of adolescents, to prevent initiation of drug injecting or high-risk sexual practices is critical, but counseling should also be provided to those who already inject drugs or engage in high risk sexual behaviors about what they can do to minimize their risk of becoming infected or of transmitting infectious agents to others, including the need for vaccination against hepatitis B and, where appropriate, hepatitis A. Establishing needle exchange and other programs to increase access to sterile syringes and needles should also be considered.

Secondary Prevention

Countries with more developed economic, medical, and public health infrastructures should also develop programs to identify, counsel, and provide medical management for persons already infected to reduce their risk for developing chronic disease. The implementation of such programs is based on the identification of HCV-infected persons through routine screening of persons most likely to be infected with HCV with established protocols for providing counseling and medical management of those found to be infected. The decision on who to test should be based on various considerations, including whether there is a known epidemiologic link between a risk factor and acquiring HCV infection, the prevalence of the risk behavior or characteristic in the population, the prevalence of infection among those with a risk behavior or characteristic, and the need for persons with a recognized exposure to be evaluated for infection.

In the United States and Europe, routine testing is recommended for individuals in groups at increased risk for HCV infection and individuals with known exposure to HCV-infected blood,[75,249] including

- Anyone who ever injected illegal drugs;
- Persons who received plasma derived products known to transmit HCV infection that were not treated to inactivate viruses;
- Persons who have received blood products that might have been contaminated with HCV, including products prepared from blood that was either donated before the widespread use of second-generation EIA testing or came from a donor who later tested positive for HCV infection;
- Persons who have been on long-term hemodialysis;
- Healthcare workers after needlesticks, sharps, or mucosal exposures to HCV-positive blood;
- Children born to HCV-positive women.

It is important that all individuals found to be infected receive counseling on ways to reduce their risk for transmitting HCV to others.[75] They should be advised to not donate blood, body organs, other tissue, or semen; to not share toothbrushes, razors, or other personal care articles that might have blood on them; and to cover cuts and sores. Infected persons with a steady sex partner do not need to change sexual practices but should be advised to discuss with their partner the need for counseling and testing. The couple should be informed of available data regarding risk for HCV transmission by sexual activity to assist them in making decisions about precautions. They might decide to use barrier precautions if they want to lower the limited chance of spreading HCV to their partner. Infected persons should also be provided with information about ways to prevent further harm to their liver, primarily through the avoidance of alcohol and by vaccination against hepatitis A and, when appropriate, hepatitis B. As part of these programs, it is also critical that protocols are in place to ensure that infected individuals receive appropriate medical evaluation for chronic liver disease and possible treatment.

ABBREVIATIONS

CDC   Centers for Disease Control and Prevention
EIA   enzyme immunoassay
HCV   hepatitis C virus
HIV   human immunodeficiency virus
MSM   men who have sex with men
STD   sexually transmitted disease

REFERENCES

1. WHO. Global surveillance and control of hepatitis C. Report of a WHO Consultation organized in collaboration with the Viral Hepatitis Prevention Board, Antwerp, Belgium. J Viral Hepat 1999;6:35–47
2. Dow BC, Coote I, Munru H, et al. Confirmation of hepatitis C virus antibody in blood donors. J Med Virol 1993;41:215–220
3. Mutimer DJ, Harrison RF, O'Donnell KB, et al. Hepatitis C virus infection in the asymptomatic British blood donor. J Viral Hepat 1995;2:47–53
4. Atrah HI, Ala FA, Ahmed MM, et al. Unexplained hepatitis C virus antibody seroconversion in established blood donors. Transfusion 1996;36:339–343
5. Mathiesen UL, Karlsson E, Foberg U, et al. Also with a restrictive transfusion policy, screening with second-generation anti-hepatitis C virus enzyme-linked immunosorbent assay would have reduced posttransfusion hepatitis C after open-heart surgery. Scand J Gastroenterol 1993;28:581–584
6. Nordoy I Schrumpf E, Elgjo K, et al. Liver disease in anti-hepatitis C virus-positive Norwegian blood donors. Scand J Gastroenterol 1994;29:77–81
7. Hennig H, Haase D, Kirchner H. Prevalence of hepatitis C virus in blood donors and comparison of 4 different anti-HCV differentiation tests. Beitr Infsuionsther Transfuisonsmed 1996;33:231–234
8. Riggert J, Schwartz DW, Uy A, et al. Risk of hepatitis C virus (HCV) transmission by anti-HCV-negative blood components in Austria and Germany. Ann Hematol 1996;72:35–39
9. Caspari G, Gerlich WH, Beyer J, Schmitt H. Non-specific and specific anti-HCV results correlated to age, sex, transaminase, rhesus blood group and follow-up in blood donors. Arch Virol 1997;142:473–489
10. Ranger S, Martin P, Roussane MC, Denis F. Prevalence of hepatitis C virus antibodies in the general population and in selected groups of patients in Limoges, France. Gut 1993;34(2 Suppl):S50-S51
11. Kleinman S, Alter H, Busch M, et al. Increased detection of hepatitis C virus (HCV)-infected blood donors by a multiple-antigen HCV enzyme immunoassay. Transfusion 1992;32:805–813
12. Murphy EL, Bryzman S, Williams AE, et al. Demographic determinants of hepatitis C seroprevalence among blood donors. JAMA 1996;275:996–1000
13. Zhang YY, Guo LS, Hao LJ, et al. Antibodies to hepatitis C virus and hepatitis C virus RNA in Chinese blood donors determined by ELISA, recombinant immunoblot assay and polymerase chain reaction. Chin Med J 1993;106:171–174
14. Garcia Z, Taylor L, Ruano A, et al. Evaluation of a pooling method for routine anti-HCV screening of blood donors to lower the cost burden on blood banks in countries under development. J Med Virol 1996;49:218–222
15. Pita-Ramirez L, Torres-Ortiz GE. Prevalence of viral antibodies and syphilis serology in blood donors from a hospital. Rev Invest Clin 1997;49:475–480
16. Ayala Gaytan JJ, Guerra Avalos FJ, Brondo Mora P, Casillas Roma A. Prevalence of viral markers for hepatitis B, C and human immunodeficiency virus in volunteer blood donors in Northeast Mexico. Rev Gastroenterol Mexico 1997;62:250–253

17. Guerrero-Romero JF, Castaneda A, Rodriguez-Moran M. Prevalence of risk factors associated with hepatitis C in blood donors in the municipality of Durango, Mexico. Salud Publica Mex 1996;38:94–100

18. Munoz G, Velasco M, Thiers V, et al. Prevalence and genotypes of hepatitis C virus in blood donors and in patients with chronic liver disease and hepatocarcinoma in a Chilean population. Rev Med Chile 1998;126:1035–1042

19. Mison LM, Young IF, O'Donoghue M, et al. Prevalence of hepatitis C virus and genotype distribution in an Australian volunteer blood donor population. Transfusion 1997;37:73–78

20. Triki H, Said N, Ben Salah A, et al. Seroepidemiology of hepatitis B, C and delta viruses in Tunisia. Trans R Soc Trop Med Hyg 1997;91:11–14

21. Abid S, Fkih S, Khlass B, et al. Screening and confirmation of anti-HCV antibodies in Tunisian blood donors. Transfus Clin Biol 1997;4:221–226

22. Soni PN, Tait DR, Kenoyer DG, et al. Hepatitis C virus antibodies among risk groups in a South African area endemic for hepatitis B virus. J Med Virol 1993;40:65–68

23. Vasconcelos HC, Yoshida CF, Vanderborght BO, Schatzmayr HG. Hepatitis B and C prevalences among blood donors in the south region of Brazil. Mem Inst Oswaldo Cruz 1994;89:503–507

24. Edelenyi-Pinto M, Carvalho AP, Nogueira C, et al. Prevalence of antibodies to hepatitis C virus in populations at low and high risk for sexually transmitted diseases in Rio de Janeiro. Mem Inst Oswaldo Cruz 1993;88:305–307

25. Hadziyannis SJ, Giannoulis G, Hadziyannis E, et al. Hepatitis C virus infection in Greece and its role in chronic liver disease and hepatocellular carcinoma. J Hepatol 1993;17(Suppl 3):S72-S77

26. Mihaljevic I, Feldbauer J, Delajlija M, Grgicevic D. Antibodies to hepatitis C virus in Croatian blood donors and polytransfused patients. Vox Sang 1992;63:236

27. Gloskowska-Moraczewska Z, Kacperska E, Seyfried H. Evaluation of screening and complementary tests for anti-HCV antibodies. Acta Haematol Pol 1993;24:273–280

28. Lai ME, Mazzoleni AP, Farci P, et al. Markers of hepatitis C virus infection in Sardinian blood donors: relationship with alanine aminotransferase levels. J Med Virol 1993;41:282–288

29. Abdourakhamanov DT, Hasaev AS, Castro FJ, Guardia J. Epidemiological and clinical aspects of hepatitis C virus infection in the Russian Republic of Daghestan. Eur J Epidemiol 1998;14:549–553

30. Barna TK, Ozsvar Z, Szendrenyi V, Gal G. Hepatitis C virus antibody in the serum of blood donors. Orvosi Hetilap 1996;137:507–511

31. Al-Faleh FZ, Ramia S, Arif M, et al. Profile of hepatitis C virus and the possible modes of transmission of the virus in the Gizan area of Saudi Arabia: a community-based study. Ann Trop Med Parasitol 1995;89:431–437

32. El Guneid AM, Gunaid AA, O'Neill AM, et al. Prevalence of hepatitis B, C and D virus markers in Yemeni patients with chronic liver disease. J Med Virol 1993;40:330–333

33. Panigrahi AK, Panda SK, Dixit RK, et al. Magnitude of hepatitis C virus infection in India: prevalence in healthy blood donors, acute and chronic liver diseases. J Med Virol 1997;51:167–174

34. Jaiswal SP, Chitnis DS, Naik G, et al. Prevalence of anti-HCV antibodies in central India. Indian J Med Res 1996;104:177–181

35. Irshad M, Acharya SK, Josha YK. Prevalence of hepatitis C virus antibodies in the general population and in selected groups of patients in Delhi. Indian J Med Res 1995;102:162–164

36. Frommel D, Tekle-Haimanot R, Berhe N, et al. A survey of antibodies to hepatitis C virus in Ethiopia. Am J Trop Med Hyg 1993;49:435–439

37. Wansbrough-Jones MH, Frimpong E, Cant B, et al. Prevalence and genotype of hepatitis C virus infection in pregnant women and blood donors in Ghana. Trans R Soc Trop Med Hyg 1998;92:496–499

38. Lo BB, Meymouna M, Boulahi MA, et al. Prevalence of serum markers of hepatitis B and C virus in blood donors of Nouakchott, Mauritania. Bull Soc Pathol Exot 1999;92:83–84

39. Develoux M, Boni G, Aguessy Ahyi B, et al. The prevalence of anti-hepatitis C antibodies in pregnant women and blood donors in Benin. Bull Soc Pathol Exot 1995;88:115–116

40. Jeannel D, Fretz C, Traore Y, et al. Evidence for high genetic diversity and long-term endemicity of hepatitis C virus genotypes 1 and 2 in West Africa. J Med Virol 1998;55:92–97

41. Ilako FM, McLigeyo SO, Riyat MS, et al. The prevalence of hepatitis C virus antibodies in renal patients, blood donors and patients with chronic liver disease in Kenya. East Afr Med J 1995;72:362–364

42. Hayashi J, Furusyo N, Sawayama Y, et al. Hepatitis G virus in the general population and in patients on hemodialysis. Dig Dis Sci 1998;43:2143–2148

43. Nakashima K, Kashiwagi S, Hayashi J, et al. Prevalence of hepatitis C virus infection among female prostitutes in Fukuoka, Japan. J Gastroenterol 1996;31:664–668

44. Sakugawa H, Nakasone H, Nakayoshi T, et al. High proportion of false positive reactions among donors with anti-HCV antibodies in a low prevalence area. J Med Virol 1995;46:334–338

45. Yamaguchi K, Kiyokawa H, Machida J, et al. Seroepidemiology of hepatitis C virus infection in Japan and HCV infection in haemodialysis patients. FEMS Microbiol Rev 1994;14:253–258

46. Wang Y, Tao QM, Zhao HY, et al. Hepatitis C virus RNA and antibodies among blood donors in Beijing. J Hepatol 1994;21:634–640

47. Wu X. Investigation on anti-HCV antibody in Shashi District. Chin J Epidemiol 1993;14:331–333

48. Tang S. Seroepidemiological study on hepatitis C virus infection among blood donors from various regions in China. Chin J Epidemiol 1993;14:271–274

49. Zhang YY, Hansson BG, Widell A, Nordenfelt E. Hepatitis C virus antibodies and hepatitis C virus RNA in Chinese blood donors determined by ELISA, recombinant immunoblot assay and polymerase chain reaction. APMIS 1992;100:851–855

50. Duraisamy G, Zuridah H, Ariffin MY. Prevalence of hepatitis C virus antibodies in blood donors in Malaysia. Med J Mal 1993;48:313–316

51. Kuperan P, Choon AT, Ding SH, Lee G. Prevalence of antibodies to hepatitis C virus in relation to surrogate markers in a blood donor population in Singapore. Southeast Asian J Trop Med Pub Health 1993;24(Suppl 1):127–129

52. Apichartpiyakul C, Apichartpiyakul N, Urwijitaroon Y, et al. Seroprevalence and subtype distribution of hepatitis C virus among blood donors and intravenous drug users in northern/northeastern Thailand. Jpn J Infect Dis 1999;52:121–123

53. Songsivilai S, Jinathongthai S, Wongsena W, et al. High prevalence of hepatitis C infection among blood donors in northeaster Thailand. Am J Trop Med Hyg 1997;57:66–69

54. Sawanpanyalert P, Boonmar S, Maeda T, et al. Risk factors for hepatitis C virus infection among blood donors in an HIV-epidemic area in Thailand. J Epidemiol Commun Health 1996;50:174–177

55. Darmadi S, Soetjipto, Handajani R, et al. Hepatitis C virus infection-associated markers in sera from blood donors in Surabaya, Indonesia. Microbiol Immunol 1996;40:401–405

56. Soetjipto, Handajani R, Lusida MI, et al. Differential prevalence of hepatitis C virus subtypes in healthy blood donors, patients on maintenance hemodialysis and patients with hepatocellular carcinoma in Surabaya, Indonesia. J Clin Microbiol 1996;34:2875–2880

57. Saleh MG, Pereira LM, Tibbs CJ, et al. High prevalence of hepatitis C virus in the normal Libyan population. Trans R Soc Trop Med Hyg 1994;88:292–294

58. Bassily S, Hyams KC, Fouad RA, et al. A high risk of hepatitis C infection among Egyptian blood donors: the role of parenteral drug abuse. Am J Trop Med Hyg 1995;52:503–505

59. Darwish MA, Raouf TA, Rushdy P, et al. Risk factor associated with ahigh seroprevalence of hepatitis C virus infection in Egyptian blood donors. Am J Trop Med Hyg 1993;49:440–447

60. Attia MA, Zekri AR, Goudsmit J, et al. Diverse patterns of recognition of hepatitis C virus core and nonstructural antigens by antibodies present in Egyptian cancer patients and blood donors. J Clin Microbiol 1996;34:2665–2669

61. Alter MJ, Kruszon-Moran D, Nainan OV, et al. Prevalence of hepatitis C virus infection in the United States, 1988–1994. N Engl J Med 1999;341:556–562

62. Lowe D, Cotton R. Hepatitis C: a review of Australia's response. Publications Production Unit, Commonwealth Department of Health and Aged Care, Commonwealth of Australia, Canberra, 1999

63. Farrell GC, Weltman M, Dingley J, Lin R. Epidemiology of hepatitis C virus infection in Australia. Gastroenterol Jpn 1993; 28(Suppl 5):32–36

64. Armstrong GL, Alter MJ, McQuillan GM, et al. The past incidence of hepatitis C virus infection: implications for the future burden of chronic liver disease in the United States. Hepatology 2000;31:777–782

65. Alter MJ. Epidemiology of hepatitis C. Hepatology 1997;26: 62S–65S

66. Tanaka E, Kiyosawa K, Sodeyama T, et al. Prevalence of antibody to hepatitis C virus in Japanese school children: comparison with adult blood donors. Am J Trop Med Hyg 1992;46:460–464

67. Ishibasi M, Shinzawa H, Kuboki M, Tsuchida H, Takahashi T. Prevalence of inhabitants with anti-hepatitis C virus antibody in an area following an acute hepatitis C epidemic: age and area-related features. J Epidemiol 1996;6:1–7

68. Guadagnino V, Stroffolini T, Rapicetta M, et al. Prevalence, risk factors, and genotype distribution of hepatitis C virus infection in the general population: a a community-based survey in Southern Italy. Hepatology 1997;26:1006–1011

69. Stroffolini T, Menchinelli M, Taliani G, et al. High prevalence of hepatitis C virus infection in a small central Italian town: lack of evidence of parenteral exposure. Ital J Gastroenterol 1995;27: 235–238

70. Abdel-Wahah MF, Zakaria S, Kamel M, et al. High seroprevalence of hepatitis C infection among risk groups in Egypt. Am J Trop Med Hyg 1994;51:563–567

71. Mohamed MK, Hussein MH, Massoud AA, et al. Study of the risk factors for viral hepatitis C infection among Egyptians applying for work abroad. J Egypt Public Health Assoc 1996;71: 113–142

72. Villano SA, Vlahov D, Nelson KE, Lyles CM, Cohn S, Thomas DL. Incidence and risk factors for hepatitis C among injection drug users in Baltimore, Maryland. J Clin Microbiol 1997;35: 3274–3277

73. Garfein RS, Doherty MC, Monterroso ER, Thomas DL, Nelson KE, Vlahov D. Prevalence and incidence of hepatitis C virus infection among young adult injection drug users. J Acquir Immune Defic Syndr Hum Retrovirol 1998;18(Suppl 1):S11–S19

74. Crofts N, Hopper JL, Bowden DS, Breschkin AM, Milner R, Locarnini SA. Hepatitis C virus infection among a cohort of Victorian injecting drug users. Med J Aust 1993;159:237–241

75. Centers for Disease Control and Prevention. Recommendations for prevention and control of hepatitis C virus (HCV) infection and HCV-related chronic disease. MMWR Morb Mortal Wkly Rep 1998;47:1–33

76. Tanaka H, Tsukuma H, Hori Y, et al. The risk of hepatitis C virus infection among blood donors in Osaka, Japan. J Epidemiol 1998;8:292–296

77. Mele A, Sagliocca L, Manzillo G, et al. Risk factors for acute non-A, non-B hepatitis and their relationship to antibodies for hepatitis C virus: a case-control study. Am J Public Health 1994;84:1640–1643

78. Chiaramonte M, Stroffolini T, Lorenzoni U, et al. Risk factors in community-acquired chronic hepatitis C virus infection: a case-control study in Italy. J Hepatol 1996;24:129–134

79. Conry-Cantilena C, VanRaden M, Gibble J, et al. Routes of infection, viremia, and liver disease in blood donors found to have hepatitis C virus infection. N Engl J Med 1996;334:1691–1696

80. Lillienfeld AM, Lilienfeld DE. Foundations of Epidemiology. New York: Oxford University Press, 1980

81. Conry-Cantilena C, Melpolder JC, Alter HJ. Intranasal drug use among volunteer whole-blood donors: results of survey C. Transfusion 1998;38:512–513

82. Alter MJ. Epidemiology of hepatitis C in the West. Semin Liver Dis 1995;15:5–14

83. Aach RD, Stevens CE, Hollinger FB, et al. Hepatitis C virus infection in post-transfusion hepatitis. An analysis with first- and second-generation assays. N Engl J Med 1991;325:1325–1329

84. Elia GF, Magnani G, Belli L, et al. Incidence of anti-hepatitis C virus antibodies in non-A, non-B post-transfusion hepatitis in an area of northern Italy. Infection 1991;19:336–339

85. Mattsson L, Grillner L, von Sydow M, et al. Seroconversion to hepatitis C virus antibodies in patients with acute posttransfusion non-A, non-B hepatitis in Sweden. Infection 1991;19: 309–312

86. Goncales FL Jr, Pedro R de J, Da Silva LJ, et al. Post-transfusional hepatitis in the city of Campinas SP, Brazil. I. Incidence, etiological agents and clinico-epidemiological aspects of hepatitis C. Rev Inst Med Trop Sao Paulo 1993;35:53–62

87. Jullien AM, Courouce AM, Massari V, et al. Impact of screening donor blood for alanine aminotransferase and antibody to hepatitis B core antigen on the risk of hepatitis C virus transmission. Eur J Clin Microbiol Infect Dis 1993;12:668–672

88. Donahue JG, Munoz A, Ness PM, et al. The declining risk of post-transfusion hepatitis C virus infection. N Engl J Med 1992;327:369–373

89. Nelson KE, Ahmed F, Ness P, et al. Comparison of first and second generation ELISA screening tests in detecting HCV infections in transfused cardiac surgery patients [abstract]. Program and Abstracts of the International Symposium on Viral Hepatitis and Liver Disease, 1993, p. 50

90. Takano S, Nakamura K, Kawai S, et al. Prospective assessment of donor blood screening for antibody to hepatitis C virus by first- and second-generation assays as a means of preventing posttransfusion hepatitis. Hepatology 1996;23:708–712

91. Gonzalez A, Esteban JI, Madoz P, et al. Efficacy of screening donors for antibodies to the hepatitis C virus to prevent transfusion-associated hepatitis: final report of a prospective trial. Hepatology 1995;22:439–445

92. Japanese Red Cross Non-A Non-B Hepatitis Research Group. Effect of screening for hepatitis C virus antibody and hepatitis B core antibody on incidence of post-transfusion hepatitis. Lancet 1991;338:1040–1041

93. Schreiber GB, Busch MP, Kleinman SH, et al. The risk of transfusion-transmitted viral infections. N Engl J Med 1996;334: 1685–1690

94. Alter MJ, Coleman PJ, Alexander WJ, et al. Importance of heterosexual activity in the transmission of hepatitis B and nonA, nonB hepatitis. JAMA 1989;262:1201–1205

95. Alter MJ, Gerety RJ, Smallwood L, et al. Sporadic non-A, non-B hepatitis: frequency and epidemiology in an urban United States population. J Infect Dis 1982;145:886–893

96. Louie M, Low DE, Feinman SV, et al. Prevalence of bloodborne infective agents among people admitted to a Canadian hospital. Can Med Assoc J 1992;146:1331–1334

97. Kelen GD, Green GB, Purcell RH, et al. Hepatitis B and hepatitis C in emergency department patients. N Engl J Med 1992; 326:1399–1404

98. Barham WB, Figueroa R, Phillips IA, Hyams KC. Chronic liver disease in Peru: role of viral hepatitis. J Med Virol 1994;42: 129–132

99. Bile K, Aden C, Norder H, et al. Important role of hepatitis C virus infection as a cause of chronic liver disease in Somalia. Scand J Infect Dis 1993;25:559–564

100. Guyer B, Bradley DW, Bryan JA, Maynard JE. Non-A, non-B hepatitis among participants in a plasmapheresis stimulation program. J Infect Dis 1979;139:634–40

101. Schvarcz R, Johansson B, Nystra;uom, Sönnerborg A. Nosocomial transmission of hepatitis C virus. Infection 1997;25:74–77

102. Allander T, Gruber A, Naghavi M, et al. Frequent patient-to-patient transmission of hepatitis C virus in a haematology ward. Lancet 1995;345:603–607

103. Widell A, Christensson B, Wiebe T, et al. Epidemiologic and molecular investigation of outbreaks of hepatitis C virus infection on a pediatric oncology service. Ann Intern Med 1999;130: 130–134

104. Bronowicki JP, Venard V, Botte C, et al. Patient to patient transmission of hepatitis C virus during colonoscopy. N Engl J Med 1997;337:237–240

105. Niu MT, Coleman PJ, Alter MJ. Multicenter study of hepatitis C virus infection in chronic hemodialysis patients and staff. Am J Kidney Dis 1993;22:568–573

106. Conlon PJ, Walshe JJ, Smyth EG, et al. Lower prevalence of anti-hepatitis C antibody in dialysis and renal transplant patients in Ireland. Irish J Med Sci 1993;162:145–147

107. Bukh J, Wantzin P, Krogsgaard K, et al. High prevalence of hepatitis C virus (HCV) RNA in dialysis patients: failure of commercially available antibody tests to identify a significant number of patients with HCV infection. J Infect Dis 1993;168:1343–1348

108. Kolho E, Oksanen K, Honkanen E, et al. Hepatitis C antibodies in dialysis patients and patients with leukaemia. J Med Virol 1993;40:318–321

109. Nordenfelt E, Lofgren B, Widell A, et al. Hepatitis C virus infection in hemodialysis patients in Southern Sweden: epidemiological, clinical, and diagnostic aspects. J Med Virol 1993;40:266–270

110. Medin C, Allander T, Roll M, et al. Seroconversion to hepatitis C virus in dialysis patients: a retrospective and prospective study. Nephron 1993;65:40–45

111. Almroth G, Ekermo B, Franzen L, Hed J. Antibody responses to hepatitis C virus and its modes of transmission in dialysis patients. Nephron 1991;59:232–235

112. Hardy NM, Sandroni S, Danielson S, Wilson WJ. Antibody to hepatitis C virus increases with time on hemodialysis. Clin Nephrol 1992;38:44–48

113. Zeldis JB, Depner TA, Kuramoto IK, et al. The prevalence of hepatitis C virus antibodies among hemodialysis patients. Ann Intern Med 1990;112:958–960

114. Jeffers LJ, Perez GO, DeMedina MD, et al. Hepatitis C infection in two urban hemodialysis units. Kidney Int 1990;38:320–322

115. Forseter G, Wormser GP, Adler S, et al. Hepatitis C in the health care setting. Seroprevalence among hemodialysis staff and patients in suburban New York City. Am J Infec Control 1993;21:5–8

116. Kallinowski B, Theilmann L, Gmelin K, et al. Prevalence of antibodies to hepatitis C virus in hemodialysis patients. Nephron 1991;59:236–238

117. Schlipkoter U, Roggendorf M, Ernst G, et al. Hepatitis C virus antibodies in haemodialysis patients [letter]. Lancet 1990;335: 1409

117. Tokars JI, Alter MJ, Favero MS, et al. National surveillance of dialysis associated diseases in the United States, 1993. ASAIO J 1996;42:219–229

119. Hayashi J, Yoshimura E, Nabeshima A, et al. Seroepidemiology of hepatitis C virus infection in hemodialysis patients and the general population in Fukuoka and Okinawa, Japan. J Gastroenterol 1994;29:276–281

120. Fujiyama S, Kawano S, Sato S, et al. Changes in prevalence of anti-HCV antibodies associated with preventive measures among hemodialysis patients and dialysis staff. Hepatogastroenterology 1995;42:162–165

121. Tsuyuguchi M. Prevalence of hepatitis C virus infection among chronic hemodialysis patients. Hokkaido J Med Sci 1994;69: 1178–1188

122. DiLallo D, Miceli M, Petrosillo N, et al. Risk factors of hepatitis C virus infection in patients on hemodialysis: a multivariate analysis based on a dialysis register in Central Italy. Eur J Epidemiol 1999;15:11–14

123. Covic A, Iancu L, Apetrei C, et al. Hepatitis virus infection in haemodialysis patients from Moldavia. Nephrol Dial Transplant 1999;14:40–45

124. Fabrizi F, Lunghi G, Pagliari B, et al. Molecular epidemiology of hepatitis C virus infection in dialysis patients. Nephron 1997;77:190–196

125. Halfon P, Khiri H, Feryn JM, et al. Prospective virolocial follow-up of hepatitis C infection in a haemodialysis unit. J Viral Hepat 1998;5:115–121

126. Forns X, Fernandez-Llama P, Pons M, et al. Incidence and risk factors of hepatitis C virus infection in a haemodialysis unit. Nephrol Dial Transplant 1997;12:736–740

127. Fabrizi F, Martin P, Dixit V, et al. Detection of de novo hepatitis C virus infection by polymerase chain in hemodialysis patients. Am J Nephrol 1999;19:383–388

128. Jadoul M, Cornu C, Van Ypersele de Strihou C, UCL Collaborative Group. Incidence and risk factors for hepatitis C seroconversion in hemodialysis: a prospective study. Kidney Int 1993;44:1322–1326

129. Muller GY, Zabaleta ME, Arminio A, et al. Risk factors for dialysis-associated hepatitis C in Venezuela. Kidney Int 1992;41: 1055–1058

130. Irie Y, Hayashi H, Yokozeki K, et al. Hepatitis C infection unrelated to blood transfusion in hemodialysis patients. J Hepatol 1994;20:557–559

131. Noguchi S, Sata M, Suzuki H, Mizokami M, Tanikawa K. Routes of transmission of hepatitis C virus in an epidemic rural area of Japan. Molecular epidemiologic study of hepatitis C virus infection. Scand J Infect Dis 1997;29:23–28

132. Kiyosawa K, Tanaka E, Sodeyama T, et al. Transmission of hepatitis C in an isolated area in Japan: community-acquired infection. Gastroenterology 1994;196:1596–1602

133. Ito S, Ito M, Cho M-J, Shimotohno K, Tajima K. Massive seroepidemiological survey of hepatitis C virus: clustering of carriers on the Southwest coast of Tsushima, Japan. Jpn J Cancer Res 1991;82:1–3

134. Frank C, Mohamed MK, Strickland GT, et al. The role of anti-schistosomal therapy in the spread of hepatitis C virus in Egypt. Lancet 2000;355:887–891

135. Hutin YJF, Harpaz R, Drobeniuc, et al. Injections given in healthcare settings as a major source of hepatitis B virus infection in Moldova. Int J Epidemiol 1999;28:782–786

136. Luby SP, Qamruddin K, Shah AA, et al. The relationship between therapeutic injections and high prevalence of hepatitis C infection in Hafizabad, Pakistan. Epidemiol Infect 1997;119:349–356

137. Centers for Disease Control and Prevention. Frequency of vaccine-related and therapeutic injections—Romania, 1998. MMWR Morb Mortal Wkly Rep 1999;48:271–274

138. Esteban JI, Gomez J, Martell M, et al. Transmission of hepatitis C virus by a cardiac surgeon. N Engl J Med 1996;334:555–560

139. Duckworth GJ, Heptonstall J, Aitken C, et al. Transmission of hepatitis C virus from a surgeon to a patient. Commun Dis Public Health 1999;2:188–192

140. Blackmore TK, Stace NH, Maddocks P, et al. Prevalence of antibodies to HCV in patients receiving renal replacement therapy, and in the staff caring for them. Aust NZJ Med 1992;22:353–357

141. Thomas DL, Factor SH, Kelen GD, et al. Viral hepatitis in health care personnel at The Johns Hopkins Hospital. Arch Intern Med 1993;153:1705–1712

142. Polish LB, Tong MJ, Co RL, et al. Risk factors for hepatitis C virus infection among health care personnel in a community hospital. Am J Infect Control 1993;21:196–200

143. Germanaud J, Barthez JP, Causse X. The occupational risk of hepatitis C infection among hospital employees. Am J Public Health 1994;84:122

144. Campello C, Majori S, Poli A, et al. Prevalence of HCV antibodies in health-care workers from northern Italy. Infection 1992;20:224–226

145. Nakashima K, Kashiwagi S, Hayashi J, et al. Low prevalence of hepatitis C virus infection among hospital staff and acupuncturists in Kyushu, Japan. J Infect 1993;26:17–25

146. Struve J, Aronsson B, Frenning B, et al. Prevalence of antibodies against hepatitis C virus infection among health care workers in Stockholm. Scand J Gastroenterol 1994;29:360–362

147. Puro V, Petrosillo N, Ippolito G, Italian Study Group on Occupational Risk of HIV and Other Bloodborne Infections. Risk of hepatitis C seroconversion after occupational exposures in health care workers. Am J Infect Control 1995;23:273–277

148. Lodi G, Porter SR, Teo CG, Scully C. Prevalence of HCV infection in health care workers of a UK dental hospital. Br Dental J 1997;183:329–332

149. Petrosilla N, Puro V, Ippolito G, the Italian Study Group on Blood-borne Occupational Risk in Dialysis. Prevalence of hepatitis C antibodies in health-care workers. Lancet 1994;343:1618–1620

150. Cooper BW, Krusell A, Tilton RC, et al. Seroprevalence of antibodies to hepatitis C virus in high-risk hospital personnel. Infect Control Hosp Epidemiol 1992;13:82–85

151. Panlilio AL, Shapiro CN, Schable CA, et al. Serosurvey of human immunodeficiency virus, hepatitis B virus, and hepatitis C virus infection among hospital-based surgeons. J Am Coll Surg 1995;180:16–24

152. Shapiro CN, Tokars JI, Chamberland ME, the American Academy of Orthopedic Surgeons Serosurvey Study Committee. Use of hepatitis B vaccine and infection with hepatitis B and C among orthopedic surgeons. J Bone Joint Surg Am 1996;78:1791–1800

153. Thomas DL, Gruninger SE, Siew C, Joy ED, Quinn TC. Occupational risk of hepatitis C infections among general dentists and oral surgeons in North America. Am J Med 1996;100:41–45

154. Lanphear BP, Linnemann CC, Cannon CG, et al. Hepatitis C virus infection in health care workers: risk of exposure and infection. Infect Control Hosp Epidemiol 1994;15:745–750

155. Mitsui T, Iwano K, Masuko K, et al. Hepatitis C virus infection in medical personnel after needlestick accident. Hepatology 1992;16:1109–1114

156. Sartori M, La Terra G, Aglietta M, et al. Transmission of hepatitis C via blood splash into conjunctiva. Scand J Infect Dis 1993;25:270–271

157. Ippolito G, Puro V, Petrosillo N, De Carli G, Micheloni G, Magliano E, Coordinating Centre of the Italian Study on Occupational Risk of HIV Infection. Simultaneous infection with

158. Aizaki H, Saito A, Kusakawa I, et al. Mother-to-child transmission of a hepatitis C virus variant with an insertional mutation in its hypervariable region. J Hepatol 1996;25:608–613

159. Catalano D, Pollio F, Ercolano S, et al. Maternal-fetal transmission of HCV. Role of HIV as a risk factor. Min Ginecol 1999;51:117–119

160. Fischler B, Lindh G, Lindgren S, et al. Vertical transmission of hepatitis C virus infection Scand J Infect Dis 1996;28:353–356

161. Giacchino R, Picciotto A, Tasso L, et al. Vertical transmission of hepatitis C. Lancet 1995;345:1122–1123

162. Granovsky M, Minkoff HL, Tess BH, et al. Hepatitis C virus infection in the Mothers and Infants Cohort Study. Pediatrics 1998;102:355–359

163. Kudesia G, Ball G, Irving WL. Vertical transmission of hepatitis C. Lancet 1995; 345:1122–1125

164. Lam JPH, McOmish F, Burns SM, et al. Infrequent vertical transmission of hepatitis C virus. J Infect Dis 1993;167:572–576

165. Latt N, Collins E, Spencer J, et al. Hepatitis C virus infection in pregnant injecting drug users—possible vertical tranmission to babies. Proceeding of National Methadone Conference, Sydney, 1994

166. Lin HH, Kao JH, Hsu HY, et al. Possible role of high-titer maternal viremia in perinatal transmission of hepatitis C virus. J Infect Dis 1994;169:638–641

167. Maccabruni A, Bossi G, Caselli D, et al. High efficiency of vertical transmission of hepatitis C virus among babies born to human immunodeficiency virus-negative women. Pediatr Infect Dis J 1995;14:921–922

168. Manzini P, Saracco G, Cerchier A, et al. Human Immunodeficiency virus infection as risk factor for mother-to-child hepatitis C virus tranmission; persistence of anti-hepatitis C virus in children is associated with the mother's anti-hepatitis C virus immunoblotting pattern. Hepatology 1995;21:328–332

169. Marcellin P, Bernuau J, Martinot-Peignoux M, et al. Prevalence of hepatitis C virus infection in asymptomatic anti-HIV1 negative pregnant women and their children. Dig Dis Sci 1993;38:2151–2155

170. Mast EE, Hwang LY, Seto D, et al. Perinatal hepatitis C virus transmission: maternal risk factors and optimal timing of diagnosis. Hepatology 1999;30(Suppl., Part 2):499A

171. Moriya T, Sasaki F, Mizui M, et al. Transmission of hepatitis C virus from mother to infants: its frequency and risk factors revisited. Biomed Pharmacother 1995;49:59–64

172. Ni YH, Lin HH, Chen PJ, et al. Temporal profile of hepatitis C virus antibody and genome in infants born to mother infected with hepatitis C virus but without human immunodeficiency virus coinfection. J Hepatol 1994;20:641–645

173. Novati R, Thiers V, D'Arminio Monforte A, et al. Mother-to-child transmission of hepatitis C virus detected by nested polymerase chain reaction. J Infect Dis 1992;165:720–723

174. Ohto H, Terazawa S, Sasaki N, et al. Transmission of hepatitis C virus from mothers to infants. N Engl J Med 1994;330:744–750

175. Paccagnini S, Principi N, Massironi E, et al. Perinatal transmission and manifestation of hepatitis C virus infection in a high risk population. Pediatr Infect Dis J 1995;14:195–199

176. Palomba E, Manzini P, Fiammengo P, et al. Natural history of perinatal hepatitis C virus infection. Clin Infect Dis 1996;23:47–50

177. Papaevangelou V, Pollack H, Rochford G, et al. Increased transmission of vertical hepatitis C virus (HCV) infection to human immunodeficiency virus (HIV)-infected infants of HIV- and HCV-coinfected women. J Infect Dis 1998;178:1047–1052

178. Pipan C, Amici S, Astori G, et al. Vertical transmission of hepatitis C virus in low-risk pregnant women. Eur J Clin Microbiol Infect Dis 1996;14:116–120

HIV and hepatitis C virus following occupational conjunctival blood exposure. JAMA 1998;280:28

179. Reinus JF, Leikin EL, Alter HJ, et al. Failure to detect vertical transmission of hepatitis C virus. Ann Intern Med 1992;117:881–886

180. Resti M, Azzari C, Lega L, et al. Mother-to-infant transmission of hepatitis C virus. Acta Paediatr 1995;84:251–255

181. Roudot-Thoraval F, Pawlotsky J-M, Thiers V, et al. Lack of mother-to-infant transmission of hepatitis C virus in human immunodeficiency virus-seronegative women: a prospective study with hepatitis C virus RNA testing. Hepatology 1993;17:722–777

182. Sabatino G, Ramenghi LA, Di Marzio M, Pizzigallo E. Vertical transmission of hepatitis C virus: an epidemiological study on 2980 pregnant women in Italy. Eur J Epidemiol 1996;12:443–447

183. Soto B, Rodrigo L, Garcia Bengoechea M, et al. Heterosexual transmission of HCV and the possible role of coexistent human immunodeficiency virus infection in the index case. A multicentre study of 432 pairings. J Intern Med 1994; 236:515–519

184. Spencer JD, Latt N, Beeby PJ, et al. Transmission of hepatitis C virus to infants of human immunodeficiency virus-negative intravenous drug-using mothers: rate of infection and assessment of risk factors for transmission. J Viral Hepat 1997;4:395–409

185. Thomas DA, Villano SA, Riester KA, et al. Perinatal transmission of hepatitis C virus from human immunodeficiency virus type 1-infected mothers. Women and Infants Transmission Study. J Infect Dis 1998;177:1480–1488

186. Uehara S, Abe Y, Saito T, et al. The incidence of vertical transmission of HCV. Tohoku J Exp Med 1993;171:195–202

187. Wejstal R, Anders W, Mansson AS, et al. Mother-to-infant transmission of hepatitis C virus. Ann Intern Med 1992;117:887–890

188. Zanetti AR, Tanzi E, Paccagnini S, et al. Mother-to-infant transmission of hepatitis C virus. Lancet 1995;345:289–291

189. Zuccotti GV, Ribero ML, Giovannini M, et al. Effect of hepatitis C genotype on mother-to-infant transmission of virus. J Pediatr 1995; 127:278–280

190. Mast EE, Alter MJ. Hepatitis C. Semin Pediatr Infect Dis 1997;8:17–22

191. Thomas DL, Zenilman JM, Alter HJ, et al. Sexual transmission of hepatitis C virus among patients attending Baltimore sexually transmitted diseases clinics—an analysis of 309 sex partnerships. J Infect Dis 1995;171:768–775

192. Osmond DH, Charlebois E, Sheppard HW, et al. Comparison of risk factors for hepatitis C and hepatitis B virus infection in homosexual men. J Infect Dis 1993;167:66–71

193. Corona R, Prignano G, Mele A, et al. Heterosexual and homosexual transmission of hepatitis C virus: relation with hepatitis B virus and human immunodeficiency virus type 1. Epidemiol Infect 1991;107:667–672

194. Quaranta JF, Delaney SR, Alleman S, et al. Prevalence of antibody to hepatitis C virus (HCV) in HIV 1 infected patients (Nice SEROCO cohort). J Med Virol 1994;42:29–32

195. Weinstock HS, Bolan G, Reingold AL, Polish LB. Hepatitis C virus infection among patients attending a clinic for sexually transmitted diseases. JAMA 1993;269:392–394

196. Thomas DL, Cannon RO, Shapiro CN, et al. Hepatitis C, hepatitis B, and human immunodeficiency virus infections among non-intravenous drug-using patients attending clinics for sexually transmitted diseases. J Infect Dis 1994;169:990–995

197. van Doornum GJJ, Hooykaas C, Cuypers MT, et al. Prevalence of hepatitis C virus infections among heterosexuals with multiple partners. J Med Virol 1991;35:22–27

198. Mast EE, Darrow WW, Witte J, et al. Hepatitis C virus infection among prostitutes: evidence for sexual transmission and protective efficacy of condoms [abstract]. Program and Abstracts of the Third International Symposium on HCV, Strasbourg, 1991, p. 95

199. Gutierrez P, Orduna A, Bratos MA, et al. Prevalence of anti-hepatitis C virus antibodies in positive FTA-ABS non-drug abusing female prostitutes in Spain. Sex Trans Dis 1992;19:39–40

200. Daikos GL, Lai S, Fischl MA. Hepatitis C virus infection in a sexually active inner city population. The potential for heterosexual transmission. Infection 1994;22:72–76

201. Hershow RC, Kalish LA, Sha B, et al. Hepatitis C virus infection in Chicago women with or at risk for HIV infection: evidence for sexual transmission. Sex Trans Dis 1998;25:527–532

202. Mesquita PE, Hernandez Granato CF, Castelo A. Risk factors associated with hepatitis C virus (HCV) infection among prostitutes and their clients in the city of Santos, Sao Paulo state, Brazil. J Med Virol 1997;51:338–343

203. Lissen E, Alter HJ, Abad MA, et al. Hepatitis C virus infection among sexually promiscuous groups and the hetersexual partners of hepatitis C virus infected index cases. Eur J Clin Micro biol Infect Dis 1993;12:827–831

204. Tedder RS, Gilson RJ, Briggs M, et al. Hepatitis C virus: evidence for sexual transmission. BMJ 1991;302:1299–1302

205. Donahue JG, Nelson KE, Munoz A, et al. Antibody to HCV among cardiac surgery patients, homosexual men, and intravenous drug users in Baltimore, Maryland. Am J Epidemiol 1991;134:1206–1211

206. Hyams KC, Phillips IA, Tejada A, et al. Three year incidence study of retroviral and viral hepatitis transmission in a Peruvian prostitute population. J AIDS 1993;6:1353–1357

207. Osella AR, Massa MA, Joekes S, et al. Hepatitis B and C virus sexual transmission among homosexual men. Am J Gastroenterol 1998;93:49–52

208. Gasparini, V, Chiaramonte M, Moschen ME, et al. Hepatitis C virus infection in homosexual men: A seroepidemiological study in gay clubs in north-east Italy. Eur J Epidemiol 1991;7:665–669

209. Westh H, Worm AM, Jensen BL, et al. HCV antibodies in homosexual men and intravenous drug users in Denmark. Infection 1993;21:115–117

210. Sonnerborg A, Abebe A, Strannegard O. HCV infection in individuals with or without human immunodeficiency virus type 1 infection. Infection 1990;18:347–351

211. Williams CL, Mast EE, Coleman PJ, et al. Risk factors for sexual transmission of hepatitis C virus among non injecting-drug-using female prostitutes in the United States [abstract]. 36th Annual Meeting of the Infectious Disease Society of America, Denver, CO, 1998

212. Bresters D, Mauser-Bunschoten EP, Reesink HW, et al. Sexual transmission of hepatitis C virus. Lancet 1993;342:210–211

213. Meisel H, Reip A, Faltus B, et al. Transmission of hepatitis C virus to children and husbands by women infected with contaminated anti-D immunoglobulin. Lancet 1995;345:1209–1211

214. David XR, Blanc P, Pageaux GP, et al. Familial transmission of HCV. Gastroenterol Clin Biol 1995;19:150–155

215. Deny P, Roulot D, Asselot C, et al. Low rate of hepatitis C virus (HCV) transmission within the family. J Hepatol 1992;14:409–410

216. Wyld R, Robertson JR, Brettle RP, et al. Absence of hepatitis C virus transmission but frequent transmission of HIV-1 from sexual contact with doubly-infected individuals. J Infect 1997;35:163–166

217. Sachithanandan S, Fielding JF. Low rate of HCV transmission from women infected with contaminated anti-D immunoglobulin to their family contacts. Ital J Gastroenterol Hepatol 1997;29:47–50

218. Pachucki CT, Lentino JR, Schaaff D, et al. Low prevalence of sexual transmission of hepatitis C virus in sex partners of seropositive intravenous drug users. J Infect Dis 1991;164:820–821

219. Eyster ME, Alter HJ, Aledort LM, et al. Heterosexual co-transmission of hepatitis C virus (HCV) and human immunodeficiency virus (HIV). Ann Intern Med 1991;115:764–768

220. Gordon SC, Patel AH, Kulesza GW, et al. Lack of evidence for the heterosexual transmission of hepatitis C. Am J Gastroenterol 1992;87:1849–1851

221. Tong MJ, Lai PPC, Hwang SH, et al. Evaluation of sexual transmission in patients with chronic hepatitis C infection. Clin Diagn Virol 1995;3:39–47

222. Scully LJ, Mitchel S, Gill P. Clinical and epidemiologic characteristics of hepatitis C in a gastroenterology/hepatology practice in Ottawa. Can Med Assoc J 1993;148:1173–1177

223. Diaz Morant V, De La Mata M, Costan G, et al. A low prevalence of antibodies to the hepatitis C virus in stable heterosexual couples. Gastroenterol Hepatol 1995;18:111–113

224. Garcia Bengoechea M, Cortes A, Lopez P, et al. Intrafamilial spread of HCV infection. Scand J Infect Dis 1994;26:15–18

225. Soto B, Rodrigo L, Garcia Bengoechea M, et al. Heterosexual transmission of HCV and the possible role of coexistent human immunodeficiency virus infection in the index case. A multicentre study of 432 pairings. J Intern Med 1994;236:515–519

226. Napoli N, Fiore G, Vella F, et al. Prevalence of antibodies to hepatitis C virus among family members of patients with chronic hepatitis C. Eur J Epidemiol 1993;9:629–632

227. Gabrielli C, Zannini A, Corradini R, et al. Spread of HCV among sexual partners of HCVAb positive intravenous drug users. J Infect 1994;29:17–22

228. Coltorti M, Caporaso N, Morisco F, et al. Prevalence of HCV infection in the household contacts of patients with HCV-related chronic liver disease. Infection 1994;22:183–186

229. Guadagnino V, Stroffolini T, Foca A, et al. Hepatitis C virus infection in family setting. Eur J Epidemiol 1998;14:229–232

230. Brusaferro S, Barbone F, Andrian P, et al. A study on the role of the family and other risk factors in HCV transmission. Eur J Epidemiol 1999;15:125–132

231. Caporaso N, Ascione A, Stroffolini T, et al. Spread of hepatitis C virus within families. J Viral Hepat 1998;5:67–72

232. Mondello P, Patti S, Vitale MG, et al. Anti-HCV antibodies in household contacts of patients with cirrhosis of the liver—preliminary results. Infection 1992;20:51–52

233. Bellobuono A, Zanella A, Petrini G, et al. Intrafamilial spread of hepatitis C virus. Transfusion 1991;31:475

234. Scaraggi FA, Lomuscio S, Perricci A, et al. Intrafamilial and sexual transmission of hepatitis C virus. Lancet 1993;342:1300–1301

235. Saltoglu N, Tasova Y, Burgut R, Dundar IH. Sexual and non-sexual intrafamilial spread of hepatitis C virus: intrafamilial transmission of HCV. Eur J Epidemiol 1998;14:225–228

236. Oshita M, Hayashi N, Kasahara A, et al. Prevalence of HCV in family members of patients with hepatitis C. J Med Virol 1993;41:251–255

237. Setoguchi Y, Kajihara S, Hara T, et al. Analysis of nucleotide sequences of HCV isolates from husband-wife pairs. J Gastroenterol Hepatol 1994;9:468–471

238. Nakashima K, Ikematsu H, Hayashi J, et al. Intrafamilial transmission of hepatitis C virus among the population of an endemic area of Japan. JAMA 1995;274:1459–1461

239. Kao JH, Chen PJ, Yang PM, et al. Intrafamilial transmission of HCV: The important role of infections between spouses. J Infect Dis 1994;170:1128–1133

240. Kim YS, Chi HS, Ahn YO, et al. Lack of familial clustering of hepatitis C virus infection. Int J Epidemiol 1998;27:525–529

241. Brackmann SA, Gerritzen A, Oldenburg J, et al. Search for intrafamilial transmission of HCV in hemophilia patients. Blood 1993;81:1077–1082

242. Camarero C, Martos I, Delgado R, et al. Horizontal transmission of hepatitis C virus in households of infected children. J Pediatr 1993;123:98–99

243. Vegnente A, Iorio R, Saviano A, et al. Lack of intrafamilial transmission of hepatitis C virus in family members of children with chronic hepatitis C infection. Pediatr Infect Dis J 1994;886–889

244. Kaldor JM, Archer GT, Buring ML, et al. Risk factors for hepatitis C virus infection in blood donors: a case-control study. Med J Australia 1992;157:227–230

245. Sun DX, Zhang FG, Geng YQ, et al. Hepatitis C transmission by cosmetic tattooing in women. Lancet 1996;347:541

246. Tumminelli, F, Marcellin P, Rizzo S, et al. Shaving as a potential source of hepatitis C virus infection. Lancet 1995;345:658

247. Mele A, Corona R, Tosti ME, et al. Beauty treatments and risk of parenterally transmitted hepatitis: results from the hepatitis surveillance system in Italy. Scand J Infect Dis 1995;27:441–444

248. Balasekaran R, Bulterys M, Jamal M, et al. A case-control study of risk factors for sporadic hepatitis C virus infection in the southwestern United States. Am J Gastroenterol 1999;94:1341–1346

249. EASL International Consensus Conference on Hepatitis C. Consensus statement. J Hepatol 1999;30:956–961

Recovery, Persistence, and Sequelae in Hepatitis C Virus Infection: A Perspective on Long-Term Outcome

HARVEY J. ALTER, M.D. and LEONARD B. SEEFF, M.D.

ABSTRACT *Hepatitis C has emerged in recent years as the most common basis for liver disease in the United States, having infected an estimated 3.9 million people in this country and an estimated 170 million worldwide. Currently, it is the predominant reason for undergoing liver transplantation. The disease it causes is characterized by silent onset in most infected individuals, a high rate of viral persistence, and the potential for development of ever-worsening chronic liver disease, ranging from chronic hepatitis to cirrhosis and occasionally to hepatocellular carcinoma. Such progression, when it occurs, is also most commonly a silent process that may take 20–40, and occasionally even more, years to reach its end point. Because of these characteristics, it has been exceedingly difficult to accurately assess the natural history. Efforts to accomplish this have consisted of retrospective, prospective, and cohort studies. The most concerning data have derived from the retrospective study approach, generally performed at tertiary referral centers. Because these centers commonly attract persons with existing chronic liver disease, they have tended to describe a high rate of progression to cirrhosis and cancer. This "referral bias" is avoided in the prospective and cohort study approach, and data derived from these studies indicate a lower rate of progression and a correspondingly higher rate of either recovery or minimal liver disease. In this review, we briefly describe potential mechanisms of viral persistence; present detailed information on outcomes that have derived from retrospective, prospective, and cohort studies, involving both adults and children; examine the data regarding progression of fibrosis and of progression to hepatocellular carcinoma; consider cofactors that might enhance liver disease progression; and report the emerging data that suggest that spontaneous viral clearance may be higher than is currently believed. We conclude with the view that severe, life-threatening, progressive liver disease clearly occurs in a sizable minority (perhaps 30%) of chronically infected persons but speculate that fibrosis progression is neither linear or inevitable and hence that most hepatitis C virus carriers will have either a stable nonprogressive course or such indolent pro-*

Objectives

Upon completion of this article, the reader should recognize: 1) the influence of study design on estimates of HCV disease severity; 2) that the rate of spontaneous recovery from HCV infection is higher than previously considered; 3) that fibrosis progression is not linear and is influenced by cofactors, particularly alcohol; 4) that it is likely that the majority of HCV infected individuals will not develop cirrhosis or other life threatening complications of their infection; and 5) that although the individual risk of developing severe complications may be less than 30%, the societal burden of HCV infection is very high because of the high prevalence and global distribution of the agent.

Accreditation

The Indiana University School of Medicine is accredited by the Accreditation Council for Continuing Medical Education to sponsor continuing medical education for physicians. The Indiana University School of Medicine takes responsibility for the contents, quality, and scientific integrity of this activity.

Credit

The Indiana University School of Medicine designates this educational activity for a maximum of 1.0 hours credit toward the AMA Physicians Recognition Award in category one. Each physician should claim only those hours of credit that he/she actually spent in the educational activity.

Disclosure

Statements have been obtained regarding the authors' relationships with financial supporters of this activity. There is no apparent conflict of interest related to the context of participation of the author of this article.

From the Department of Transfusion Medicine, Warren Grant Magnuson Clinical Center, and Section of Digestive Diseases and Nutrition, NIDDK, NIH, Bethesda, Maryland.

Reprint requests: Dr. H.J. Alter, Dept. Transfusion Medicine, Bldg. 10, Rm. 1C-711, NIH, 10 Center Drive, MSC 1184, Bethesda, MD 20894.

gression that they will die from an unrelated disease before the severe sequelae of hepatitis C become manifest or will have a sustained "curative" response to therapy. Although this view provides reasonable hope to the hepatitis C virus-infected individual, it does not deny the enormous burden this infection presents as the result of its high prevalence and global distribution. The sheer magnitude of the infected population will result in a large number with severe life-threatening liver disease even if the proportion of infected individuals that develop progressive disease is relatively small.

KEY WORDS: HCV, chronic hepatitis, fibrosis, cirrhosis

As the chronic consequences of hepatitis C virus (HCV) infection receive increased attention from patient advocate groups, public health advisories, and the lay press and as patient concern escalates, it is important to reexamine the natural history of this infection and to place disease outcomes in proper perspective. This is not an easy task because the disease process is indolent and outcomes may not be known for many decades. Thus, studies with 10-year or even 20-year follow-up that provide definitive outcome assessments for most diseases may not be adequate to fully assess the chronic sequelae of HCV infection. At present, there are considerable data regarding 20-year outcomes in HCV infection, but with few exceptions, extrapolations are required beyond that point. In addition to the slow evolution of disease, a balanced perspective must take into account variables such as the age at onset and cofactors, particularly alcohol. Further, one must examine both the disease burden for the infected individual and the disease burden for society. Based on currently available data, it would appear that the societal burden is considerable because of the high prevalence of the infection, but for most HCV-infected individuals, the infection has both low morbidity and low mortality. The problem is that we cannot predict the 20–30% of individuals who will sustain more dire outcomes.

In this review, we examine the evidence that HCV infection has serious and sometimes mortal consequences and, paradoxically, the evidence that this infection can be largely silent and compatible with uncompromised longevity. Specifically, we attempt to provide the framework within which the clinician can address the most common concerns of the HCV-infected individual, namely, "What is the likelihood that I will die of this disease?" "How sick will I become?" "Can I be cured?"

The clinician cannot provide definitive answers to these questions for the individual patient, but by presenting balanced data from natural history studies and treatment options, the physician can render a perspective that can reduce patient anxiety and offer realistic hope that the hepatitis will not progress rapidly, may not progress at all, may be compatible with a normal lifespan, and may respond to therapy.

HISTORICAL PERSPECTIVE

When first recognized, non-A, non-B hepatitis was regarded as a relatively mild illness that generally lacked the typical clinical manifestations of hepatitis A or B.[1] Speculation abounded as to whether non-A, non-B was a distinct viral illness or a nonspecific transaminitis related to postoperative events. The issue was resolved when non-A, non-B hepatitis was linked to needlestick injuries in health workers and, particularly, when human inocula were shown to transmit non-A, non-B hepatitis to chimpanzees.[2–5] Nonetheless, it required an additional 15 years before this nebulous transmissible agent was identified as HCV.[6]

The initial equanimity about the condition gave way to concern when it became apparent that about 50% of those infected had persistence of raised serum enzyme values even though most continued to have no symptoms.[7] Subsequently, liver biopsies established that the chronic asymptomatic hepatitis was accompanied by moderate to marked fibrosis or cirrhosis in about 20% of cases. Concern escalated when sporadic reports began to appear linking hepatocellular carcinoma (HCC) to previous episodes of non-A, non-B hepatitis.[8] The association between non-A, non-B/HCV and both cirrhosis and HCC was then confirmed in multiple studies.[9–12]

Later, epidemiologic studies of anti-HCV positive blood donors[13] and patients with community-acquired hepatitis C[14] revealed that 75–85% of HCV-infected individuals failed to resolve their infection, and population surveys determined that the prevalence of HCV infection in the United States was close to 2.0%, suggesting that almost 4 million people were chronically infected in the United States alone.[15]

Increasingly, the accrued evidence indicates that HCV infection, despite its generally mild clinical presentation, is a problem of considerable magnitude leading to persistent infection and chronic hepatitis in most and to cirrhosis and end-stage liver disease in some. Further, hepatitis C has now become the most frequent reason for hepatologic consultation and the single leading indication for hepatic transplantation, accounting for 30% of such procedures in the United States.[16] Thus, from obscure beginnings as a mild infection of unknown etiology, hepatitis C has ascended to international eminence as a leading cause of major liver disease. Nonetheless, the proportion of infected patients who reach these well-publicized deleterious outcomes remains poorly defined, and recent data suggest that such dire outcomes are less frequent than commonly feared.

MECHANISMS OF VIRAL PERSISTENCE AND THE PATHOGENESIS OF CHRONIC HEPATITIS

Although viral persistence is a fundamental prerequisite of chronic hepatitis, the mechanisms of viral persistence and liver injury may be distinct. It appears that the primary determinant of persistence is the quasispecies nature of the virus. HCV, like other RNA viruses, exists as a family of closely related but immunologically distinct variants that have been termed the quasispecies. More than 20 strains of HCV have been cloned from a single patient at a single point in time, and this is an underestimate of the total number of variants actually present. Thus, even if the host mounts a neutralizing immune response to the predominant HCV strain, any of the other variants already present could escape the immune attack and replicate to become the new predominant strain. By inoculating chimpanzees with mixtures of known infectious inocula and human sera obtained at various time points after the onset of infection, it has been shown that humans develop neutralizing antibodies to HCV but that these antibodies are highly strain specific and incapable of preventing the emergence of viral variants that can maintain the infection.[17]

Similar conclusions have been reached using in vitro systems that measure the uptake or binding of HCV to cultured cells.[18,19] Recently, Farci et al.[20] measured both the number of strain variants (complexity) and the number and breadth of nonsynonymous nucleic acid substitutions (diversity) that occur during the first 16 weeks of HCV infection and showed that the extent of viral diversity predicts whether HCV infection will resolve or become chronic. It appears that in most HCV-infected patients, the development of antibody exerts immune pressure that drives the quasispecies and leads to an increasingly complex population that can elude the immune attack and result in viral persistence.

The importance of antibody in driving viral diversity is further illustrated in patients with agammaglobulinemia, in whom it has been shown that in the absence of antibody the viral population remains homogeneous (see Farci and Purcell in this issue). Despite the correlation between viral diversity early in HCV infection and

the subsequent development of chronic hepatitis,[20] it is clear that humoral immune pressure and escape variants are not the only mechanisms determining persistent infection. Bukh et al.[20a] showed in the chimpanzee model that two animals, although infected with the identical full-length monotypic infectious clone, nonetheless had diverse outcomes, with one recovering and the other developing chronic infection. Other speculative mechanisms for viral persistence include the potential that HCV has mechanisms to decrease the effectiveness of antiviral cytokines, to increase the resistance of infected cells to cytotoxic T lymphocyte (CTL)-mediated killing, to infect immunologically privileged sites, or to induce immunologic tolerance.[21]

The net result of this host–virus interplay is that despite the development of antibodies to proteins expressed along the entire HCV genome, most patients are unable to eradicate the virus and manifest persistent infection usually with evidence of chronic liver disease. Further, the immune responses are so highly strain specific that even patients or animals that recover from HCV are susceptible to reinfection.[17,22]

Studies of cell-mediated immunity to HCV are just beginning to emerge, and the role of cell-mediated immunity in viral clearance and liver cell damage is still inconclusive but probably fundamentally important. Of interest, studies of intrahepatic CTL responses in chimpanzees have shown that viral variants can escape the CTL response just as they escape the humoral antibody response.[23] The influence of cell-mediated immunity on viral persistence will be comprehensively reviewed by Rehermann in the next issue of *Seminars*.

The mechanisms of cell death in HCV infection are not fully elucidated. Clearly, liver cell damage is not solely due to viral cytopathic effects because very high titers of virus within the liver and in serum are compatible with minor cell damage. Similarly, it is not clear that cytotoxic T cells are responsible because the worst degrees of liver disease are often observed in patients who are immunodeficient, particularly patients coinfected with human immunodeficiency virus (HIV).[24] Liver cell damage is probably a complex interplay of direct viral injury, cell mediated cytotoxicity, cytokine effects, apoptotic events, and other intracellular events that have not been elucidated.

HEPATITIS C OUTCOME BASED ON PATIENTS REFERED FOR CHRONIC LIVER DISEASE

As might be expected, the most severe outcomes of HCV infection have been observed in retrospective studies that assess persons with already established chronic hepatitis and attempt to define the rate of development of adverse sequelae by tracing the chronic disease back in time to the moment of acute onset (Table 1).

Kiyosawa et al.[9] conducted a retrospective evaluation of 231 patients with chronic non-A, non-B hepatitis (96 with chronic hepatitis, 81 with cirrhosis, and 54 with HCC) of whom approximately 90% were HCV related and 30–50% had been previously transfused. Serial liver biopsies in some documented the sequential progression from stages of increasingly severe inflammation and fibrosis to cirrhosis and, ultimately, to HCC. When frequent serial biopsies were available, cirrhosis was always found to precede HCC.

Similar data on clinical outcomes of transfusion-associated hepatitis C came from a report by Tong et al.[10] These investigators conducted a retrospective evaluation with short-term follow-up of 131 individuals from a group of 213 patients with chronic hepatitis C referred to their hospital. All 131 selected individuals had received blood transfusion on a single occasion. Initial liver biopsies in 101 patients revealed chronic hepatitis in 21%, chronic active hepatitis in 23%, cirrhosis in 51%, and HCC in 5%. Follow-up over a mean duration of 3.9 years (range, 1–15 years) demonstrated that an additional 7 patients (5%) developed HCC and 20 (15%) died, 8 from complications of cirrhosis, 11 from HCC, and 1 from pneumonia.

Yano et al.[25] examined histologic progression in 70 noncirrhotic patients who had 2–10 liver biopsies (mean, 3.9) obtained over the course of 5–26 years of follow-up. During follow-up, 50% developed cirrhosis,

including all patients who had a high histologic grade on a prior biopsy; the rapidity of progression correlated directly with the histologic grade. This important study clearly demonstrates the potentially serious nature of this chronic infection, particularly among Japanese patients. However, again this was a retrospective study of referred cases and had an inherent selection bias. A small number of patients were selected from a large patient base (70/2,000) without specific reasons being offered for their selection.

Niederau et al.,[26] from Germany, conducted a follow-up study of 838 HCV RNA positive patients referred to their tertiary-care center for therapy. The duration of follow-up ranged from 6 to 122 months (median, 50.2 months). At study entry, 141 (16.8%) patients had cirrhosis, mostly classified as Childs' A cirrhosis. A total of 62 patients (3.7%) died during the course of the study, 18 from cirrhosis, 13 from HCC, and 31 from other causes. Mortality was strongly related to the presence of cirrhosis and estimated duration of infection. Importantly, among the 696 patients without cirrhosis, mortality was no greater than that of the general population regardless of duration of infection. All patients who developed HCC either had cirrhosis at entry or developed cirrhosis later.

These studies (Table 1) conducted by referral centers unequivocally demonstrate the severe outcomes that can derive from HCV infection. However, because of referral bias, such studies do not assess the broad spectrum of outcomes that might occur if the entire HCV-infected populations were fully evaluated. Thus, referral-based studies do not determine the proportion of patients who

TABLE 1. Long-term Outcome of HCV Infection According to the Method of Study

Method of Study	Author (Reference)	Country	No. Patients	Interval from Exposure (mean or range of means, yr)*	Cirrhosis (%)	HCC (%)	Liver Death (%)
Retrospective†	Kiyosawa (9)	Japan	231	10–29	35.1	23.4	NR
	Tong (10)	USA	131	14–28	51.0	10.6	15.3
	Yano (25)	Japan	70	NR	50.0	NR	NR
	Niederau (26)	Germany	838	9–22	16.8	2.0	3.7
	Gordon (62)	USA	215‡	19	55.0	3.7	NR
	Gordon (62)	USA	195§	20	21.0	1.0	NR
Prospective‖	DiBisceglie (27)	USA	65	9.7	12.3	0	3.7
	Koretz (28)	USA	80	16.0	7.0	1.3	1.3
	Mattson (29)	Sweden	61	13.0	8.0	NR	1.6
	Tremolada (30)	Italy	135	7.6	15.6	0.7	3.7
Cohort¶	Seeff (38)	USA	103	20	15**	1.9	2.7
	Seeff (40)	USA	17	45–50	5.9	0.0	5.9
	Kenny-Walsh (43)	Ireland	376	17	2.0	0.0	0.0
	Vogt††(45)	Germany	458	17	0.3	0.0	0.0

*Based on interval from transfusion or initial use of intravenous drugs when that date was known.
†Based on referrals to tertiary care centers for persons with established liver disease.
‡Exposure through transfusion.
§Exposure through intravenous drug use
‖Long-term follow-up of persons studied from the time of acute infection.
¶Recall of patients diagnosed with acute hepatitis in prior prospective transfusion studies followed by renewed prospective follow-up with non-hepatitis controls.
††Study in children.

spontaneously recover from infection, the proportion who have mild disease and do not seek medical attention, or the proportion who die of intercurrent illnesses before their HCV status can be assessed. Thus, by their very design, such selective referral-based studies demonstrate only the more severe outcomes of HCV infection and represent a "worst-case" scenario. It is critically important to know that such severe outcomes occur but equally important to realize that retrospective studies provide incomplete information on the frequency with which progressively severe liver disease occurs in the entire universe of HCV-infected individuals.

OUTCOME BASED ON LONG-TERM FOLLOW-UP OF ACUTE HEPATITIS C

The original indication that acute non-A, non-B hepatitis progressed to chronic hepatitis in a large proportion of cases emanated from the long-term follow-up of patients enrolled in prospective studies of transfusion-associated hepatitis.[27–30] These studies, originally designed to investigate the incidence and causes of transfusion-associated hepatitis, were extended when it was observed that many patients still had elevated alanine aminotransferase (ALT) levels at the end of their designed 6-month follow-up (Table 1).

Patients originally enrolled in the NIH prospective transfusion-associated hepatitis studies[31] were reassessed for evidence of chronic liver disease by Di Bisceglie et al.[27]; 65 patients, 53 (82%) of whom had hepatitis C, were evaluated 1–24 years (mean, 9.7 years) after onset of acute non-A, non-B transfusion-associated hepatitis. Forty-five of the 53 (65%) developed chronic hepatitis, of whom 33 consented to liver biopsy. The study described these 33 patients plus 6 others with chronic non-A, non-B transfusion-associated hepatitis who were not enrolled in the original prospective study. When initially biopsied, 4 of 39 (10%) already had cirrhosis. Twenty of the 39 patients were rebiopsied at varying intervals, at which time 4 additional patients had histologic evidence of cirrhosis. Thus, cirrhosis was found in 20% of the 39 patients biopsied, or 12.3% of the total 65 patients assessed; none had HCC. Eleven patients died during follow-up, but only 2 from liver failure. Thus, liver-related death occurred in 2 of 45 (4%) of those with chronic hepatitis.

Koretz et al.[28] followed 80 patients who had developed acute transfusion-associated hepatitis approximately 16 years earlier, 64 (80%) of whom were HCV-infected based on enzyme immunoassay (EIA). Fifty-five of the 80 (69%) had biochemical evidence of chronic hepatitis. Liver biopsies were obtained in only 10 patients and were based on clinical severity; 5 (50%) had cirrhosis. Liver failure after 16 years of follow-up,

primarily the development of hypersplenism, developed in 22% of those with chronic hepatitis C. Approximately one third of the cases died during follow-up, but only one (1.3%) from liver disease (HCC).

Mattson et al.[29] reported a 13-year follow-up of 39 of 61 patients who had developed acute transfusion-associated non-A, non-B hepatitis. Serologic and molecular screening of archived blood samples identified acute hepatitis C in 24. Follow-up examination revealed that all 24 were still anti-HCV positive 13 years later and that 16 (66%) continued to have detectable HCV RNA. Most of the patients in follow-up (79%) continued to show abnormal serum enzyme levels whether or not HCV RNA could be detected, whereas 21% seemed to have recovered. Liver biopsies showed the presence of cirrhosis in 8%. One patient (1.6%) died as a consequence of liver disease.

Tremolada et al.[30] reported a follow-up study (mean, 7.6 years) among 135 patients with transfusion-associated non-A, non-B hepatitis, most having undergone cardiac surgery. Almost all cases were a consequence of HCV infection. Chronic hepatitis evolved in 104 (77%). Thirteen percent had splenomegaly and 5%, esophageal varices. Sixty-five patients were biopsied and 21 (32.3%) were found to have cirrhosis. This represents a cirrhosis frequency of 21% among those with chronic hepatitis and 15.6% among all of those diagnosed with acute hepatitis C. Among the 104 with chronic hepatitis, 5 (4.8%) died from liver disease (3, bleeding; 1, liver failure; 1, HCC). Thus, 5 (3.7%) of the original 135 HCV-infected group died as a consequence of liver disease.

Less severe outcomes were noted in the follow-up of community-acquired hepatitis C cases in the Center for Disease Control and Prevention's Sentinel Counties Study.[14] Among 130 identified hepatitis cases, 106 (82%) were diagnosed as hepatitis C, of whom 62% advanced to chronic hepatitis. Liver biopsies were performed in 30 of the 60 individuals with chronic hepatitis; 10 (33%) had "chronic active hepatitis," 1 of whom also had cirrhosis; 13 (43%) had "chronic persistent hepatitis"; and 6 (20%) had chronic lobular hepatitis. Thus, cirrhosis was found in only 1% of the 106 community-acquired hepatitis C cases followed over this relatively short interval. No patient with hepatitis C died over the course of the study.

Thus, these five prospective studies identified that progression from acute to chronic hepatitis C was common, that during the time periods of follow-up (approximately 4–16 years) cirrhosis, when sought, was identified in between 1 and 20% of the cases, that development of HCC was rare, and that liver-related mortality was modest in frequency, ranging from 0 to 3.7%. These prospective studies, which focus on entire populations with an identified episode acute hepatitis C, provide a more balanced portrait of hepatitis C outcomes than do the retrospective studies that concentrate on patients with already established chronic hepatitis. However, these prospective studies also have their failings in that they were not initially designed to study the chronic sequelae of hepatitis and had no mechanism for systematic liver biopsies. Biopsies thus tended to be performed on those who had the most severe biochemical abnormalities or physical evidence of chronic liver disease, and thus biopsy data are skewed to detect those with more severe liver disease. These studies are also flawed in that the dramatic interplay between hepatitis C and alcoholism was not established at the time the studies were conducted and data on coexistent alcoholism were sparse. Thus, these studies generally underestimate the role of alcohol and attribute all outcomes to the viral infection per se. Although this does not invalidate the outcome data, it confounds the interpretation of the natural history of uncomplicated hepatitis C infection. Finally, these prospective studies do not provide data on long-term clinical outcomes in control patients who did not develop hepatitis and do not extend their follow-up into what may prove to be the critical third and fourth decades of this infection.

OUTCOME BASED ON COHORTS STUDIED LONG AFTER A DEFINED PARENTERAL EXPOSURE

Four studies were designed to investigate the clinical and histologic outcomes of HCV infection in cohorts infected 17–40 years earlier (Table 1). The unique feature of these studies is that the HCV status of the subjects at or near the time of initial exposure was known and that an attempt was made to recall all known positives at least 15 years later. This design allows assessment not only of those who developed chronic infection and severe liver disease, but also those that cleared infection and/or had benign outcomes. In essence, this study design has some characteristics of a prospective study but allows long-term follow-up that rarely can be achieved in prospective studies.

The "concurrent-prospective" approach is illustrated by the collaborative Veterans Administration (VA) study of transfusion-associated hepatitis conducted by Seeff et al.[32] This study assessed long-term mortality after transfusion-associated non-A, non-B hepatitis using data from five separate prospective studies of transfusion-associated hepatitis performed between 1967 and 1980 (two VA studies[33,34]), an NIH study,[31] the national Transfusion-Transmitted Viruses study,[35] and a study conducted at the Walter Reed Army Hospital.[36]

A total of 1,552 of the 6,438 persons who entered the original studies were included in the follow-up study, 568 patients with non-A, non-B hepatitis and 984

matched controls.[32] At initiation of follow-up, an average of 18 years after transfusion, all-cause mortality was 51% in both non-A, non-B hepatitis cases and controls and was related primarily to the cardiac diseases that necessitated the original open-heart surgery. Liver-related mortality occurred in 3.3% of the non-A, non-B cases and in 1.5% of controls ($p = 0.02$). Cirrhosis as the cause of liver death occurred in 1.9% of the non-A, non-B cases and 1.0% of the controls. In the first 18 years of study, death due to HCC occurred in only one patient with non-A, non-B hepatitis (0.2%) and in two control patients (0.2%). Medical records could be examined for alcohol history in 28 of the 34 patients with a liver-related cause of death; among these, 78% of cases and 60% of controls were identified as heavy drinkers. Hence, liver-related mortality was generally low and, when found, strongly correlated with alcohol abuse.

In a follow-up report adding an additional 5 years of evaluation,[37] life-table analysis of all-cause mortality showed an increase among the non-A, non-B hepatitis cases to 69.1% and to 69.4% for the controls ($p = 0.67$). Liver-related death for the entire cohort was 4.0% for the cases and 1.7% for the controls ($p = 0.009$); for cases identified as HCV-related, liver-related death was 2.7% for the cases and 1.5% among their controls ($p = 0.31$) (Table 1). Thus, over the course of 23 years after exposure, most deaths could be ascribed to the underlying disease that initiated transfusion rather than to liver disease; though the proportion who died of liver disease was small, there was a trend toward increasing liver-related death among the non-A, non-B hepatitis cases with increasing time from exposure; the development of HCC was rare; and alcoholism alone or in combination with chronic viral hepatitis appeared to be the primary determinant of liver-related death. The number of deaths in HCV-infected patients in the absence of alcohol was extremely small.

In a separate analysis of this same multicenter cohort, long-term morbidity was assessed by recalling living patients for whom an archived blood sample was available for HCV testing.[38] Of the 146 living patients with a prior episode of transfusion-associated hepatitis, 103 (71%) had detectable HCV markers in a sample obtained during the course of their original hepatitis. An assessment of the 103 HCV-related cases approximately 20 years after disease onset revealed that 74% were still HCV RNA positive, 16% were HCV RNA negative on at least two determinations but had persistent anti-HCV antibody, and 10% had no residual markers of their HCV infection. One half of the viremic patients had biochemical evidence of chronic hepatitis, whereas the other half had normal serum enzymes. By protocol, biopsies were restricted to those with abnormal ALT values. Among these with persistent HCV RNA and ALT elevations, 30% had histologically defined cirrhosis. On the assumption that cirrhosis would occur in no more than 5% of those with HCV RNA and persistently normal ALT and in less than 1% in those repeatedly HCV RNA negative, an extrapolation to the entire group of HCV-related cases projected that less than 15% of acute hepatitis C cases would develop cirrhosis in 20 years.

Combining the mortality and morbidity data from this large, controlled, ~20-year follow-up study, it appeared that 25% of patients had spontaneously recovered from their HCV infection as evidenced by the loss of HCV RNA and in 10%, the concomitant loss of HCV serologic markers; 75% had persistent infection. Within the full cohort who developed acute hepatitis C, 3.5% subsequently died from liver disease and an additional 15% of living patients had cirrhosis. Thus, severe progressive chronic liver disease occurred in 15–20% of transfusion-related HCV-infected persons. The remaining 55% of the cohort had stable generally asymptomatic chronic hepatitis. The ultimate outcome of those with stable chronic liver disease over the first two decades of infection will determine the true severity of chronic hepatitis C. One can only speculate at present whether the disease will be inexorably progressive over time or whether a significant proportion of patients with chronic hepatitis C will, in the absence of alcohol excess, maintain an indolent nonprogressive infection that will have no impact on mortality and minimal impact on morbidity. It is critical that such cohorts continue in follow-up through the third and fourth decades of their infection.

The high mortality unrelated to liver disease, the inclusion of older patients, and the relatively restricted duration of follow-up in these transfusion studies has detracted from their acceptance as fully valid indicators of the natural history of hepatitis C infection. Some of these concerns could be addressed subsequently when it became possible to test a repository of 10,000 frozen sera that had been drawn from Air Force recruits between 1948 and 1954.[39] Outcome data could be ascertained in 8,568 of these individuals, all of whom were tested for anti-HCV and, when positive, tested by a confirmatory recombinant immunoblot (RIBA) assay and by polymerase chain reaction (PCR) for HCV RNA.[40] Outcome was determined using VA and Medicare files and Social Security and National Death Index tapes. Only 17 of 8,568 (0.2%) were confirmed to be anti-HCV positive in the repository sample; 11 of the 17 (65%) were HCV RNA positive. The average age at initial detection of HCV was 23 years. Over the almost 50-year interval from the first detection of anti-HCV until outcome tracing, mortality in the HCV-positive group (7/17, 41%) was significantly higher than that in the negative group (26%), but only one of the seven deaths was related to chronic liver disease. No HCV-infected patient died of HCC compared with 9 of 8,557 (0.1%) HCC-related deaths in the large population that was

HCV negative in the repository sample. Although the sample size was very small, this unique almost 50-year follow-up study of HCV-positive individuals revealed only one death from liver disease and no cases of HCC.

Milder outcomes are also observed in individuals whose HCV infection is detected incidentally during donor screening or other routine evaluation. In an NIH study of anti-HCV-positive blood donors,[41] 15% appeared to have recovered from their HCV infection based on the finding of RIBA-confirmed antibody but repeatedly negative PCR determinations for HCV RNA. Of those with persistent infection, peak ALT level exceeded two times the upper limit of normal in only 16%, and clinical symptoms were minimal. Liver biopsies were initially performed on 60 patients.[42] In 20 donors with persistently normal ALT, the mean histologic activity index (HAI) score was 5.4 and the mean fibrosis score 0.3; the corresponding HAI and fibrosis scores for donors with ALT levels between one and two times the upper limit of normal were 7.7 and 0.6 and for those with ALT levels more than twice normal, 9.0 and 1.2. Only one patient had cirrhosis, that patient being in the high ALT group. The number of biopsies in this population has now been expanded to 94 (Ghany M, Hoofnagle J, Alter HJ, unpublished data). No patients have severe inflammatory changes (HAI 15–18), 13% have stage 3 fibrosis, and 2% have cirrhosis after an average duration of infection of 19 years based on a defined parenteral exposure. Thus, this study of blood donors corroborates the findings in the Seeff study,[38] indicating that at least 15% of HCV-infected individuals spontaneously recover and that less than 15% have severe histologic lesions during the first two decades of infection.

To determine the progression of histologic lesions over time, repeat biopsies were obtained 5 years after the initial biopsy in 47 of 60 patients initially reported. Fibrosis progression over that interval was minimal. The mean fibrosis score increased from 0.5 to 0.9 in 13 donors with normal ALT, remained constant in 19 with ALT levels one to two times the upper limit of normal, and decreased from 1.4 to 0.8 in 15 donors with high ALT levels. Overall, no patients developed severe inflammatory changes or progressed to cirrhosis in the 5-year interval, which brought the average follow-up time since exposure to 24 years.

Two very important outcome studies were derived from the inadvertent administration of HCV-contaminated Rh immune globulin. Kenny-Walsh et al.[43] recently described clinical outcomes 17 years after HCV infection that resulted from the use of contaminated lots of anti-D immune globulin in Ireland in 1977. Eight batches of HCV-contaminated Rh immune globulin were thought to have been administered. A national inquiry organized tracing of recipients of these contaminated lots. Of 62,667 women who presented for screening, 704 were found to be anti-HCV positive, of whom

390 (55%) were also HCV RNA positive. Extensive evaluation was accomplished for 376 (96%) of those HCV RNA positive persons. Analysis revealed that the mean age at exposure was 28 years, that all genotyped as type 1, that about one third had at least one other hepatitis C risk factor, and that 5% had a history of heavy alcoholism. Serum ALT values were normal in 45%, slightly elevated (40–99 IU/mL) in 47%, and exceeded 100 IU/mL in 8%. The median ALT concentration was 42 IU/mL. Liver biopsies were performed on 363 of the 376 subjects enrolled in the recall evaluation. No inflammation was found in 2%, grade 1–3 inflammation in 41%, grade 4–8 in 52%, and grade 9–18 in 4%. Strikingly, 49% had no fibrosis, 34% showed periportal or portal fibrosis (stage 1), 15% had portal to portal or portal to central bridging (stage 3), and 2%, probable or definite cirrhosis (stage 4). Two of the seven women with cirrhosis were also heavy alcohol drinkers.

These results were quite similar to those of a study in Germany that involved 152 women who also had received HCV-contaminated Rh immune globulin[44]; approximately 15 years after exposure, none of these women had evidence of chronic active hepatitis or cirrhosis. Although the duration of follow-up in these two studies of contaminated Rh immune globulin was only 15–17 years, it is striking that fewer than 2% of HCV infected subjects had cirrhosis and less than 10% had severe inflammation or fibrosis. The relatively benign outcome in these studies may reflect the small size of the viral inoculum, the young age at the time of infection, less rapid progression in females, or simply insufficient duration of follow-up. Nonetheless, these findings substantiate that of the other cohort studies cited above and studies in children cited below, each of which suggest that when the entire HCV-infected population is followed, only a small percentage have severe outcomes during the first two decades of infection. Indeed, in the Air Force study, relatively benign outcomes were observed over five decades of follow-up.

Outcome in Children

Data from studies of infants and children are just beginning to emerge. Hepatitis C infection is not common in children because perinatal spread is uncommon and because needle exposures are generally limited to blood transfusion. The National Health and Nutrition Epidemiologic Survey shows that the prevalence of anti-HCV in children aged 6–11 is only 0.2% and rises to only 0.4% in those aged 12–19.[15] One of the most comprehensive outcome studies in children was conducted by Vogt et al. in Germany,[45] who enrolled 458 children who had cardiac surgery before the implementation of blood donor screening (Table 1). The patients had undergone cardiac surgery a mean of 17 years

(range, 12–27 years) earlier at a mean age at first operation of 2.8 years. None had received prior or subsequent transfusions and none had mothers with detectable HCV infection. An age- and sex-matched control group from the general population was also studied. Anti-HCV was detected in 67 (14.6%) patients compared with 3 (0.7%) among the controls. At follow-up evaluation, 37 patients (55%) were HCV RNA positive and 45% appeared to have spontaneously cleared the infection. All but one patient was found to have normal ALT values, and this single patient had severe right-sided congestive heart failure. Of the 17 patients who underwent liver biopsy, only 2 had histologic evidence of portal fibrosis, and both these patients had chronic congestive heart failure that might have accounted for the observed changes. One additional patient had "micronodular" cirrhosis, but this person was co-infected with the hepatitis B virus (HBV), and the relative role of HCV in the pathogenesis of the cirrhosis could not be established.

The study of Vogt et al. is the largest reported outcome study in children and describes a relatively benign course for transfusion-associated hepatitis C over a period of near 20 years. Importantly, they also found that almost one half of the infected children had spontaneously cleared HCV over this interval. The authors concluded that the natural history of chronic hepatitis C in childhood is either more benign or more slowly progressive than in adults.

Losasciulli et al[46] reported serologic and molecular follow-up data on 114 children with childhood leukemia of whom 56 (49%) were HCV RNA positive at the end of chemotherapy. Seventeen year follow-up of the HCV RNA positive cohort revealed that all were asymptomatic, that ALT values were normal in 71%, and that 16 of the 56 (29%) had spontaneously cleared their viremia. No liver biopsy data was reported in this study. A small study by Garcia-Monzon et al.[47] compared the outcome in 24 HCV-infected children and 22 HCV-infected adults. After a mean follow-up of 11 years, the comparative outcomes for children versus adults were as follows: mean viral load 3.6×10^5 versus 5.6×10^5 copies/mL, histologic grade (scale 0–4) 0.6 ± 0.7 versus 3.2 ± 1.1, and histologic stage (scale 0–4) 0.5 ± 0.5 versus 2.6 ± 1.2. Thus, despite similar viral loads, both hepatic inflammation and fibrosis were markedly less in children than adults.

Luban et al.[48] recently provided an interim report of a look-back study of 5,446 pediatric recipients of blood administered between 1982 and 1992. The mean age at transfusion was 1.0 year (range, birth to 10.7 years). The mean age at testing was 11 years (range, 4–17 years). Of 1,753 recipients thus far tested, 36 (2.0%) are confirmed anti-HCV positives compared with 0.3% of an age-matched nontransfused control population. Of the 36 HCV-positive children, all are asymptomatic. The range of ALT was 29–140 IU/L and 80% had at least one ALT value greater than 1.5 times the upper limit of normal. Thus far, only 7 of the 36 have been biopsied. After a mean interval of 13.6 years since exposure to blood, six patients showed only mild inflammation without fibrosis and one patient had mild inflammation with early bridging fibrosis.

Thus, although data from pediatric follow-up studies are still sparse, the available data consistently show mild outcomes over the first two decades of infection with a high rate of spontaneous recovery (29–45%) as assessed by the loss of HCV RNA. Nonetheless, it is unclear whether hepatitis C is actually milder in children or just more slowly progressive. If the latter, then the long-anticipated lifespan of infected children would allow them to eventually reach the same levels of cirrhosis and HCC as persons infected later in life. It is critical that these childhood cohorts continue to be followed and reported and that additional studies be undertaken among children infected 10 or more years ago.

Fibrosis Progression and Interval to Development of Cirrhosis and HCC

Although retrospective studies do not provide the full spectrum of outcomes, they do provide insight into the interval between the presumed causative exposure and disease development. This is generally achieved by

tracing back to a single transfusion episode or to a limited period of intravenous drug use. Both the Kiyosawa study[9] and the Tong study[10] related histologic diagnosis to the date of prior transfusion. In the Kiyosawa study[9] (Fig.1), transfusions had been received a mean of 10, 21.9, and 29 years earlier in patients with chronic hepatitis, cirrhosis, and HCC, respectively. Among the 21 patients with HCC, transfusions had been received as recently as 15 years earlier and as remotely as 60 years earlier. In the Tong study,[10] the mean interval from the date of transfusion to the diagnosis of chronic hepatitis was 13.7 years, to cirrhosis, 20.6 years, and to HCC, 28.3 years (Fig. 1). These two classic studies have led to the useful approximations that the interval to development of histologically recognized chronic hepatitis, cirrhosis, and HCC are 10, 20, and 30 years, respectively.

The rate of fibrosis progression to cirrhosis was evaluated in a large multicenter histologic analysis conducted by Poynard et al.[49] A total of 2,235 patients were recruited from three large population-based studies performed in France. Fibrosis progression was determined as a ratio between the fibrosis stage (scale of 0–4 METAVIR units) and the estimated duration of infection in years. The METAVIR scoring system incorporated fibrosis staging and activity grading using carefully defined parameters. Most data were derived from single biopsies, although 70 patients had paired biopsy samples. The median rate of fibrosis progression was

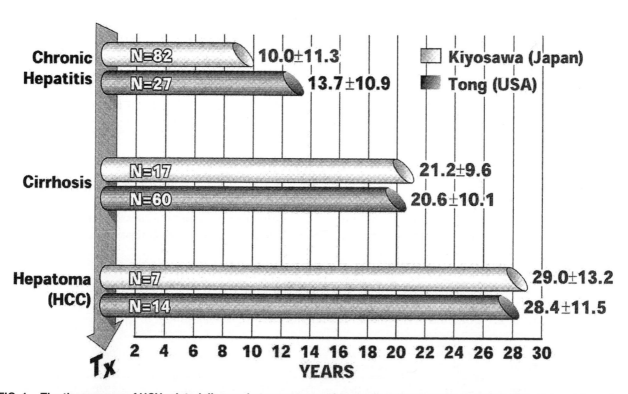

FIG. 1. The time course of HCV-related disease in two retrospective studies[9,10] that performed liver biopsies on referred patients with a past history of blood transfusion. The indicated duration of disease was based on the interval from the time of transfusion to the time of liver biopsy.

0.133 units/year. Thus, if fibrosis progression were linear, it would require 7.5 years to progress from one fibrosis stage to another and a median of 30 years to progress from no fibrosis to cirrhosis. By incorporating other variables in fibrosis progression, Poynard et al. estimated that the development of cirrhosis would range from a median of 13 years among men who were infected over the age of 40 and drank more than 50 g of alcohol/day to a median of 42 years for women infected under the age of 40 who did not drink. Because the rate of fibrosis progression was not normally distributed, they considered it likely that there are three separate populations with regard to outcome: rapid fibrosers, intermediate fibrosers, and slow fibrosers. These data prompted their view that about one third of HCV-infected persons will advance to cirrhosis in less than 20 years and that another one third would either never develop cirrhosis or would do so over a span of at least 50 years. These estimates are very consistent with the progression intervals defined by Tong et al.[10] and Kiyosawa et al.[9] and also with the observations of the previously cited prospective studies of transfusion-associated hepatitis.[27–30]

Outcome After the Development of Cirrhosis

An important and somewhat unexpected observation was that of the long duration of survival even after the development of cirrhosis. Fattovich et al.[50] conducted a retrospective follow-up study of 384 patients with compensated HCV-related cirrhosis to assess morbidity and mortality (Table 2). Fifty-one patients (13.3%) died during follow-up, 17 from HCC, 16 from liver failure, 6 from bleeding, and 15 from causes unrelated to cirrhosis. Thus, 9% died from liver-related causes 9–124 months (mean, 50 months) after study entry. Survival probability was 96% at 3 years, 91% at 5 years, and 79% at 10 years unless decompensation ensued, in which case survival fell to 50% at year 5. The annual mortality rate was 1.9% during the first 5 years. Multivariate analysis identified elevated bilirubin, physical evidence of cirrhosis and portal hypertension,

older age, and low platelet count as independent risk factors for survival. Treatment with interferon was not identified to be an independent prognostic factor for survival.

HCC developed in 29 (8%) patients over periods of 7–134 months (mean, 48 months), the cumulative probability of its occurrence being 4% at 3 years after recognition of cirrhosis, 7% at 5 years, and 14% at 10 years. The calculated yearly incidence of HCC development was 1.4%. Among the remaining 355 patients, 65 (18%) developed evidence of decompensation at a mean interval of 37 months. Overall, most patients with documented cirrhosis in the Fattovich study survived for more than 10 years without evidence of hepatic decompensation or HCC.

A similar analysis was undertaken by Serfaty et al.[51] (Table 2). Among 668 patients with HCV infection referred to a tertiary care institution in Paris, 103 (15.4%) had cirrhosis. These patients were followed for a median period of 40 months (range, 6–72 months). Fifty-nine of the 103 were treated with interferon-α, six of whom developed normal ALT and three, a sustained virologic response. Twenty-six (25%) of the 103 patients with cirrhosis developed hepatic complications, consisting of HCC in 11 patients and hepatic decompensation without HCC in 15. HCC developed in 3% after 2 years and 11.5% after 4 years for a calculated annual incidence of 3.3%. The cumulative probability of decompensation without HCC at 2 and 4 years was 15% and 20%, respectively. Sixteen percent of patients died in follow-up, all but one from hepatic causes (liver failure, HCC, bleeding), and three patients underwent transplantation. The annual incidence of death or transplantation was 5.5%, and conversely, the cumulative probabilities of survival were 96% at 2 years and 84% at 4 years. In contrast to the Fattovich study,[50] interferon therapy was shown to reduce the risk of hepatic decompensation and HCC in patients with established cirrhosis.

HCV and HCC

Although the data for a causal relationship between HCV and HCC are not as compelling as for HBV, they

---

TABLE 2.   Outcome in HCV-infected Patients after the Development of Cirrhosis

Author (Reference)	No. Patients	Mean Follow-up (mo)	Hepatic Decompensation	HCC (%)	HCC Annual Rate (%)	Liver Death (%)	Annual Death Rate (%)
Fattovich (50)	384	61	18.0	8.0	1.4	9.0*	1.9
Serfaty (51)	103	40	14.5	10.6	3.3	16.0	5.5

*Survival probability 91% at 5 years and 79% at 10 years unless decompensation ensued, in which case survival fell to 50% at 5 years.

nonetheless strongly suggest that HCV plays a major role in the evolution of HCC, usually through the intermediary development of cirrhosis. Although cirrhosis may not be an absolute prerequisite to the evolution of HCC, it has been substantiated that HCC develops in the setting of cirrhosis in at least 90% of cases. Because HCV does not integrate into the host genome, it is commonly speculated that malignant transformation is the byproduct of the numerous mitotic events that accompany compensatory hepatic regeneration in the face of progressive viral and immune-mediated hepatocellular destruction and fibrosis. This is clearly a simplistic explanation of complex extra- and intracellular events, but it provides a common foundation for the development of HCC in a variety of viral and nonviral diseases that affect the liver.

Although an association between HCV and HCC has been recognized throughout the world, the strongest evidence emanates from Japan, where HCC is the leading cause of cancer death in men. The association has been weaker in Western counties, particularly the United States, and has been more difficult to evaluate in areas such as China, Southeast Asia, and sub-Saharan Africa where HBV is highly endemic and is the leading cause of primary liver cell cancer.

One of the earliest clues to the relationship between HCV and HCC came from the study of Kiyosawa et al.,[9] who performed HCV serology on 54 HBsAg-negative patients with HCC; 94% were shown to have antibody to HCV. Most convincing in this study was the fact that serial biopsies were available from 21 patients who developed HCC at varying intervals after an established episode of transfusion-associated non-A, non-B hepatitis. In cases with frequent biopsies, the sequential progression from acute hepatitis to chronic persistent hepatitis to chronic active hepatitis to cirrhosis and then to HCC was well documented. In those with less frequent biopsies, histologic evidence of cirrhosis was documented before the onset of HCC in 18 of 21 (86%). The transfusion event that was the presumed source of HCV infection occurred 17–60 years earlier and most commonly occurred more than 30 years before the diagnosis of HCC.

A study of HCV seroprevalance among 105 HBV-negative HCC cases was undertaken in five districts of Japan[52]; 76% were found anti-HCV positive by first generation assays compared with 1% of donors in these same districts. A history of blood transfusion was found in 40% of the HCV-positive cases compared with only 5% of those with HCC related to HBV or of unknown cause. Hence, both transfusion and HCV infection were strongly associated with the occurrence of HCC in this population.

Also in Japan, Kato et al.[53] estimated the cumulative risk for HCC development in patients with cirrhosis related to HCV, HBV or a presumed non-ABC (cryptogenic) agent. Although the diagnosis of HCC was initially made using imaging techniques, most patients had histologic confirmation of the cancerous lesion. Based on clinical diagnosis, the 5-year and 10-year cumulative incidence of HCC was 25% and 57%, respectively. During follow-up of approximately 4 years, HCC was recognized in 38% of patients in the HBV group, 44% in the HCV group, and only 13% in the cryptogenic group. The cumulative risk for HCC was slightly, but not significantly, higher in HCV-infected patients compared with HBV-infected patients with a yearly incidence of 7–14%.

A recent representative study from Japan is that of Yoshida et al.[54] that focused on the effect of interferon in the prevention of HCC. This was a multicenter retrospective cohort study of 2,890 patients with chronic hepatitis C who had undergone liver biopsy since 1986; 2,400 (83%) were treated with interferon. HCC developed in 89 interferon-treated patients (3.7%) and in 59 of 490 (12%) untreated patients. Among untreated patients, the annual incidence of HCC increased with the degree of liver fibrosis from 0.5% in those with stage 0 or stage 1 fibrosis to 7.9% in those with cirrhosis. The cumulative incidence of HCC in treated patients was significantly ($p < 0.001$) less than that in untreated subjects for those who had stage 2 or 3 fibrosis at the time of enrollment. Overall, the risk of HCC during the follow-up period of 4.3 years was significantly affected by both the initial stage of fibrosis and treatment with interferon. In a multivariate analysis, the adjusted risk ratio for the interferon-treated group was 0.516 ($p < 0.001$) and 0.197 for the subset who had a sustained virologic response to treatment. Thus, this very large study confirms the progression from chronic hepatitis C to HCC, relates progression to the stage of fibrosis, and demonstrates that successful treatment with interferon can block both fibrosis progression and malignant transformation.

Although most studies on the relationship of HCV to HCC have derived from Japan, to various degrees there is confirmation of this association throughout the world. In Italy, Colombo et al.[12] found anti-HCV in 64 of 91 (70%) HBsAg-negative patients with HCC and in 22 of 41 (54%) patients with HCC who were HBsAg positive. Because the prevalence was similar in HBsAg-positive and -negative cases and because all anti-HCV-positive/HBsAg-negative cases were also anti-HBc positive, it was difficult in this study to isolate the impact of HCV in HCC causation. Nonetheless, the authors concluded that HCV was an important factor in the development of HCC and postulated that combined infection with HCV and HBV would be more likely to result in serious outcomes. In contrast, Chen and Chen,[55] who studied HCC in Taiwan, showed that patients coinfected with HCV and HBV were on the average 10 years older than HCC patients infected only with HBV. The authors interpreted this observation to indicate that HCV did not accelerate the occurrence of HCC among HBV carriers. In another area of high HBV endemicity, Hadzyannis et al.[56] studied 65 cases of HCC in Greece and compared seroprevalance for HBV and HCV with that of age- and sex-matched controls with benign conditions. In a logistic regression model of HCC cases versus controls, the odds ratio for cases being HBsAg positive was 18.8 (CI, 8.2–43.2) and for being anti-HCV positive was 7.7 (CI, 1.7–35.1). In a study of 380 South African blacks with HCC, Kew et al.[57] found anti-HCV in 110 patients (29%) and in only 1 of 110 controls. However, only 27 (7%) had anti-HCV in the absence of markers for current or past HBV infection. Overall, in areas of high HBV prevalence, it appears that HCV plays a causal role in HCC pathogenesis, but the precise impact is difficult to ascertain because of the more predominant and confounding role of HBV.

In contrast to Japan where HCC is a leading cause of cancer death and where most cases appear related to HCV, in the United States, HCC accounts for only 2% of cancer deaths and the role of HCV in cancer causation is less well defined. Yu et al.[58] studied 51 patients with HCC in Los Angeles County; 15 of 51 (29%) patients with HCC had anti-HCV and the relative risk of HCC in those anti-HCV positive was 10.5. Based on combined HCV and HBV markers, it was estimated that of the 51 cases, 9% were related to HCV alone, 20% to HBV alone, and 18% to co-infection with HCV and HBV. Hence, most cases had no identified viral etiology. Di Bisceglie et al.[59] studied HCV prevalence in 99 consecutive cases of HCC and compared that with 98 cases with other malignant tumors. Anti-HCV was found in 13% of HCC patients and in 2% of controls, and the relative risk of HCC for those anti-HCV positive was 7.3. In this same study, 15% of cases were thought related to HBV infection, and the relative risk for HBsAg positive individuals was 17.3. Together, HCV and HBV accounted for only 28% of HCC cases. Thus, in these U.S. studies, HCV-infected patients have a definite increased risk of developing HCC, but the proportion of HCC cases due solely to HCV is low (13–17%). Most cases were unrelated to either HCV or HBV, implicating other viral or nonviral etiologies.

Two other U.S. studies, both involving patients from the Miami area, demonstrated a stronger association with HCC. Hassan et al.[60] retrospectively studied 59 patients with HCC, 90% of whom had biopsy-proven cirrhosis; 53% had anti-HCV by first generation assays and none had other risk factors for HCC. A high proportion (36%) of patients with HCC was negative for both HCV and HBV markers. Liang et al.[61] performed a molecular and serologic analysis of 112 patients with HCC referred to the University of Miami. None of the patients had nonviral risk factors for HCC and 95% had

documented cirrhosis. HBsAg was found in 21 (19%) patients. Of the 91 HBsAg negative HCC cases, 29 (32%) had isolated HBV DNA in serum and/or liver and thus probably represent cryptic HBV cases, 42 (46%) were anti-HCV positive, and an additional 8 (9%) were HCV RNA positive in the absence of anti-HCV; 13% had no identified viral marker. Thus, 50 of the 91 HBsAg negative cases (55%) had serologic and/or molecular evidence of HCV infection. In addition, HCV markers were found in 6 of 21 (29%) HBsAg positive cases. HCV RNA was amplified from the liver tissue of seven of nine HBsAg negative cases; three of these patients had no HCV markers in their serum.

This study provides the most compelling evidence that HCV plays a prominent role in HCC pathogenesis in the United States as well as in Japan. Indeed, it has been argued that the differences in the incidence of HCV-related HCC in the United States and Japan is a reflection of time rather than pathogenesis. The average age of Japanese patients with HCC is 10–20 years greater than U.S. patients, raising the possibility that the HCV "endemic" began in Japan 10–20 years earlier than in the United States and that decades from now the United States will experience the same high rates of HCC as now seen in Japan. Alternately, there may be genetic factors or environmental cofactors present in Japan that either accelerate the progression to cirrhosis, providing the backdrop for malignant transformation, or that play a more direct oncogenic role. Only time will resolve this issue.

Cofactors as Determinants of Severity

The outcomes of HCV infection vary so widely from patient to patient that codeterminants of disease progression have long been suspected. Differences in outcome could relate to viral factors (viral load, viral genotype, multiplicity of quasispecies); host factors (age at infection, duration of infection, gender, immune deficiency, genetic susceptibility, co-infection with other viruses such as HBV and HIV, comorbid conditions such as hemochromatosis and iron overload); or external factors (chronic alcoholism, diet, smoking, medicines, established hepatotoxins, or undefined environmental contaminants).

Gordon et al.[62] studied whether the mode of HCV transmission affected long-term outcomes (Table 1). They found that 19–20 years after acquiring hepatitis C, the cumulative risk of developing cirrhosis in 215 patients who had been transfused was 55% compared with 21% among 195 persons who had been exposed through intravenous drug use ($p = 0.001$). The authors concluded that the risk of liver failure was more closely related to the mode of transmission than to other risk factors evaluated, including age and duration of infection.

Of the viral factors, HCV genotypes 1a and 1b appear to be associated with more severe disease and clearly are more resistant to therapy.[63,64] In contrast, there has been no reproducible relationship between viral load and disease outcome.[65] Although a prospective study has shown that the degree of diversity of the viral quasispecies during the first 4 months of HCV infection predicts whether the patient will recover or develop chronic liver disease,[20] there is no apparent relationship between viral diversity and disease outcome once chronic infection is established.

Of host factors, age at the onset of infection appears to be an important determinant of disease progression and severity. As indicated above, infected children seem to have a more benign outcome than infected adults. Also, the mildest outcomes in adults have been observed in those infected under the age of 40, as seen in the study of Air Force recruits[40] and the studies of HCV-contaminated Rh immune globulin[43] described above. Poynard et al.[49] assessed fibrosis progression in relation to nine factors: age at biopsy, estimated duration of infection, sex, age at infection, alcohol consumption, HCV genotype, hepatitis C viremia, cause of infection, and histologic activity grade. Only three factors were independently associated with fibrosis progression: age at infection (older than 40 years), daily alcohol consumption of 50 g or more, and male sex. Niederau et al.[26] also performed a multivariate regression analysis of factors that affected survival in HCV-infected individuals. Older age was a significant independent variable in decreased survival, as was cirrhosis, long disease duration, chronic alcoholism, and intravenous drug abuse. Age, however, is a complex variable to interpret. It is important to distinguish age at the onset of infection from age at the time of diagnosis. Older age at the time of diagnosis may simply reflect duration of infection, and it is clear that for many patients, the longer the duration of infection, the more severe the observed sequelae. In this respect, even though those infected at a younger age appear to do better, they also have a longer anticipated lifespan in which severe outcomes may ultimately emerge. Finally, there is the complex issue of whether there are elements of old age that will accelerate formerly stable disease independent of the duration of infection. Basically, do age-related changes in the host, such as depression of the immune system, accelerate the course of the disease? Unfortunately, it is difficult to design studies that clearly distinguish the influence of disease duration from the influence of age itself.

Hepatitis C progression appears to be more rapid in patients with hypogammaglobulinemia, most of whom have been exposed through contaminated lots of intravenous immunoglobulin. Rates of progression to cirrhosis of 31% and 35% have been observed within 10 years of exposure in two Swedish studies.[66,67] The immuno-suppression associated with HIV infection also appears to influence outcome, though the data differ according to the source of infection. In hemophiliacs, who were frequently infected with both HCV and HIV before the viral inactivation of clotting factor concentrates, those coinfected with HIV had more severe histologic changes and higher liver related mortality than those infected with HCV alone.[24,68–70] Although there is a general correlation between low CD4 count, the level of HCV viremia, and disease severity in these studies, the exact mechanism by which HIV adversely influences the outcome of HCV infection is not well elucidated. In intravenous drug abusers co-infected with HIV and HCV, there is a clear inverse relationship between CD4 count and the level of HCV RNA but no consistent relationship between HIV infection and the severity of coexistent hepatitis C.[71]

Genetic factors may also influence the outcome of HCV infection through their effect on the immune response or other susceptibility factors. Although specific human leukocyte antigen alleles, particularly class II DR and DQ loci,[72,73] have been associated with disease progression, there has been no consistent genetic link to the outcome of HCV infection. Active investigations continue in this area, particularly in search of genetic links unrelated to HLA.

Of these potential cofactors, the relationship of alcohol to disease severity is the most clearcut and has been consistently demonstrated in multiple studies. In a unique study, designated the Dionysios study, Bellentani et al.[74] attempted to determine the extent and causes of chronic liver disease in the entire population of two small Northern Italian towns. The study enrolled 6,917 of 10,151 inhabitants (69%) and undertook medical and epidemiologic histories, physical exams, and serologic and biochemical testing. Among 1,211 patients diagnosed with chronic liver disease, 58% were attributed to alcohol abuse (>60 g/day), 16% to HCV infection, 3% to alcohol plus HCV, and 7% to HBV. The remaining cases were thought to be due to medications or other rare events. A different pattern emerged when serious liver disease was evaluated. Among 78 cases with cirrhosis, 28% were HCV related, 26% alcohol related, 9% HBV related, and 11% due to combinations of alcohol and virus; the remaining cases were hereditary or cryptogenic. Important to this analysis, among HCV- or HBV-infected patients who did not drink excessively, 11.5% and 8.7%, respectively, developed cirrhosis or HCC. In contrast, among HCV- or HBV-infected patients who drank excessively, 31.2% developed cirrhosis or HCC ($p < 0.001$).

The role of alcohol in exacerbating viral infection was dramatically demonstrated in a study by Corrao and Arico[75] wherein they compared lifetime teetotalers with alcohol abusers (175 g/day) according to HCV status

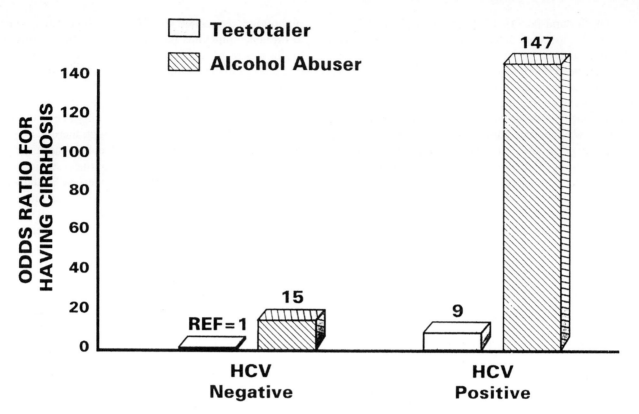

FIG. 2. Comparison of the risk of developing cirrhosis in relation to both alcohol abuse and HCV status. Persons who do not drink and are HCV negative are the referent group. Abusing alcohol in the absence of HCV imposes a 15-fold increased risk of cirrhosis. A nine-fold increased risk was observed in persons who were HCV-infected but abstained from alcohol. A marked increased risk (147-fold) was observed in patients who were HCV-infected and drank excessively. Thus, the combined deleterious effects of alcohol and HCV infection were substantially more than additive.

(Fig. 2). Subjects who did not drink and were HCV negative served as the reference population. The relative risk for developing cirrhosis in alcohol abusers who were not HCV infected was 15 and that for persons HCV infected who did not drink was 9. In contrast, in patients who were both HCV infected and abused alcohol, the relative risk of developing cirrhosis was 147. These studies, and others,[76–78] have led to the accepted conclusion that HCV-infected patients should abstain from alcohol or limit their intake to no more than one drink per day.

CONCLUSIONS

There is an incontestable association between HCV infection and the subsequent development of cirrhosis, HCC, and end-stage liver disease. At present, 30% of liver transplants in the United States are a consequence of underlying HCV-related cirrhosis. These are somber associations that are well publicized and create considerable fear in those diagnosed with hepatitis C, even though most such individuals have a clinically silent infection. It is important to provide this "silent majority" with a balanced perspective that incorporates probabili-

ties not only of dire outcomes, but also long-term survival and successful therapy. When these elements are balanced, the patient is not only better informed but also generally relieved.

Although HCV infection is rarely encountered in the acute stages, it is important to ascertain outcome in those who are recognized during incipient infection. It has become increasingly clear that at least 15% of HCV-infected individuals have a spontaneous recovery, generally within the first year. The 15% recovery rate, based on the absence of HCV RNA in sequential samples and normalization of ALT, has been documented in prospective studies[7] and confirmed in population-based screening.[41] This spontaneous recovery in HCV infection is as unequivocal as is the progression to cirrhosis. Further, data now suggest that spontaneous recovery rates may be even higher than initially described. When cohorts known to have been HCV infected from a defined exposure are recalled decades later, the percent that maintain antibody but have lost HCV RNA has ranged from 26% to 45% (Table 3). It is probable that on average the recovery rate in acute HCV infection is closer to 20% than to the commonly cited 15%. The key issue then becomes the clinical outcome in the 80% who develop persistent HCV infection. There is an accumu-

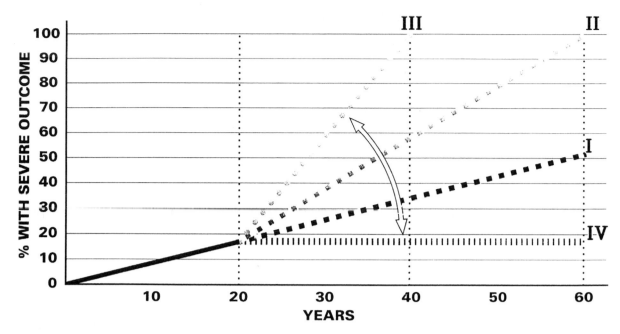

FIG. 3. Projection of the severe outcomes of HCV infection. The percent with severe outcomes in the first two decades of infection is based on a considerable body of evidence (see text) and appears to be less than 20%. Curve I assumes that the development of severe disease (fibrosis progression) will be linear and that approximately 50% of infected individuals will have severe outcomes 60 years after the onset of infection. Curves II and III assume that every HCV-infected individual will develop severe liver disease if they do not die of another illness in the 40–60 years that might be required for this indolent progression. Curve IV assumes that if severe disease has not developed in 20 years, it generally will not occur. The relative probabilities of these assumptions are discussed in the text, and it is the author's speculation that the "true" outcome will reside below curve I.

lating and consistent body of evidence that during the first two decades of HCV infection, fewer than 20% of patients followed prospectively from the time of acute infection or recalled subsequent to a known exposure have evidence of severe liver disease (Table 1). Indeed, in persons infected as children and young adults, the proportion with severe liver disease in the first two decades appears to be less than 5%.

Thus, at the end of 20 years, approximately 80% of HCV-infected individuals have either recovered, have stable chronic hepatitis, or have died of an intercurrent illness. To estimate the long-term outcome of HCV infection, attention must focus on the majority of infected

TABLE 3. Studies Indicating High Rates of Spontaneous Recovery* in HCV Infection

Author (Reference)	Country	Percent Recovery*	Setting
Alter (15)	USA	26	Population survey (NHANES III)
Kenny-Walsh (43)	Ireland	45	Contaminated Rh immune glob.
Seeff (38)	USA	26	TAH—Adult
Vogt (45)	Germany	45	TAH—Pediatric

*Recovery based on the sustained loss of HCV RNA, generally with normalization of ALT and persistence of RIBA-confirmed antibody. TAH, transfusion-associated hepatitis; NHANES III, National Health and Nutrition Epidemiologic Survey III.

individuals who have apparent stable or very slowly progressive liver disease. Figure 3 is databased for the first 20 years, showing a less than 20% incidence of severe disease during this interval, and then projects a series of potential long-term outcomes. In projection I, progression of liver disease is considered linear, advancing at a constant pace so that after 60 years of HCV infection, approximately 50% will have developed severe liver disease. Projections II and III assume an acceleration of fibrosis after the first 20 years of infection, in which case every HCV-infected individual would ultimately develop severe liver disease if they survived 40–60 years from the onset of infection. Projection IV makes a very different assumption, namely that if severe disease has not occurred in 20 years, it may never occur. The dilemma is to decide where the truth lies in these assumptions that project beyond our database? Conclusions drawn from these projections are clearly speculative and tenuous, but worthy of comment.

Is HCV-related liver disease linear in its progression as depicted in curve I? The dramatically variable outcomes among HCV-infected patients argues against linear progression as do studies in blood donors,[42] blood recipients,[7,38] or unique cohorts.[40] The large METAVIR analysis of fibrosis progression by Poynard et al.[49] derives fibrosis units that assume a linearity of progression. Nonetheless, the authors recognize that fibrosis progression is neither linear nor normally distributed.

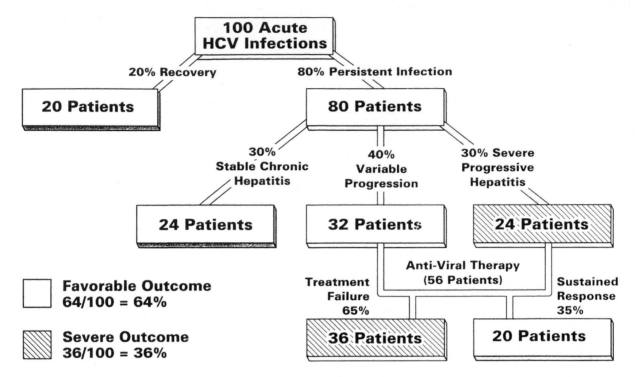

FIG. 4. Projected outcome in a hypothetical cohort of 100 individuals with acute HCV infection. Existing data (see text) suggests that 20% will spontaneously resolve their acute infection. Natural history studies suggest that of the residual 80 patients, 30% would manifest progressively severe liver disease, 30% would have stable chronic hepatitis that did not progress to cirrhosis, and 40% would have a variable outcome that might or might not eventuate in cirrhosis. The natural history of HCV infection is now tempered by therapeutic intervention. Because the ultimate outcome in an individual patient cannot be predicted accurately , most patients with chronic hepatitis are now being treated. The figure projects that of the 56 patients who might have advanced to cirrhosis during the natural history of their infection, 35% (20 patients) will be "cured" by existing combination therapy. The figure assumes that the 24 patients with stable chronic hepatitis will do well whether or not they are treated. Hence, of the total population of 100 acutely infected individuals, 64% will have a favorable outcome either through spontaneous recovery, an inherently stable chronic hepatitis, or a sustained treatment response.

They considered the likelihood that there are three populations consisting of rapid fibrosers, intermediate fibrosers, and slow fibrosers (we would add a category of nonfibrosers). Based on this, the investigators projected that about one third of HCV-infected individuals would advance to cirrhosis in 20 years, that a third would advance more slowly, and that a third would either never develop cirrhosis or require 50 or more years to do so. When combined, this even distribution of diverse outcomes could give the impression of a linearity that does not indeed exist. It is of interest that the METAVIR projections are not inconsistent with the ultimate outcome predicted by curve I wherein 50% would develop severe disease in 60 years.

Is there reason to suspect that liver disease progression will accelerate after the first 20 years due to increasing duration of infection or age-related changes in the host environment? Clearly, as indicated in this review, there is an established relationship between disease duration and disease severity and evidence that liver disease is more severe in the elderly.[9,49] Increasing disease severity over time is indeed integral to the assumptions of slope I (Fig. 3). In contrast, scenarios II

and III are predicated on acceleration, a distinct change in the slope of the curve, at some point in time. Although this could occur, to date, there has been no published evidence to support an acceleration of fibrosis progression after any given number of years of infection or any given age. Rather there are early data that the liver disease can be nonprogressive for up to 50 years.[40] Overall, curve I appears more likely and more evidence based than curves II or III.

Curve IV suggests that patients who have not demonstrated progression to more intense inflammatory activity or fibrosis by 20 years may never do so. There is little published evidence to support the flat trajectory depicted in curve IV, but anecdotally, long-term follow-up of HCV-infected patients in NIH prospective studies has demonstrated that some have late spontaneous normalization of ALT levels and diminution in anti-HCV reactivity despite the continued presence of HCV RNA and others have persistently normal or near-normal ALT with minimal histologic lesions in repeat biopsies obtained over the course of two decades. More detailed studies are required to determine if there is a true "burnout" or complete long-term stabilization of HCV-related liver disease, as also suggested in the METAVIR analysis.[49] Based on the above considerations, it is our speculation that in the absence of treatment, the natural history of HCV infection will lie somewhere between curves I and IV, perhaps closer to curve I. Successful treatment would, of course, lower the slope as it improves outcome; highly effective therapy would flatten the curve.

Clearly, these long-term projections are speculative, but it seems reasonable, based on the data in this review, to conclude that of 100 persons acutely infected with HCV (Fig. 4), 20% (20 patients) will spontaneously recover and 80% (80 patients) with develop persistent infection. Of the 80 persons with persistent infection (chronic hepatitis C), based on the composite data presented in this review, it would appear that up to 30% (24 patients) will have progressively severe liver disease culminating in cirrhosis and/or HCC and another 30% (24 patients) will have stable liver disease that will not progress to cirrhosis and its serious sequelae whether or not treatment is given. The remaining 40% of those chronically infected (32 patients) will have a slowly evolving infection whose outcome cannot be predicted (Fig. 4). This results in 56 patients who are either highly likely to progress to cirrhosis or who have a variable and unpredictable likelihood of fibrosis progression. Of these 56 patients, approximately 35% (20 patients) can be "cured" by existing combination therapy,[79] leaving only 36 (36%) from this theoretic cohort of 100 acutely infected individuals who will have progressive HCV-related liver disease not responsive to therapy. In addition, the slow pace of HCV progression will allow time for the development of improved treatments that will further diminish long-term morbidity and mortality.

Although this perspective allows reasonable hope for the individual HCV-infected patient, it is not intended to ignore the large number of persons who may die or require liver transplantation as a result of HCV infection. This individualized perspective is also not intended to diminish the enormous global impact of HCV infection engendered by the sheer magnitude of the infected population. The absolute number of dire events on a global scale is staggering even if the proportion that encounters those events is encouragingly small.

ABBREVIATIONS

ALT	alanine aminotransferase
CTL	cytotoxic T lymphocyte
HAI	histologic activity index
HBV	hepatitis B virus
HCC	hepatocellular carcinoma
HCV	hepatitis C virus
HIV	human immunodeficiency virus

PCR	polymerase chain reaction
RIBA	recombinant immunoblot
VA	Veterans Administration

REFERENCES

1. Dienstag JL. Non-A, non-B hepatitis. I. Recognition, epidemiology and clinical features. Gastroenterology 1983;85:439–462
2. Seeff LB. Hepatitis C from a needlestick injury. Ann Intern Med 1991;115:411
3. Alter HJ, Purcell RH, Holland PV, Popper H. Transmissible agent in non-A, non-B hepatitis. Lancet 1978;1:459–463
4. Tabor E, Gerety RJ, Drucker JA, et al. Transmission of non-A, non-B hepatitis from man to chimpanzee. Lancet 1978;1: 463–466
5. Tabor E, Purcell RH, Gerety RJ. Primate animal models and titered inocula for the study of human hepatitis A, B, and non-A, non-B hepatitis. J Med Primatol 1981;1:305–318
6. Choo Q-L, Kuo G, Weiner AJ, Overby LR, Bradley DW, Houghton M. Isolation of cDNA clone derived from bloodborne non-A, non-B viral hepatitis genome. Science 1989;244: 359–362
7. Alter HJ. Chronic consequences of non-A, non-B hepatitis. In: Seeff LB, Lewis JH, eds. Hepatology: Festschrift for Hyman J. Zimmerman, M.D. New York: Plenum Press, 1989, pp. 83–97
8. Gilliam JH III, Geisinger KR, Richter JE. Primary hepatocellular carcinoma after chronic non-A, non-B post-transfusion hepatitis. Ann Intern Med 1984;101:794–794
9. Kiyosawa K, Sodeyama T, Tanaka E, et al. interrelationship of blood transfusion, non-A, non-B hepatitis and hepatocellular carcinoma: Analysis by detection of antibody to hepatitis C virus. Hepatology 1990;12:671–675
10. Tong MJ, El-Farra NS, Reikes AR, Co RL. Clinical outcomes after transfusion-associated hepatitis C. N Engl J Med 1995;332: 1463–1466
11. Bruix J Barrera JM, Calvet X, et al. Prevalence of antibody to hepatitis C virus in Spanish patients with hepatocellular carcinoma and hepatic cirrhosis. Lancet 1989;2:1004–1006
12. Colombo M, Kuo G, Choo QL, et al. Prevalence of antibodies to hepatitis C virus in Italian patients with hepatocellular carcinoma. Lancet 1989;2:1006- 1008
13. Alter HJ, Conry-Cantilena C, Melpolder J, Tan D, Van Raden M, Herion D, Lau D, Hoofnagle JH. Hepatitis C in asymptomatic blood donors. Hepatology 1997;26(Suppl 1):29S–33S
14. Alter MJ, Margolis HS, Krawczynski K, et al. The natural history of community-acquired hepatitis C in the United States. N Engl J Med 1992;327:1899–1905
15. Alter MJ, Kruszon-Moran D, Nainan OV, McQuillan GM, Gao F, Moyer LA, Kaslow RA, Margolis HS. The prevalence of hepatitis C virus infection in the United States, 1988 through 1994. N Engl J Med 1999;341:556–562
16. Pessoa MG, Wright TL. Hepatitis C infection in transplantation. Clin Liver Dis 1997;1:663–690
17. Farci P, Alter HJ, Govindarajan S, et al. Lack of protective immunity against reinfection with hepatitis C virus. Science 1992;258:135–140
18. Shimizu YK, Yoshikuta H, Hijikata M, Iwamoto A, Alter HJ, Purcell RH.Neutralizing antibodies against hepatitis C virus and the emergence of neutralization escape mutants. J Virol 1994;68:1494–1500
19. Rosa D, Campagnoli S, Moretto C, et al. A quantitative test to estimate neutralizing antibodies to the hepatitis c virus: Cytofluorometric assessment of envelop glycoprotein 2 binding to target cells. Proc Natl Acad Sci USA 1996 93;1759–1763

20. Farci P, Shimoda A, Coiana A, et al. The outcome of acute hepatitis C predicted by the evolution of the viral quasispecies. Proc Natl Acad Sci USA (in press)

20a. Bukh J, Yanagi M, Emerson SU, Purcell RH. Course of infection and evolution of monoclonal hepatitis C virus (HCV) strain H77 in chimpanzees transfected with RNA transcripts from an infectious cDNA clone. Hepatology 1998;28:319A.

21. Cerny A, Chisari FV. Pathogenesis of chronic hepatitis C: Immunological features of hepatic injury and viral persistence. Hepatology 1999;30:595–601.

22. Lai ME, Mazzoleni AP, Argiolu F, De Virgilis S, Balastrieri A, Purcell RH, Farci P. Hepatitis C virus in multiple episodes of acute hepatitis in polytransfused thalassaemic children. Lancet 1994;343:388–390

23. Weiner A, Erickson AL, Kansopon J, et al. Persistent hepatitis C virus infection in a chimpanzee is associated with emergence of a cytotoxic T lymphocyte escape variant. Proc Natl Acad Sci USA 1995;92:2755–2759

24. Eyster ME, Diamondstone LS, Lien JM. Natural history of hepatitis C virus infection in multitransfused hemophiliacs: Effect of coinfection with human immunodeficiency virus. The Multicenter Hemophilia Cohort Study. J Acquir Immune Def Syndr 1993;6:602–610

25. Yano M, Kumada H, Kage M, et al. The long-term pathological evolution of chronic hepatitis C. Hepatology 1996;23:1334–1340

26. Niederau C, Lange S, Heintges T, et al. Prognosis of chronic hepatitis C: Results of a large, prospective cohort study. Hepatology 1998;28:1687–1695

27. Di Bisceglie AM, Goodman ZD, Ishak KG, Hoofnagle JH, Melpolder JJ, Alter HJ. Long-term clinical and histopathological follow-up of chronic posttransfusion hepatitis. Hepatology 1991;14:969–974

28. Koretz RL, Abbey H, Cloeman E, Gitnick G. Non-A, non-B post-transfusion hepatitis: Looking back in the second decade. Ann Intern Med 1993;119:110–115

29. Mattson L, Sonnerborg A, Weiland O. Outcome of acute asymptomatic non-A, non-B hepatitis: A 13-year follow-up study of hepatitis C virus markers. Liver 1993;13:274–278

30. Tremolada F, Casarin C, Albert A, Drago C, Tagger A, Ribero ML, Realdi G. Long-term follow-up of non-A, non-B (type C) post-transfusion hepatitis. J Hepatol 1992;16:273–281

31. Alter HJ, Purcell RH, Feinstone SM, Holland PV, Morrow AG. Non-A/non-B hepatitis: A review and interim report of an ongoing prospective study. In: Vyas GN, Cohen SN, Schmid R, eds. Viral Hepatitis: A Contemporary Assessment of Etiology, Epidemiology, Pathogenesis and Prevention. Philadelphia: Franklin Institute Press, 1978, pp. 359–369

32. Seeff LB, Buskell-Bales Z, Wright EC, et al. Long-term mortality after transfusion-associated non-A, non-B hepatitis. N Engl J Med 1992;327:1906–1911

33. Seeff LB, Zimmerman HJ, Wright EC, et al. A randomized, double-blind, controlled trial of the efficacy of immune serum globulin in the prevention of post-transfusion hepatitis: A Veterans Administration cooperative study. Gastroenterology 1977;72: 111–121

34. Seeff LB, Wright EC, Zimmerman HJ, et al. Posttransfusion hepatitis, 1973–1975: A Veterans Administration cooperative study. In: Vyas GN, Cohen SN, Schmid R, eds. Viral Hepatitis: A Contemporary Assessment of Etiology, Epidemiology, Pathogenesis and Prevention. Philadelphia: Franklin Institute Press, 1978, pp. 371–381

35. Aach RD, Szmuness W, Mosley JW, et al. Serum alanine aminotransferase of donors in relation to risk of non-A, non-B hepatitis in recipients: The Transfusion-Transmitted Viruses Study. N Engl J Med 1981;304:989–994

36. Knodell RG, Conrad ME, Ginsberg AL, Bell CJ, Flanery EP. Efficacy of prophylactic gamma-globulin in preventing non-A, non-B hepatitis. Lancet 1976;1:557–561

37. Wright EC, Seeff LB, Hollinger FB, Alter HJ, Buskell-Bales Z, Cain C, the NHLBI Study Group. Updated long-term mortality of transfusion- associated hepatitis (TAH), non-A, non-B and C. Hepatology 1998;28:272A

38. Seeff LB, Hollinger FB, Alter HJ, Wright EC, Bales ZB, the NHLBI Study Group. Long-term morbidity of transfusion-associated hepatitis (TAH) C. Hepatology 1998;28:407A

39. Denny FW, Wannamaker LW, Brink WR, Rammelkamp H. Prevention of rheumatic fever, treatment of preceding streptococcic infection. JAMA 1950:143:151–153

40. Seeff LB, Miller RN, Rabkin CS, Bales ZB, Smoak BL, Johnson LD, Kaplan EL. 45-Year follow-up of hepatitis C virus infection in healthy young adults. Ann Intern Med 2000;132:105–111

41. Conry-Cantilena C, VanRaden M, Gibble J, et al. Routes of infection, viremia, and liver disease in blood donors found to have hepatitis C virus infection. N Engl J Med 1996;334: 1691–1696

42. Shakil AO, Conry-Cantilena C, Alter HJ, et al. Volunteer blood donors with antibody to hepatitis C virus: Clinical, biochemical, virologic and histologic features. Ann Intern Med 1995;123: 330–337

43. Kenny-Walsh E for the Irish Hepatology Research Group. Clinical outcomes after hepatitis infection from contaminated anti-globulin. N Engl J Med 1999;340:1228–1233

44. Muller R. The natural history of hepatitis C: Clinical experiences. J Hepatol 1996;24(Suppl):52–54

45. Vogt M, Lang T, Frosner G, et al. Prevalence and clinical outcome of hepatitis C infection in children who underwent cardiac surgery before the implementation of blood-donor screening. N Engl J Med 1999;341:866–870

46. Locasciulli A, Testa M, Pontisso P, et al. Prevalence and natural history of hepatitis C infection in patients cured of childhood leukemia. Blood 1997;11:4628–4633

47. Garcia-Monzon C, Jara P, Fernandez-Bermejo M, et al. Chronic hepatitis C in children: A clinical and immunohistochemical comparative study with adults. Hepatology 1998;28: 1696–1701

47. Luban N, Post J, Glymph C. Transfusion associated hepatitis C and G in pediatric patients identified through a universal lookback approach. Transfusion 1999;106(Suppl):110S

49. Poynard T, Bedossa P, Opolon P, for the OBSVIRC, METAVIR, CLINIVIR, and DOSVIRC groups. Natural history of liver fibrosis progression in patients with chronic hepatitis C. Lancet 1997;349:825–832

50. Fattovich G, Giustina G, Degos F, et al. Morbidity and mortality in compensated cirrhosis type C: A retrospective follow-up study of 384 patients. Gastroenterology 1997;112:463–472

51. Serfaty L, Aumaitre H, Chazouilleres O, Bonand A-M, Rosmorduc O, Poupon RE, Poupon R. Determinants of outcome of compensated hepatitis C virus-related cirrhosis. Hepatology 1998; 27:1435–1440

52. Nishioka K, Watanabe J, Furuta S, et al. A high prevalence of the antibody to hepatitis C virus with hepatocellular carcinoma in Japan. Cancer 1991;67:429–433

53. Kato Y, Nakata K, Omagari K, et al. Risk of hepatocellular carcinoma in patients with cirrhosis in Japan: Analysis of infectious hepatitis viruses. Cancer 1994;74:2234–2238

54. Yoshida H, Shiratori Y, Moriyama M, et al. Interferon therapy reduces the risk for hepatocellular carcinoma: National Surveillance Program of cirrhotic and noncirrhotic patients with chronic hepatitis C in Japan. Ann Int Med 1999;131:174–181

55. Chen P-J, Chen D-S. Hepatitis B virus and hepatocellular carcinoma. In: Okuda K, Tabor E, eds. Liver Cancer. New York: Churchill Livingstone, 1997, pp. 29–37

56. Hadziyannis S, Tabor E, Kaklamani E, et al. A case-control study of hepatitis B and C virus infections in the etiology of hepatocellular carcinoma. Int J Cancer 1995;60:627–631

None of the 94 babies of mothers with anti-HCV alone became infected with HCV.

Paccagnini et al.[12] studied 70 women with HCV infection; 76% were found to have HIV co-infection. The frequency of HCV transmission was 12% (2 of 17) in infants born to HIV-negative mothers and 23% (12 of 53) in infants of HIV-positive mothers. One third of the infants (4 of 12) who developed HCV infection and were born to women with HIV co-infection also developed HIV co-infection.

Thomas et al.[13] prospectively followed 155 mothers co-infected with HCV and HIV and their infants. Thirteen (8.4%) of 155 infants were infected with HCV. Six of these 13 infants were also co-infected with HIV. The median concentration of plasma HCV RNA was higher among the 13 mothers of HCV-infected infants (2.0 × 106 copies/mL) than among the 142 mothers with HCV-negative infants (3.5 × 105 copies/mL; $p < 0.001$).

Breast-feeding

HCV infection of the mother is not a contraindication to breast-feeding according to the Public Health Service guidelines.[14] The American Academy of Pediatrics (AAP) Committee on Infectious Disease recommends that "HCV-infected women who wish to breast-feed their infants should be counseled that although there appears to be no increased risk of transmission, HCV RNA has been detected in breast milk, and the data are limited."[15]

In the first study specifically addressing the role of breast-feeding on transmission, Lin et al.[16] studied 11 women who were infected with HCV and breast-fed their infants for a mean duration of 2 months. Four of the 11 women had HCV RNA detectable in their colostrum at levels of 1.25×10^2 to 1.25×10^4 copies/mL. None of the 11 infants had anti-HCV antibody or HCV RNA present in their serum at 12 months of age.

Others studies examined transmission of HCV via breast-feeding as a secondary outcome. The study by Ohto et al.[5] found that infected infants were breast-fed longer than noninfected infants, but this difference did not reach statistical significance. In the study by Zannetti et al.,[11] mothers with abnormal aminotransferases or co-infection with HIV were directed not to breast-feed their infants. The authors did note, however, that 23 breast-fed infants born to mothers who were HCV RNA positive remained uninfected.

In a study published after the AAP guidelines, Kumar and Shahul[17] enrolled 65 pregnant women that were anti-HCV positive, HCV RNA positive, and anti-HIV negative. The women all had normal serum alanine aminotransferase (ALT) levels. All the women breast-fed their infants, and HCV RNA was found in the colostrum of all 65 women. By 3 months postpartum, 5 of the 65 women developed symptomatic liver disease, and three of their infants subsequently developed acute viral hepatitis C. The mothers of the three infected infants had high serum titers of HCV RNA (2.25- to × 4.25 × 10^9 copies/mL). In the remaining 60 mother–infant pairs, breast-feeding was continued for a mean duration of 8.2 months. None of the 60 infants developed HCV infection by 12 months of age.

Summary of Maternal–Infant Transmission

The larger studies of maternal–infant transmission estimate the rate to be between 3% and 8% in unselected HIV-negative pregnant populations. In infants who acquire HCV infection, HCV RNA can be undetectable and aminotransferase levels can be normal. Thus, HCV infection probably cannot be excluded in infants with one-time testing.[9] Transmission rates are higher for HIV co-infected mothers, perhaps as a consequence of higher viral loads. For all women, transmission is largely restricted to those with detectable HCV viremia during pregnancy or delivery. Therefore, it is reasonable to reassure pregnant women in whom HCV RNA cannot be detected that the transmission risk is exceedingly low.[18] Although the maternal–infant transmission rate is low, because of the reduction in parenteral transmission, maternal–infant transmission is likely to be a major route of childhood infection. Studies to date have been too small to accurately assess the timing of infection, the importance of genotype, the effect of mode of delivery, and the role of breast-feeding. A randomized clinical trial would have to include more than 800 mother–infant pairs to detect a twofold increase in transmission with 80% power.[18]

In mothers with HCV infection, HCV RNA has been widely documented in colostrum. However, the risk of HCV transmission by breast-feeding is low in asymptomatic HCV carrier mothers without HIV co-infection. Nevertheless, active symptomatic maternal liver disease and high levels of HCV RNA may increase the risk of transmission.

SCREENING AND COUNSELING

The AAP recommends screening of all persons with risk factors for HCV infection, including transfusion of at least one unit of blood or blood products before 1992, hemodialysis, or injection drug use.[15] Screening is not recommended for all pregnant women. This recommendation is unlikely to change until there is a means of decreasing vertical transmission. However, all babies born to women who are known to be HCV positive should be tested for infection. Testing for anti-HCV should be delayed for 12 to 18 months to allow for maternally derived IgG to clear from the blood of the infant.

All children should receive the hepatitis B vaccine. Because children with HCV are at increased for severe disease with hepatitis A infection, they should also be immunized against hepatitis A. Adolescents with HCV infection need to be counseled to abstain completely from ethanol consumption. Furthermore, they should be counseled about the possibility of transmission of HCV to sexual partners.

NATURAL HISTORY OF HEPATITIS C IN CHILDREN

In adults, acute HCV infection is usually asymptomatic. Jaundice occurs in approximately 25%. Nonspecific symptoms such as anorexia, malaise, or abdominal pain have been reported in 10% of patients. Fulminant hepatic failure due to HCV is rare. However, only 20% of patients will resolve their infection. In the remaining 80% of people, HCV infection runs a chronic course. Cirrhosis is believed to develop in 20% of people with chronic infection. Once cirrhosis is established, hepatocellular carcinoma (HCC) develops at a rate of 1–4% per year.

Studies of Natural History in Children

The natural history of hepatitis C infection in children is not fully characterized. The important differences in the pediatric age group are likely to be the mode of acquisition and the age at acquisition. The age at infection may play a role in the host response and development of tolerance. There may also be a difference in the ability of the immune system to clear the infection. One important issue is the outcome of perinatally acquired HCV as compared with parenterally transmitted HCV.

Chang et al.[19] reported on the outcome of children infected with HCV from differing sources; five were chronically transfused for hemolytic anemia, two received blood products during cardiac surgery, and three had maternal–infant transmission of HCV. Acute hepatitis occurred in five of the seven children with parenteral transmission and none of the three infants born to mothers infected with HCV. In 6 of the 10 children, the disease ran a chronic course with persistently positive HCV RNA. Only three had persistently elevated ALT levels. The other major studies of natural history in children have looked at populations with the same mode of acquisition.

Outcome of Maternal–Infant Transmission

Palomba et al.[20] prospectively followed seven infants with maternal–infant transmission of HCV infection from birth to a mean age of 65 months. The mother of each child was co-infected with HIV, but the subjects studied were restricted to infants with only HCV infection. Serum ALT levels varied widely during the follow-up. All had HCV RNA present in their serum during the first year of life, and it was still present at the last follow-up examination. All children had normal physical examinations and growth throughout the study period. Two children developed autoantibodies. Chronic hepatitis developed in each of the seven cases of perinatal HCV infection.

Bortolotti et al.[21] prospectively followed 14 infants with vertically transmitted HCV infection born to women not co-infected with HIV. All the infants were asymptomatic during the study period. All had elevated serum ALT levels and HCV RNA present in their serum during the first year of life. Ten children were followed beyond 12 months for as long as 48 months. Eight of these 10 remained viremic throughout follow-up. Two patients had normalization of serum ALT and disappearance of HCV RNA. Progression to chronicity occurred in most cases.

Outcome of Parenteral Transmission

Matsuoka et al.[22] identified 29 Japanese children who developed HCV hepatitis from blood and plasma transfusions at a mean age of 3.2 years during open-heart surgery. The patients were followed for a mean of 7.1 years. All 29 children were asymptomatic despite elevated serum ALT level posttransfusion. In 13 (45%) of the 29, the elevated ALT persisted throughout follow-up. Only 14 (48%) of the 29 had detectable HCV RNA. Thus, approximately one half of the children appeared to clear the infection.

Garcia-Monzon et al.[23] retrospectively evaluated 15 children who acquired HCV infection from blood transfusions in the neonatal period. All children had been referred for abnormal ALT; thus, the study did not capture patients with normal aminotransferase levels. The mean duration of infection was 11 years. The children's disease was mild compared with a control population of adults with posttransfusion chronic HCV for a mean duration also of 11 years. The children had mild ALT elevation, low but detectable viremia, and mild liver inflammation and fibrosis.

Bortolotti et al.[24] studied 57 children with known hepatitis C infection who were being followed with a previous diagnosis of non-A, non-B hepatitis. The children had a mean age of 4.4 years at presentation and were followed for a mean of 6 years. At presentation, only 22% were symptomatic. All had normal growth and development throughout the study. During the observation period, 11 of 57 complained of anorexia or abdominal pain and 11 of 40 cases had histologic features of active hepatitis. Two patients had severe hepatitis associated with cirrhosis. In 51 (89%) of the 57 children, abnormal serum ALT persisted.

Locasciulli et al.[25] prospectively followed 114 children in Italy who were cured of leukemia. At chemotherapy withdrawal, 56 patients were HCV RNA positive, often without detectable anti-HCV. Patients were then followed-up for a mean duration of 17 years after chemotherapy withdrawal. Forty patients were persistently HCV RNA positive in serum, whereas 16 (29%) initially viremic patients became HCV RNA negative during follow-up. At the end of the observation period, a persistent aminotransferase elevation was detected only in four HCV RNA-positive cases. Despite the years of follow-up and the high rate of infection, no patients developed signs or symptoms of severe liver disease.

In a large study of natural history, Vogt et al.[26] studied 458 patients who had received blood transfusions during cardiac surgery at a mean age of 2.8 years. When examined 17 years after surgery, 67 (14.6 %) were positive for antibodies to HCV. At a mean interval of 19.8 years after the first operation, 37 (55%) of the 67 patients who were anti-HCV positive had detectable serum HCV RNA. The subjects had serial testing over 2 years to avoid any false negatives due to the potential for fluctuation in HCV RNA levels. Therefore, the authors were able to conclude that HCV infection was cleared in 30 (45%) of the 67 patients. For those patients who were still infected, only one had elevated aminotransferase levels. Liver biopsies were performed in 17 patients with HCV infection of genotype 1. In 14 of these 17 patients there was only mild inflammation, whereas 2 had periportal fibrosis and 1 had micronodular cirrhosis. Each child with more severe disease had risk factors in addition to hepatitis C.

Liver Transplantation

McDiarmid et al.[27] described their experience with 13 children who developed hepatitis C infection de novo after orthotopic liver transplantation (OLT). The mean time to diagnosis after OLT was 8.1 years. The liver biopsy specimen showed chronic active or chronic persistent hepatitis in 11 children, cirrhosis in 1 child, and nonspecific changes in 1 child. Twelve children were treated with interferon-2α(IFN-2α) Four patients developed rapidly progressive liver failure while receiving IFN therapy and required urgent retransplantation. Three of the four children developed histologic evi-

dence of recurrent HCV 4–6 months after the second OLT, and all three died of HCV-induced liver failure. Of the other eight children treated with IFN, only two had a sustained biochemical response and one became HCV RNA negative. Overall mortality for de novo HCV hepatitis was 23%. Seventy-five percent of children who received a second transplant for HCV hepatitis had early histologic recurrence that led to liver failure and death. IFN resulted in sustained improvement in ALT in only 15% of children.

Histopathology

The studies of natural history have principally addressed symptoms and levels of HCV RNA and aminotransferases, but not histopathology. The development of cirrhosis, liver failure, and HCC are ultimately the most important determinants of long-term outcome. Therefore, several investigators have systematically assessed liver biopsy specimens in children with HCV infection. Guido et al.[28] studied 80 children aged 1–19 years with chronic hepatitis C infection. The diagnosis was based on the presence of antibodies to HCV in serum for longer than 6 months and abnormal ALT values on at least one occasion. None of these children had underlying systemic disease. The children had biochemical evidence of hepatitis for a mean duration of 42 months. Chronic hepatitis was mild in most cases but had high-grade activity in 17 children (21%). Fibrosis was absent in 22 cases (28%), mild in 44 (55%), and moderate in 13 (16%). Only one patient had cirrhosis. A significant relationship was detected between fibrosis scores and the duration of disease ($p < 0.002$), suggesting that children may be at risk for more severe liver disease over time.

In a study by Kage et al.,[29] most children with chronic hepatitis C infection had only mild fibrosis. They examined the liver histology in 109 children aged 4–14 years with HCV infection. The mean duration of serum aminotransferase elevation before biopsy was 30 months. None of the children had cirrhosis. In 105 (97%) of the 109 patients, the fibrosis was stage 1 or 2.

Badizadegan et al.[30] presented the liver histopathology for 40 children aged 2–18 years with chronic HCV infection. In the 24 children where it was known, the mean duration of infection to biopsy was 6.8 years. Portal fibrosis was present in 78% of the biopsies, including fibrous portal expansion (26%), portal bridging (22%), bridging with architectural distortion (22%), and cirrhosis (8%). There was an association between the extent of fibrosis and age ($p = 0.032$) and extent of fibrosis and duration of infection ($p = 0.046$). All three children with cirrhosis had stainable iron.

Summary of Natural History

Most children with perinatally acquired HCV seem to develop chronic infection. However, they remain asymptomatic and have normal or only mildly elevated aspartate aminotransferase (AST). In large prospective studies of children receiving HCV-infected blood products, between 30% and 50% of infected children are able to spontaneously clear the infection. Most patients who have chronic HCV infection have normal ALT. When a preselected referral population of children with parenterally acquired HCV is studied, there is a high prevalence of elevated aminotransferase levels. Despite the persistence of abnormal ALT, the disease still remains mild in most patients. However, a few children do develop cirrhosis. Whether this requires a second insult such as autoimmune hepatitis remains unknown. The studies of histopathology confirm that the disease is mild in most children; however, fibrosis did progress with older age at infection and the duration of infection. In contrast to the other children discussed, those who develop HCV infection after OLT have a high morbidity and mortality

THERAPY OF CHRONIC HEPATITIS C IN CHILDREN

The National Institute of Health Consensus Statement on management of hepatitis C recommends treatment for patients between 18 and 60 who have persistently elevated ALT, positive HCV RNA, and a liver biopsy with either portal or bridging fibrosis and at least moderate degrees of inflammation and necrosis.[3] Initial therapy with IFN-α should be 3 million units (mu) three times per week for 12 months. Patients not responding to therapy after 3 months should not receive further treatment with IFN alone, but should be considered for combination therapy of IFN and ribavirin or for enrollment in investigational studies.

Pediatric Data

Children would seem to be ideal candidates for therapy because they typically are of young age and have a short duration of disease and mild histology. Given their young age, children with chronic hepatitis C have a long duration in which the disease might progress. Therefore there may be a strong rationale for intervention. However, IFN treatment is not U.S. Food and Drug Administration approved for patients less than 18 years of age. Furthermore, there have been few published trials of treatment with IFN for chronic HCV in children (Table 1).

Ruiz-Moreno et al.[31] studied 12 children aged 18 months to 15 years with chronic hepatitis C. All children HCV RNA present in serum; however, only five were anti-HCV positive. This pattern is atypical for immunocompetent patients. Each child received 3 MU/m^2 of recombinant IFN-αSC, three times a week for 6 months. They were followed for an additional 18 months. In 67% (8 of 12) of the children there was a virologic end of treatment response. However, only 42% (5 of 12) had a sustained biochemical response at 24 months. Most children experienced a transient influenza-like syndrome. One child had treatment suspended after 4 months because of a severe increase in serum ALT. Alopecia, leukopenia, and thrombocytopenia were also encountered.

Clemente et al.[32] conducted a controlled trial for patients aged 6–21 years with thalassemia major and chronic hepatitis C. Fourteen patients were untreated control subjects, and 51 patients received recombinant IFN-α-2b, 3 MU/m^2 SC 3 times a week for 6 months. Patients who had a biochemical response received an additional 9 months of treatment. The subjects were followed for a total of 3 years. In 21 (41%) of 51 treated patients, there was a biochemical response along with disappearance of HCV RNA from the serum. In 19 of the 21 responders, there was an improvement in liver histology. During the first year of follow-up, two responder pa-

TABLE 1.   Clinical Trials of IFN for Chronic HCV in Children

Dose (Three Times per Week)	Treated Patients	Control Patients	Complete Sustained Response (%)	Reference
3 MU/m^2 × 6 mo	12	0	?	Ruiz-Moreno
3 MU/m^2 × 6 mo	51	14	37	Clemente
5 MU/m^2 × 12 mo	14	13	43	Bortolotti
3 MU/m^2 *or* 1.75 MU/m^2 × 24 w	6	0	0	Zwiener
3 MU/m^2 × 12 mo	11	10	45	Iorio
0.1 MU/kg/day × 2 wk *then* tiw × 22 wk	13	0	31	Komatsu
5 MU/m^2 × 2 mo *then* 3 MU/m^2 × 10 mo	70	0	40	DiMarco
5 MU/m^2 × 12 mo	25	0	8	Pensati

tiw, thrice weekly.

tients had relapses. In all untreated patients and 30 of the 51 treated patients, there was no improvement in serum ALT, HCV RNA, or liver histology. Side effects included fever, fatigue, anorexia, granulocytopenia, and thrombocytopenia. Treatment had to be temporarily suspended in six children because of leukopenia.

Bortolotti et al.[33] conducted a randomized controlled pilot study of IFN therapy for chronic hepatitis C in 27 children aged 2–14 years without underlying systemic disease. All patients had ALT elevation for greater than 6 months and chronic hepatitis on liver biopsy. Twenty-six of the 27 patients were positive for HCV RNA before treatment. The children were randomly assigned to receive treatment with 5 MU/m^2 of recombinant IFN-α-2b three times per week for 12 months or no treatment. The patients were followed for 12 months beyond the treatment period. In 9 (64%) of the 14 treated patients, there was a biochemical and virologic end of treatment response. Moreover, there was a complete sustained response in 6 (43%) of the 14 patients. One patient experienced a febrile seizure. Another child had a dramatic increase in ALT level associated with the development of anti-LKM antibodies.

Zwiener et al.[34] conducted an uncontrolled pilot study on 6 boys with factor VIII deficiency and biopsy-proven chronic hepatitis C. The first 3 patients were treated with IFN-α-2b in a dosage of 3 MU/m^2 SC three times a week for 24 weeks. The second 3 patients received 1.75 MU/m^2 using the same schedule. One patient who was co-infected with HIV had therapy discontinued after 3 weeks because of a depressed CD4 count. None of the 6 children had a sustained normalization of the serum ALT or clearance of HCV RNA from serum.

Iorio et al.[35] enrolled 21 children aged 2–13 years with histologically proven chronic hepatitis C without other systemic disease for a randomized controlled study. Eleven children received treatment with lymphoblastoid IFN-α, 3 MU/m^2 SC, three times a week for 12 months. Ten children received no therapy. One child had therapy discontinued during the first month because of a marked rise in serum ALT. Two others had therapy discontinued after 6 months because of a lack of biochemical response. All treated patients had a transient influenza-like syndrome. In 5 patients, neutropenia required tapering of the IFN dose. All patients were followed for 18 months beyond the treatment period. In 5 (45%) of the 11 treated patients, there was normalization of serum ALT and disappearance of serum HCV RNA. The response was sustained throughout follow-up. In one of the untreated patients, there was a spontaneous and sustained biochemical and virologic response. All treated patients showed a significant improvement in liver histology.

Komatsu et al.[36] reported the results of a trial of IFN therapy in 13 children aged 5–17 years with acute leukemia in remission and chronic hepatitis C infection. The children were treated with natural IFN-α administered at a dose of 0.1 MU/kg daily for 2 weeks and then three times a week for an additional 22 weeks. Therapy was discontinued after 4 months for one patient who developed mild transient heart failure. The children were followed for 18 months after the completion of therapy. In 7 (54%) of the 13 patients there was normalization of serum ALT and disappearance of serum HCV RNA. However, only 4 (31%) of the 13 children had a complete sustained response.

Di Marco et al.[37] studied 70 patients, with a mean age of 14.1 years, who had beta-thalassemia major and biopsy-proven chronic hepatitis C. All subjects received IFN-α2b at a dose of 5 MU/m^2 three times weekly for 2 months. The dose was then lowered to 3 MU/m^2 for an additional 10 months. The patients were followed for a minimum of 24 months after completion of therapy. There was a complete sustained biochemical and virologic response in 28 (40%) of the 70 patients. Two patients discontinued therapy after 4 weeks because of persistent influenza-like symptoms. Another patient developed hemolytic anemia with positive direct and indirect Coombs' tests.

Pensati et al.[38] reported preliminary results for 25 children aged 3–11 years with chronic hepatitis C. The children received treatment with 5 MU/m^2 of recombinant IFN-α2b three times a week for 12 months. They were followed for an additional 21 months. Only 2 (8%) of the 25 children had sustained normalization of serum ALT and disappearance of HCV RNA.

In eight studies of treatment with IFN in children, there were a total of 172 patients treated. The study design and treatment dose used varied widely, making it difficult to accurately pool the data. The complete sustained response rate reported was 0 to 45%. Overall, 40% (69 of 172) had a biochemical and virologic response sustained for at least 6 months beyond the treatment period. Side effects of IFN treatment were commonly observed. Nearly all patients had a transient influenza-like syndrome. A small number of children had to discontinue therapy, mostly for a rise in serum ALT. Other frequent side effects were alopecia, leukopenia, and thrombocytopenia. The patients less commonly experienced serious complications including development of autoantibodies, febrile seizure, hemolytic anemia, and heart failure.

Predictors of Response

In adults with chronic hepatitis C, the main factors associated with a good response to IFN treatment are the following: female sex, young age, shorter duration of disease, absence of alcohol consumption, low hepatic iron concentration, lean body habitus, genotypes 2 and

3, and low serum HCV RNA levels. However, these factors have not been validated as pretreatment predictors that are clinically useful in the decision to treat.

In the pediatric age group, genotype and liver iron content have been evaluated as predictors of response. In the study by Bortolotti et al.,[33] response to IFN varied by genotype. A complete sustained response was observed in one of six children with HCV type 1, two of two children with HCV type 3, and two of four children with unidentifiable genotypes. In the larger study by DiMarco et al.,[37] multivariate analysis showed infection by genotype other than 1b to be associated with a complete sustained response.

In the study of Clemente et al.,[32] quantitative and qualitative assessments of the level of iron in the liver were useful in predicting response to treatment. The response to IFN therapy was inversely related ($p < 0.02$) to the liver iron burden as assessed by atomic absorption or the histologic semiquantitative method. In a prospective study, the investigators used IFN in the treatment of 34 additional patients with a low score in the semiquantitative assessment of hepatic iron stores: The percentage of responders rose to 76% of those treated. The authors hypothesized that intensive chelation therapy for patients with severe iron overload might improve the subsequent response to IFN. The study of DiMarco et al.[37] further demonstrates the importance of iron liver content. The degree of liver siderosis markedly affected the kinetics of biochemical response. Almost all patients with a complete sustained response and a mild degree of liver iron overload responded within 4 months of treatment, whereas those with more severe siderosis took as long as 10 months to respond. The authors concluded that IFN treatment for chronic HCV in patients with thalassemia major should not be stopped after 3–4 months if ALT is still raised.

Long-term Benefits of Treatment with IFN in Adults

In adults with HCV infection, there is preliminary evidence that patients with a sustained virologic response have a favorable long-term clinical and histologic outcome.[39] IFN therapy seems to reduce the incidence of HCV-related cirrhosis.[40] Furthermore, IFN may reduce the incidence of HCC.[41]

In a multicenter study, investigators retrospectively analyzed 245 patients who had chronic hepatitis C, did not have HBV infection, and had Child's A cirrhosis.[42] HCC developed in 29 (20%) of 129 untreated patients and in 6 (5%) of 116 patients treated with IFN. The patients treated with IFN appeared to have a substantial benefit despite only 15% having a sustained response to treatment. In addition, Kasahara et al.[41] conducted a nonrandomized study in Japan of 1,022 patients who had chronic hepatitis C and were treated with IFN.[41]

The patients were followed for a median duration of 36 months. Biochemical response was sustained in 313 patients, transient in 304 patients, and absent in 405 patients. HCC developed in 46 (5%) of the 1,022 patients, of whom 5 were sustained responders, 9 were transient responders, and 32 were nonresponders. The risk of HCC development was not elevated in transient responders compared with sustained responders, but the risk was 7.9-fold higher in nonresponders than in sustained responders ($p = 0.006$). Because of the relatively short duration of follow-up, it remains unclear whether treatment with IFN only delays or actually prevents HCC.

Combination Therapy with IFN and Ribavirin

Because the complete sustained response to treatment with IFN is low, additional strategies have been tested. The most promising to date is the combination of ribavirin with IFN. McHutchison et al.[43] conducted a multicenter, double blind, randomized, placebo-controlled trial with 912 patients with chronic hepatitis C who received IFN alone or in combination with ribavirin for 24 or 48 weeks. At the end of follow-up, the rate of sustained virologic response was higher among patients who received combination therapy for either 24 weeks (31%) or 48 weeks (38%) than among patients who received IFN alone for either 24 weeks (6%) or 48 weeks (13%). Late viral clearance with a subsequent sustained response was an important finding in many patients. No studies to date have tested the combination of IFN and ribavirin in the pediatric age group.

RECOMMENDATIONS FOR TREATMENT OF CHRONIC HEPATITIS C IN CHILDREN

It is possible that children may respond better to antiviral treatment than adults. However, they may also have a more benign course, and therefore in the absence of reliable therapy, a no-treatment policy may be justifiable at present. No pediatric studies have evaluated the critical outcomes of quality of life or development of cirrhosis and HCC. Currently, we are unable to accurately predict which children will progress to more serious disease. Furthermore, we do not know if the benign course described in most children will persist after 30–40 years of disease. Finally, children may have unique side effects of IFN treatment. There has been an association of high IFN levels and spastic diplegia.[44,45] It also remains to be seen if the antiproliferative effect of IFN will adversely effect growth. For the above reasons, we recommend that children with hepatitis C infection only be considered for treatment as part of a controlled clinical trial.

In the future, we need drugs that have greater specificity for HCV with less systemic toxicity. We also need markers that are predictive of the course of disease and the response to therapy. It is likely that vertical transmission will become the most common means of HCV infection in children. We therefore need antiviral therapy that is compatible with pregnancy. Finally, all pediatric treatment should take place in randomized controlled trials to properly assess not only biochemical and virologic outcomes but also quality of life and development of cirrhosis. These studies will also need to address pediatric-specific side effects such as growth and spastic diplegia.

ABBREVIATIONS

AAP American Academy of Pediatrics
ALT alanine aminotransferase
HCV hepatitis C virus
HCC hepatocellular carcinoma
HIV human immunodeficiency virus
IFN interferon
MU million units
OLT orthotopic liver transplant

REFERENCES

1. Murphy EL, Bryzman S, Williams AE, et al. Demographic determinants of hepatitis C virus seroprevalence among blood donors. JAMA 1996;275:995–1000
2. Alter MJ, Kruszon-Moran D, Nainan OV, et al. The prevalence of hepatitis C virus infection in the United States 1988 through 1994. N Engl J Med 1999;341:556–562
3. National Institutes of Health. Management of Hepatitis C. NIH Consens Statement Online 1997 Mar 24–26 [1999, September 9];15(3)1–41
4. Centers for Disease Control and Prevention. Recommendations for prevention and control of hepatitis C virus (HCV) infection and HCV-related chronic disease. Morb Mortal Wkly Rep 1998; 47:1–39
5. Ohto H, Terazawa S, Sasaki N, et al. Transmission of hepatitis C virus from mothers to infants. The Vertical Transmission of Hepatitis C Virus Collaborative Study Group. N Engl J Med 1994;330:744–750
6. Resti M, Azzari C, Lega L, et al. Mother-to-infant transmission of hepatitis C virus. Acta Paediatr 1995;84:251–255
7. La Torre A, Biadaioli R, Capobianco T, et al. Vertical transmission of HCV. Acta Obstet Gynaecol Scand 1998;77:889–892
8. Giacchino R, Tasso L, Timitillli A, et al. Vertical transmission of hepatitis C virus infection: Usefulness of viremia detection in HIV-seronegative hepatitis C virus-seropositive mothers. J Pediatr 1998;132:167–169
9. Granovsky MO, Minkoff HL, Tess BH, et al. Hepatitis C virus infection in the Mothers and Infants Cohort Study. Pediatrics 1998;102:355–359
10. Resti M, Azzari C, Mannelli F, et al. Mother to child transmission of hepatitis C virus: prospective study of risk factors and timing of infection in children born to women seronegative for HIV-1. BMJ 1998;317:437–441

11. Zanetti AR, Tanzi E, Paccagnini S, et al. Mother-to-infant transmission of hepatitis C virus. Lancet 1995;341:289–291
12. Paccagnini S, Principi N, Massironi E, et al. Perinatal transmission and manifestation of hepatitis C virus infection in a high risk population. Pediatr Infect Dis J 1995;14:195–199
13. Thomas DL, Villano SA, Riester KA, et al. Perinatal transmission of hepatitis C virus from human immunodefidiency virus type 1-infected mothers. J Infect Dis 1998;177:1480–1488
14. Centers for Disease Control and Prevention. Public Health Service inter-agency guidelines for screening donors of blood, plasma, organs, tissues, and semen for evidence of hepatitis B and hepatitis C. Morb Mortal Wkly Rep 1991;40:1–17
15. AAP Committee on Infectious Diseases. Hepatitis C virus infection. Pediatrics 1998;101:481–484
16. Lin H, Kao J, Hsu H, et al. Absence of infection in breast-fed infants born to hepatitis c virus-infected mothers. J Pediatr 1995;126:589–591
17. Kumar RM, Shahul S. Role of breast-feeding in transmission of hepatitis C virus to infants of HCV-infected mothers. J Hepatol 1998;29:191–197
18. Thomas DL. Mother-infant hepatitis c transmission: second generation research. Hepatol 1999;29:992–993
19. Chang M, Ni Y, Hwang L, et al. Long term clinical and virologic outcome of primary hepatitis C infection in children: A prospective study. Pediatr Infect Dis J 1994:13:769–773
20. Palomba E, Manzini P, Fiammengo P, et al. Natural history of perinatal hepatitis C virus infection. Clin Infect Dis 1996;23: 47–50
21. Bortolotti F, Resti M, Giacchino R, et al. Hepatitis C virus infection and related liver disease in children of mothers with antibodies to the virus. J Pediatr1997;130:990–993
22. Matsuoka S, Tatara K, Haybuchi Y, et al. Serologic, virologic, and histologic characteristics of chronic phase hepatitis C virus disease in children infected by transfusion. Pediatrics 1994;94: 919–922
23. Garcia-Monzon C, Jara P, Fernandez-Bermejo M, et al. Chronic hepatitis C in children: A clinical and immunohistochemical comparative study with adult patients. Hepatol 1998;28: 1696–1701
24. Bortolotti F, Jara P, Diaz C, et al. Posttransfusion and community-acquired hepatitis C in childhood. J Pediatr Gastroenterol Nutr 1994;18:279–283
25. Locasciulli A, Testa M, Pontisso P, et al. Prevalence and natural history of hepatitis C infection in patients cured of childhood leukemia. Blood 1997;90:4628–4633
26. Vogt M, Lang T, Frosner G, et al. Prevalence and clinical outcome of hepatitis C infection in children who underwent cardiac surgery before the implementation of blood-donor screening. N Engl J Med 1999;341:886–870
27. McDiarmid SV, Conrad A, Ament ME, et al. De novo hepatitis C in children after liver transplantation. Transplantation 1998;66: 311–318
28. Guido M, Rugge M, Jara P, et al. Chronic hepatitis C in children: The pathological and clinical spectrum. Gastroenterology 1998;115:1525–1529
29. Kage M, Fujisawa T, Shiraki K, et al. Pathology of chronic hepatitis C in children. Hepatol 1997;26:771–775
30. Badizadegan K, Jonas MM, Ott MJ, Nelson SP, Perez-Atayde AR. Histopathology of the liver in children with chronic hepatitis C viral infection. Hepatol 1998;28:1416–1423
31. Ruiz-Moreno M, Rua MJ, Castillo I, et al. Treatment of children with chronic hepatitis C with recombinant interferon-alpha: A pilot study. Hepatol 1992;16:882–885
32. Clemente MG, Congia M, Lai ME, et al. Effect of iron overload on the response to recombinant interferon-alfa treatment in transfusion-dependent patients with thalassemia major and chronic hepatitis C. J Pediatr 1994;125:123–128

33. Bortolotti F, Giacchino R, Vajro P, et al. Recombinant inter-feron-alpha therapy in children with chronic hepatitis C. Hepatol 1995;22:1623–1626

34. Zwiener RJ, Fielman BA, Cochran C, et al. Interferon-alpha-2b treatment of chronic hepatitis C in children with hemophilia. Pediatr Infect Dis J 1996;15:906–908

35. Iorio R, Pensati P, Porzio S, et al. Lymphoblastoid interferon alfa treatment in chronic hepatitis C. Arch Dis Child 1996;74: 152–156

36. Komatsu H, Fujisawa T, Inui A, et al. Efficacy of interferon in treating chronic hepatitis C in children with a history of acute leukemia. Blood 1996;87:4072–4075

37. DiMarco V, Lo Iacono O, Almasio P, et al. Long-term efficacy of alpha-interferon in beta-thalassemics with chronic hepatitis C. Blood 1997;90:2207–2212

38. Pensati P, Iorio R, Botta S, et al. Low rate sustained response to IFN therapy in children with chronic hepatitis C (CHC). Hepatol 1998;28:289A

39. Lau DTY, Kleiner DE, Ghany MG, et al. 10-Year follow-up after interferon-alpha therapy for chronic hepatitis C. Hepatol 1998; 28:1121–1127

40. Serfaty L, Aumaitre H, Chazouilleres O, et al. Determinants of outcome of compensated hepatitis C virus-related cirrhosis. Hepatol 1998;27:1435–1440

41. Kasahara A, Hayashi N, Mochizuki K, et al. Risk factors for hepatocellular carcinoma and its incidence after interferon treatment in patients with chronic hepatitis C. Hepatol 1998;27: 1394–1402

42. International Interferon-Hepatocellular Carcinoma Study Group. Effect of interferon-α on progression of cirrhosis to hepatocellular carcinoma: A retrospective cohort study. Lancet 1998;351:1535–1539

43. McHutchison JG, Gordon SC, Schiff ER, et al. Interferon alfa-2b alone or in combination with ribavirin as initial treatment for chronic hepatitis C. N Engl J Med 1998;339:1485–1492

44. Grether JK, Nelson KB, Dambrosia JM, Phillips TM. Interferons and cerebral palsy. J Pediatr 1999;134:324–332

45. Vesikari T, Nuutila A, Cantell K. Neurologic sequelae following interferon therapy of juvenile laryngeal papilloma. Acta Paediatr Scand 1988;77:619–622

Fibrosis in Patients with Chronic Hepatitis C: Detection and Significance

THIERRY POYNARD, M.D., Ph.D.,[1] VLAD RATZIU, M.D.,[1]
YVES BENMANOV, M.D.,[1] VINCENT DI MARTINO, M.D.,[1]
PIERRE BEDOSSA, M.D., Ph.D.,[2] and PIERRE OPOLON, M.D.[1]

ABSTRACT: *Estimates of the extent of hepatic fibrosis and the rate of fibrosis progression represent important surrogate end points for evaluation of the vulnerability of an individual patient and for assessment of the impact of treatment on natural history in chronic hepatitis C. Using the median fibrosis progression rate, the median expected time to cirrhosis in untreated patients is around 30 years. However, one third of patients have an expected median time to cirrhosis of less than 20 years and one third will only progress to cirrhosis in more than 50 years, if ever. Factors independently associated with fibrosis progression are duration of infection, age, male gender, consumption of alcohol, human immunodeficiency virus co-infection, and low CD4 count. Evaluation of fibrosis progression is useful to decide treatment. Among patients with sustained viral response, fibrosis regresses. Evaluation of fibrosis progression has permitted validation of the concept of suppressive therapy. Among patients without viral clearance, interferon alone or in combination with ribavirin significantly reduces fibrosis progression rate in comparison with progression before treatment and to control groups. There is a major need for noninvasive markers of liver fibrosis. None are clearly useful today for the diagnosis of early stages of fibrosis.*

KEY WORDS: fibrosis, HCV, ribavirin, liver biopsy

Worldwide, the major clinical consequence of chronic hepatitis C infection is the progression to cirrhosis and its potential complications: hemorrhage, hepatic insufficiency, and primary liver cancer.[1-4] Cumulative evidence strongly suggests that the increase in mortality due to hepatocellular carcinoma in most Western countries is due to hepatitis C infection.[5-8]

Current understanding of hepatitis C virus (HCV) infection has been advanced by the concept of liver fibrosis progression.[9-10] Fibrosis is the deleterious but variable consequence of chronic inflammation. It is characterized by the deposition of extracellular matrix components, leading to the distortion of the hepatic architecture with impairment of liver microcirculation

---

Objectives

Upon completion of this article, the reader should be able to 1) summarize the important steps in assessing the fibrosis progression rate, 2) discuss the appropriateness of liver biopsy, and 3) describe the concept of suppressive therapy in a patient with chronic hepatitis C.

Accreditation

The Indiana University School of Medicine is accredited by the Accreditation Council for Continuing Medical Education to sponsor continuing medical education for physicians. The Indiana University School of Medicine takes responsibility for the contents, quality, and scientific integrity of this activity.

Credit

The Indiana University School of Medicine designates this educational activity for a maximum of 1.0 hours credit toward the AMA Physicians Recognition Award in category one. Each physician should claim only those hours of credit that he/she actually spent in the educational activity.

Disclosure

Statements have been obtained regarding the authors' relationships with financial supporters of this activity. There is no apparent conflict of interest related to the context of participation of the author of this article.

From the [1]Service d'Hépato-Gastroentérologie, Groupe Hospitalier Pitié-Salpêtrière, Paris, and [2]Service d'Anatomie Pathologique, Hôpital de Bicètre, Paris, France.

Reprint requests: Dr. Thierry Poynard, Service d'Hépato-Gastroentérologie Groupe, Hospitalier Pitié-Salpêtrière, 47–83 Boulevard de l'-Hôpital, 75651 Paris Cedex 13, France. E-mail: tpoynard@teaser.fr

and liver cell function. HCV is usually only lethal when it leads to cirrhosis, the last stage of liver fibrosis. Therefore, an estimate of fibrosis progression represents an important surrogate end point for evaluation of the vulnerability of an individual patient and for assessment of the impact of treatment on natural history.

For hepatologists, liver biopsy is considered to be an essential procedure for making rational decisions in patients with chronic hepatitis C.[11–12] For patients and general practitioners, it can be considered as an aggressive procedure.[13,13a] The aim of this chapter is to review the different markers of liver fibrosis progression and to discuss the appropriateness of liver biopsy in comparison with other procedures in chronic hepatitis C.

FIBROSIS STAGES AND NECROINFLAMMATORY ACTIVITY GRADES

Activity (necroinflammation) and fibrosis are two major histologic features of chronic hepatitis C included in different proposed classifications.[11–17] One of the few validated scoring systems is called the METAVIR scoring system.[16,17] This system assesses histologic lesions in chronic hepatitis C using two separate scores, one for necroinflammatory grade (A for activity) and another for the stage of fibrosis (F). These scores are defined as follows; stages of fibrosis (F) (Fig. 1): F0, no fibrosis; F1, portal fibrosis without septa; F2, portal fibrosis with rare septa, F3, numerous septa without cirrhosis; F4, cirrhosis. Grade for activity (A): A0, no histologic necroinflammatory activity; A1, minimal activity, A2, moderate activity, A3, severe activity. The degree of activity was assessed by integration of the severity of the intensity of both piecemeal (periportal) necrosis and lobular necrosis as described in a simple algorithm.[17] The intra- and interobserver variations of this METAVIR scoring system are lower than those of the widely used Knodell scoring system.[16,17] For METAVIR

fibrosis stages there is an almost perfect concordance (kappa = 0.80) among pathologists.

As did others, we observed that fibrosis stage and inflammatory grade were correlated.[18–20] However, for 36% of patients, there was a discordance (178 of 500). If recommendations for treatment had been based on activity grades, 56% of patients without significant activity (119 of 214) would not have been treated despite significant fibrosis. In these patients who were infected for more than 10 years, fibrosis progression was therefore not related to significant activity, which also raises questions concerning the pathophysiology of fibrosis. The other discordant cases were 59 patients with nonsignificant fibrosis despite significant activity. This observation raises the question of the utility of treatment of significant inflammatory damages if fibrosis does not occur. To summarize, clinicians should not take "significant activity" as a surrogate marker of "severe disease."

Fibrosis stage is the result of the imbalance between synthesis and degradation of extracellular matrix components. Hepatic stellate cells are the major cell types involved in extracellular matrix production (i.e., collagens, fibronectin, and laminin). Although hepatic stellate cells produce extracellular matrix under the influence of various stimuli (growth factors, cytokines, and lipid peroxydation products), they also produce a set of matrix metalloproteinases (MMPs) that control degradation. MMPs are a family of related zinc-dependent endopeptidases capable of degrading all extracellular matrix components, playing a major role in extracellular matrix remodeling. Finally, proteolytic activity of MMPs can be inhibited by the tissue inhibitors of metalloproteinases, a group of proteins also produced by hepatic stellate cells. Activity grade, which represents necrosis is not a good predictor of fibrosis progression.[21] In fact, fibrosis alone is the best marker of ongoing fibrogenesis.[21] So far there is no study demonstrating clearly that activity grades are predictive of fibrosis progression independently of fibrosis stage.[22]

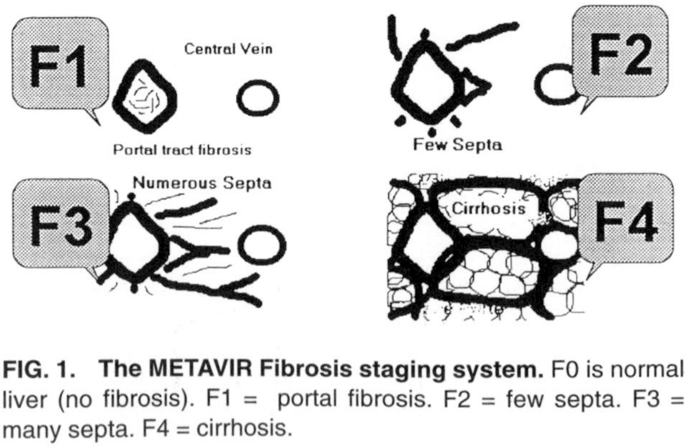

FIBROSIS AS A TIME-DEPENDENT END POINT

Because fibrosis stage summarizes the vulnerability of a patient and is predictive of the progression to cirrhosis, we looked at its association with the duration of infection and age at biopsy. The basic concept was to estimate the transition times from infection to cirrhosis and between the different stages of fibrosis (Fig. 2). An ideal assessment would have been to follow a large representative sample of patients prospectively from infection to death, with repeated liver biopsies and without treatment. Obviously, this type of study is both ethically and pragmatically impossible. The rare published studies on several biopsies were retrospective and included

FIG. 1.   The METAVIR Fibrosis staging system. F0 is normal liver (no fibrosis). F1 = portal fibrosis. F2 = few septa. F3 = many septa. F4 = cirrhosis.

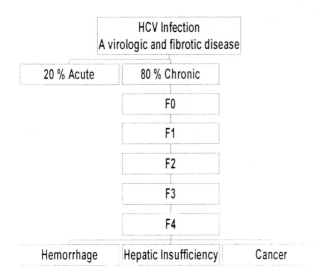

FIG. 2.   The model of fibrosis progression from infection to complications.

few and selected patients. We described the natural history of liver fibrosis progression and relevant risk factors in a cross-sectional study of single liver biopsy in a large number of patients for whom a reliable estimate of fibrosis had been performed.[9] The estimate was assessed primarily in patients for whom the duration of infection was known, but its validity had been checked by indirect estimates using age at biopsy and in two smaller longitudinal studies with repeated biopsies.[9]

This study found a strong, almost linear, correlation of fibrosis stages with age at biopsy and duration of infection. This correlation was not observed between activity grades (Fig. 3). Therefore, fibrosis stages are more representative of disease progression in comparison with activity grades. Although hepatitis C is a viral disease, it is mainly a fibrotic disease. Mortality and complications are related to cirrhosis. The clinical hallmarks of major necrosis and inflammation (i.e., severe

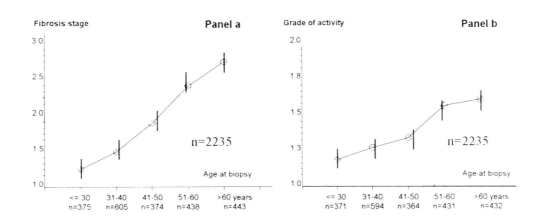

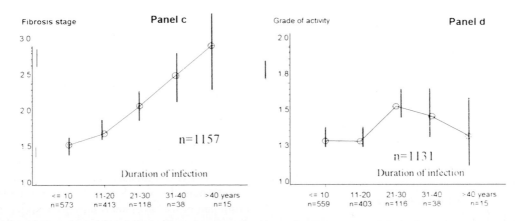

FIG. 3.   Relationship between age at biopsy and stage of fibrosis (panel a), and grade of activity (panel b), and between estimated duration of infection and stage of fibrosis (panel c) and grade of activity (panel d).

acute hepatitis and fulminant hepatitis) are very rare compared with hepatitis B. Even in immunologically compromised patients, there are very few acute flare ups in patients with chronic hepatitis C.

DYNAMIC VIEW OF FIBROSIS PROGRESSION

Because of the informative value of fibrosis stage, it is of interest for clinicians to assess the speed of the fibrosis progression. We observed that fibrosis progression rate was not normally distributed (median, 0.133 METAVIR grade per year, lower than the mean 0.252) but rather, asymmetric. The distribution suggested the presence of at least three populations: one population of "rapid fibrosers," a population of "intermediate fibrosers," and one population of "slow fibrosers." Therefore, the computation of a mean (or median) fibrosis progression rate per year and of a mean expected time to cirrhosis does not signify that the progression to cirrhosis is universal and inevitable. Using the median fibrosis progression rate, the median expected time to cirrhosis in untreated patients was 30 years; 33% of patients had an expected median time to cirrhosis of less than 20 years and 31% will progress to cirrhosis in more than 50 years, if ever (Fig. 4).

Different Estimates of Fibrosis Progression

Limitations of any estimate of fibrosis include the difficulty in obtaining paired liver biopsies, the necessity for large numbers of patients to achieve statistical power, and the sample variability in fibrosis distribution. Even in published randomized trials, fewer than 50% of included patients undergo a second liver biopsy after the end of the treatment. Because the time elapsed between biopsies is relatively short (usually between 12

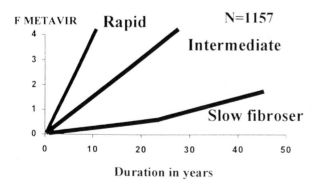

FIG. 4. Progression of liver fibrosis in patients with chronic hepatitis C.

and 24 months), the number of events (transition from one stage to another) is rare. Therefore, the comparisons between fibrosis progression rates requires a large sample size to observe significant differences. The slope of progression is difficult to assess because there is no large database with several biopsies. Therefore, the real slope is currently unknown, and even if there is a linear relationship between stages and age at biopsy or duration of infection, other models are possible.[23] Furthermore, liver biopsy has its own limitations in assessing liver fibrosis. Although it is the gold standard to score fibrosis, its value is limited by sample variability. At least a 10-mm-length biopsy is mandatory to assess fibrosis accurately.

The assessment of fibrosis progression over time can be achieved by different methods.[9,10,24] The observed (direct) fibrosis progression rate is defined as the ratio of the difference in fibrosis stages between two biopsies, expressed in METAVIR units, and the interval between the two biopsies in years. For example, for a patient with fibrosis stage 2 at the first biopsy and stage 3 at the second biopsy performed 2 years later, the fibrosis progression rate was 0.500 fibrosis units per year. The advantage of this assessment is that the exact duration is known. The limitations are that the interval between biopsies is rather short (mean, 20 months) compared with the mean time for transition between fibrosis stages (7 years) and that there is a risk of sampling and interpretation errors for both biopsies.

The estimated (indirect) fibrosis progression rate per year is defined as the ratio between the fibrosis stage in METAVIR units and the estimated duration of infection in years. In this model it is assumed that the patient has no liver fibrosis the day of infection (stage F0) and that the fibrosis progression rate is constant. For example, for a patient with fibrosis stage 2 and an 8-year duration of infection, the fibrosis progression rate was 0.250 fibrosis units per year. The advantages of this assessment are the longer duration (mean, 16 years) and the absence of variability at infection if the assumption of F0 is correct. The limitations are that the duration of infection may be unknown and, even when known, it remains an estimate (i.e., it is assumed that the first transfusion or the first intravenous drug injection was the true date of infection). It is also possible that some patients already have a degree of fibrosis (i.e., due to alcohol) on the day of infection.

Nonquantitative assessment of fibrosis progression can be obtained more simply by the percentage of patients who worsen, improve or do not change their stage between two biopsies. The advantage of this assessment is simplicity. The disadvantage is that it does not take into account the observation period and the lack of discriminant power over short durations between biopsies. If these percentages (transition probability from stage to stage) are used in Markov modelling, they have to be expressed by time units. This Markov transition modelling has been used to reconstruct HCV epidemics in France (8). This modelling was possible only because age and sex influences on fibrosis progression have been taken into account. The transition rates from normal liver at infection to the different stages can also be estimated by time dependent modelling as actuarial curves.

Factors Associated with Fibrosis Progression

Several factors clearly have been shown to be associated with fibrosis progression rate[8–9,23–26]: duration of infection, age, male gender, consumption of alcohol, human immunodeficiency virus (HIV) co-infection, and low CD4 count. The progression from infection to cirrhosis depends strongly on sex and age.[8,9] Viral factors such as genotype, viral load at the time of the biopsy, and quasispecies are not correlated with fibrosis.[8–9,23–26]

APPROPRIATENESS OF LIVER BIOPSY

In chronic liver disease, several studies have evaluated the intra- and interobserver (pathologist) concordance,[30–32] the discordances among methods,[33–36] and the sampling errors.[31,37] For chronic viral liver disease, there were significant concordances for standardized items, particularly for fibrosis staging.[18,19]

Four randomized trials have compared different biopsy methods.[33–36] For the diagnosis of cirrhosis, one trial observed better sensitivity with laparoscopy versus percutaneous biopsy[33] and another trial better sensitivity using the Tru-Cut versus the Menghini needle.[34] One

trial reported larger sampling by ultrasound-guided anterior large-bore cutting needle biopsy than with the intercostal Menghini technique,[35] and less adverse events. One trial observed fewer adverse events when ultrasound-guided biopsy was used (2 vs. 9%), whatever the needle used.[36]

It is only very recent that the histologic standards defining a normal liver have been revisited.[38] No scoring systems have so far integrated a definition of normal liver in their own definitions.

Adverse Events and Mortality of Liver Biopsy

A summary of the published articles (with more than 200 patients) assessing severe adverse events and mortality rates is given in Table 1.[39–48] There was significant heterogeneity among the observed mortality rates, with a range from 0 to 3.3/1,000. Risk factors identified were age and cirrhosis.

Indication of Liver Fibrosis Assessment in Hepatitis C

Chronic Hepatitis C

Recent consensus conferences have stated that liver biopsy is mandatory in chronic hepatitis C with abnormal alanine aminotransferase permitting grading and staging of the disease.[1,2] It is stated that liver biopsy should be performed before initiating treatment and that it is not known if and when repeat biopsy is necessary.

In chronic hepatitis C, liver biopsy is probably not mandatory in patients who need treatment whatever the

TABLE 1. Uncontrolled Observations of Adverse Events and Mortality Associated with Liver Biopsy

Publication Year	First Author	Number of Patients	Type of Biopsy	Design	Adverse Events Definition	Severe Adverse N (per thousand, 95% CI)	Mortality N (per thousand, 95% CI)
1979	Gayral	2,346	Laparoscopy, percutaneous, surgery	Retrospective	Bleeding	11 (4.7; 2.3–8.4)	4 (1.7; 0.5–4.4)
1982	Lebrec	932	Transvenous	Retrospective	Bleeding	1 (1.1; 0.3–6.0)	1 (1.1; 0.3–6.0)
1986	Piccinino	68,276	Intercostal	Retrospective	Bleeding, pneumothorax, biliary peritonitis	137 (2.0; 1.7–2.4)	5 (0.07;0.02–0.017)
1990	McGill	9,212	Percutaneous	Retrospective	Bleeding	22 (2.4; 1.5–3.6)	10 (1.1; 0.5–2.0)
1992	Maharaj	2,646	Percutaneous	Prospective	Bleeding, pneumothorax, biliary peritonitis, pain	63 (24; 18–30)	8 (3.0; 1.3–5.9)
1993	Van Thiel	12,750	Percutaneous transplant	Retrospective	"Major complications"	26 (2.0; 1.3–3.0)	0 (0.0; 0.0–0.3)
1993	Janes	405	Percutaneous outpatients	Retrospective	Admission	13 (32; 17–54)	0 (0.0; 0.0–9.1)
1995	Gilmore	1,500	Percutaneous	Retrospective	Bleeding	26 (17; 11–25)	5 (3.3; 1.1–7.8)
1998	Vivas	378	Percutaneous	Prospective	Admissions and bleeding	7 (19; 7–38)	0 (0.0; 0.0–9.7)
	Total	**98,445**				**306 (3.1; 2.8–3.5)**	**33 (0.3; 0.2–0.5)**

results of the biopsy, for example in patients who can contaminate other people or in patients who have extrahepatic manifestations impairing the quality of life. Liver biopsy assesses the rate of disease progression when the date of contamination is known (fibrosis progression rate) and improves the prediction of treatment response.

Diagnosis of Cirrhosis

Biopsy can also be viewed as necessary for the diagnosis of cirrhosis, which implies a different follow-up than in noncirrhotic patients. In a patient with cirrhosis, for example, it is necessary to screen for varices and for hepatocellular carcinoma.

When the cirrhosis is obvious, biopsy is not appropriate. There are few studies in the literature estimating the predictive values for cirrhosis of clinical, biologic,[41-42] or morphologic signs.[49-53] The following signs potentially have a high positive predictive value: firm liver, ascites, splenomegalia, spider angioma, prothrombin time lower than 60%, high serum hyaluronate, and platelet count < 100,000. With ultrasound, liver surface nodularity and reduction of portal flow velocity have the better predictive values. A reduction in the indications for biopsy could be achieved by increasing the positive predictive value and the negative predictive value of surrogate cirrhosis markers. A summary of the present informational value of cirrhosis markers in chronic hepatitis C is given in Figure 5.

Acute Hepatitis C

In acute hepatitis C, because of the effectiveness of treatment and the high (80%) spontaneous evolution to a chronic disease, a recommendation for treatment seems mandatory whatever the results of liver biopsy. Therefore, liver biopsy is not recommended when the diagnosis of acute hepatitis C is certain.

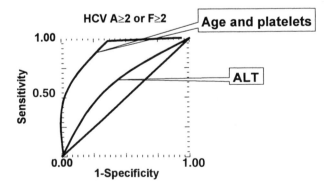

FIG. 5. Ranges of sensitivity and specificity of cirrhosis markers in patients with chronic hepatitis C.

Patients with Normal Transaminases

Another important issue is the ability to diagnose minimal disease without biopsy. Among HCV polymerase chain reaction-positive patients with sustained normal transaminases despite a low median fibrosis progression rate, only 20% have a normal liver (no activity and no fibrosis).[54] Thirteen percent of such patients have extensive fibrosis (METAVIR stage 2, 3 or 4), and for them treatment is mandatory. No surrogate markers currently permit us to identify these patients with minimal disease, and therefore we continue to biopsy such patients.

Patients with Several Causes of Liver Disease

One common issue is the influence of other risk factors on the fibrosis progression rate. It has been clearly demonstrated that a daily alcohol consumption of 50 g/day or above is highly associated with enhanced fibrosis progression rate.[9,55] Similarly, the suspicion of associated hemochromatosis, autoimmune disease, nonalcoholic steatohepatitis, or co-infection with hepatitis B should lead to liver biopsy. Liver biopsy helps clinicians to estimate the specific impact of each factor.

Patients Co-infected with HIV Virus

Several studies have demonstrated that patients coinfected with HCV and HIV have a faster fibrosis progression rate than controls even after taking into account age, sex, and alcohol consumption.[26] The prevalence of cirrhosis is three-fold higher in HIV–HCV co-infected patients than in HIV negative HCV-infected patients, and one third of co-infected patients are at risk of dying of liver disease.

The progression of fibrosis is more rapid in coinfected patients compared with matched controls infected by HCV alone. In co-infected patients, a low CD4 count ($\leq$200 cells/μL), alcohol consumption (>50 g/day), and age at HCV infection are associated with a higher liver fibrosis progression rate.

Anti-HIV treatments are often associated with increased transaminases (stavudine, didanosine, abacavir, nevirapine, protease inhibitor). When the increase is appreciable, another liver biopsy must be considered and compared with biopsy before treatment. The following factors can be involved: alcohol consumption, illicit intravenous drug injection, substitution drug toxicity, anti-HIV drug toxicity, co-infection with hepatitis B or delta virus, opportunistic liver infection, immune restoration, and sclerosing cholangitis. The impact of immune reconstitution on liver fibrosis progression is unknown.

Assessment of Liver Fibrosis Stage during or after Treatment

Together with the concept of assessing fibrosis progression rate during the natural history of chronic hepatitis C,[9] the concept of suppressive therapy has emerged as a new standard for the impact of treatments.[10,55] It is possible now to assess the impact of treatment on the fibrosis progression rate. Several studies have demonstrated that a sustained viral response, obtained by interferon alone or by the combination of ribavirin and interferon, was associated with a reduction in fibrosis progression and with stage regression.[10,24,56–57] For nonresponders (60% of patients) there is also now accumulating evidence that interferon treatment alone or in combination with ribavirin has a suppressive effect on fibrosis progression.[10,24,55] Serum markers of fibrosis or fibrogenesis have been evaluated in small studies without identifying practical predictive values.[58–67]

CONCLUSION

Liver biopsy is certainly appropriate for fibrosis staging of chronic hepatitis C. However, the appropriate role of liver biopsy in a practical diagnostic/staging algorithm should be further evaluated. Excess requirements for liver biopsy, because of its cost and risk, could actually become a barrier to treatment. By contrast, underuse of liver biopsy could also lead to inappropriateness of hepatitis treatments. There is a major need for noninvasive markers of liver fibrosis. None are useful today for the diagnosis of early stages.

ABBREVIATIONS

HCV   hepatitis C virus
HIV   human immunodeficiency virus
MMPs   matrix metalloproteinases

REFERENCES

1. WHO. Hepatitis C: global prevalence. Wkly Epidemiol Rec 1997;72:341–344
2. Seeff LB, Buskell-Bales Z, Wright EC, et al. Long-term mortality after transfusion-associated non-A non-B hepatitis. N Engl J Med 1992;327:1906–1911
3. Tong MJ, el-Farra NS, Reikes AR, Co RL. Clinical outcomes after transfusion-associated hepatitis C. N Engl J Med 1995;332:1463–1466
4. Darby SC, Ewart DW, Giangrande PLF, et al. Mortality from liver cancer and liver disease in haemophilic men and boys given blood products contaminated with hepatitis C. Lancet 1997;350:1425–1431
5. El-Serag HB, Mason A. Rising incidence of hepatocellular carcinoma in the United States. N Engl J Med 1999;34:745–750
6. Taylor-Robinson SD, Foster GR, Arora S, Hargreaves S, Thomas HC. Increase in primary liver cancer in the UK, 1979–94 [letter]. Lancet 1997;350:1142–1143
7. Deuffic S, Poynard T, Buffat L, Valleron A-J. Trends in primary liver cancer [letter]. Lancet 1998;351:214–215
8. Deuffic S, Buffat L, Poynard T, Valleron AJ. Modeling the hepatitis C virus epidemic in France. Hepatology 1999;29:1596–1601
9. Poynard T, Bedossa P, Opolon P, for the OBSVIRC, METAVIR, CLINIVIR and DOSVIRC groups. Natural history of liver fibrosis progression in patients with chronic hepatitis C. Lancet 1997;349:825–832
10. Sobesky R, Mathurin P, Charlotte F, et al. Modeling the impact of interferon alfa treatment on liver fibrosis progression in chronic hepatitis C: a dynamic view. Gastroenterology 1999;116:378–386
11. Perrillo RP. The role of liver biopsy in hepatitis C. Hepatology 1997;26:57S–61S
12. Consensus Statement. EASL International Consensus Conference on Hepatitis C. J Hepatol 1999;30:956–961
13. Poynard T, Lebrec D. The inconvenience of investigations used in hepatology: patients' and hepatologists' opinions. Liver 1982;2:369–375
13a. Scheuer PJ. Classification of chronic viral hepatitis: a need for reassessment. J Hepatol 1991;13:372–374
14. Ludwig J. The nomenclature of chronic active hepatitis: an obituary. Gastroenterology 1993;105:274–278
15. Desmet VJ, Gerber M, Hoofnagle JH, Manns M, Scheuer PJ. Classification of chronic hepatitis: diagnosis, grading and staging. Hepatology 1994;19:1513–1519
16. Bedossa P, Poynard T, the METAVIR Cooperative Group. Inter- and intra-observer variation in the assessment of liver biopsy of chronic hepatitis C. Hepatology 1994;20;1:15–20
17. Bedossa P, Poynard T. An algorithm for the grading of activity in chronic hepatitis C. The METAVIR Cooperative Study Group. Hepatology 1996; 24:289–293
18. Knodell KG, Ishak KG, Black WC, et al. Formulation and application of a numerical scoring system for assessing histological activity in asymptomatic chronic active hepatitis. Hepatology 1981;1:431–435
19. Wong VS, Wight DG, Palmer CR, Alexander GJ. Fibrosis and other histological features in chronic hepatitis C virus infection: a statistical model. J Clin Pathol 1996;49:465–469
20. Poynard T, Bedossa P. Age and platelet count: a simple index for predicting the presence of histological lesions in patients with antibodies to hepatitis C virus. METAVIR and CLINIVIR Cooperative Study Groups. J Viral Hepatol 1997;4:199–208
21. Paradis V, Mathurin P, Laurent A, et al. Histological features predictive of liver fibrosis in chronic hepatitis C infection. J Clin Pathol 1996;49:998–1004
22. Yano M, Kumada H, Kage M, et al. The long term pathological evolution of chronic hepatitis C. Hepatology 1996;23:1334–1340
23. Datz C, Cramp M, Haas T, et al. The natural course of hepatitis C virus infection 18 years after an epidemic outbreak of non-A, non-B hepatitis in a plasmapheresis centre. Gut 1999;44:563–567
24. Poynard T, McHutchison J, Davis G, Esteban-Mur R, Goodman Z, Bedossa P, Albrecht J, and the FIBROVIRC Project Group. Impact of interferon alfa-2b and ribavirin on the liver fibrosis progression in patients with chronic hepatitis C. Hepatology 1998;28:497A
25. Wiley TE, McCarthy M, Breidi L, McCarthy M, Layden TJ. Impact of alcohol on the histological and clinical progression of hepatitis C infection. Hepatology 1998;28:805–809

26. Benhamou Y, Bochet M, Di Martino V, et al. Liver fibrosis progression in human immunodeficiency virus and hepatitis C virus coinfected patients. The Multivirc Group. Hepatology 1999;30:1054–1058

27. von Frerichs. Uber den diabetes. Berlin: Hirschwald, 1884

28. Schupfer F. De la possibilité de faire "intra vitam" un diagnostic précis des maladies du foie et de la rate. Semin Méd 1907;27:229–230

29. Huard P. La ponction biopsie du foie et son utilité dans le diagnostic des affections hépatiques. Ann Anat Path 1935;12:1118–1124

30. Theodossi A, Spiegelhalter D, Portmann B, Eddleston AL, Williams R. The value of clinical, biochemical, ultrasound and liver biopsy data in assessing patients with liver disease. Liver 1983;3:315–326

31. Soloway RD, Baggenstoss AH, Schoenfield LJ, Summerskill WH. Observer error and sampling variability tested in evaluation of hepatitis and cirrhosis by liver biopsy. Am J Dig Dis 1971;16:1082–1086

32. Theodossi A, Skene AM, Portmann B. Observer variation in assessment of liver biopsies including analysis by kappa statistics. Gastroenterology 1980;79:232–241

33. Pagliaro L, Rinaldi F, Craxi A, et al. Percutaneous blind biopsy versus laparoscopy with guided biopsy in diagnosis of cirrhosis. A prospective, randomized trial. Dig Dis Sci 1983;28:39–43

34. Colombo M, Del Ninno E, de Franchis R, et al. Ultrasound-assisted percutaneous liver biopsy: superiority of the Tru-Cut over the Menghini needle for diagnosis of cirrhosis. Gastroenterology 1998;95:487–489

35. Papini E, Pacella CM, Rossi Z, et al. A randomized trial of ultrasound-guided anterior subcostal liver biopsy versus the conventional Menghini technique. J Hepatol 1991;13:291–297

36. Lindor KD, Bru C, Jorgensen RA, et al. The role of ultrasonography and automatic-needle biopsy in outpatient percutaneous liver biopsy. Hepatology 1996;23:1079–1083

37. Maharaj B, Maharaj RJ, Leary WP, et al. Sampling variability and its influence on the diagnostic yield of percutaneous needle biopsy of the liver. Lancet 1986;1:523–525

38. Crawford AR, Lin XZ, Crawford JM. The normal adult human liver biopsy: a quantitative reference standard. Hepatology 1998;28:323–331

39. Urena MA, Ruiz-Delgado FC, Gonzalez EM, et al. Assessing risk of the use of livers with macro and microsteatosis in a liver transplant program. Transplant Proc 1998;30:3288–3291

40. Gayral F, Potier M, Salmon R, Labayle D, Larrieu H. Vascular complications of needle biopsy of the liver. J Chir (Paris) 1979;116:261–264

41. Lebrec D, Goldfarb G, Degott C, Rueff B, Benhamou JP. Transvenous liver biopsy: an experience based on 1000 hepatic tissue samplings with this procedure. Gastroenterology 1982;83:338–340

42. Piccinino F, Sagnelli E, Pasquale G, Giusti G. Complications following percutaneous liver biopsy. A multicentre retrospective study on 68,276 biopsies. J Hepatol 1986;2:165–173

43. McGill DB, Rakela J, Zinsmeister AR, Ott BJ. A 21-year experience with major hemorrhage after percutaneous liver biopsy. Gastroenterology 1990;99:1396–1400

44. Maharaj B, Bhoora IG. Complications associated with percutaneous needle biopsy of the liver when one, two or three specimens are taken. Postgrad Med J 1992;68:964–967

45. Van Thiel DH, Gavaler JS, Wright H, Tzakis A. Liver biopsy. Its safety and complications as seen at a liver transplant center. Transplantation 1993;55:1087–1090

46. Janes CH, Lindor KD. Outcome of patients hospitalized for complications after outpatient liver biopsy. Ann Intern Med 1993;118:96–98

47. Gilmore IT, Burroughs A, Murray-Lyon IM, Williams R, Jenkins D, Hopkins A. Indications, methods, and outcomes of percutaneous liver biopsy in England and Wales: an audit by the British Society of Gastroenterology and the Royal College of Physicians of London. Gut 1995;36:437–441

48. Vivas S, Palacio MA, Rodriguez M, Lomo J, Cadenas F, Giganto F, Rodrigo L. Ambulatory liver biopsy: complications and evolution in 264 cases. Rev Esp Enferm Dig 1998;90:175–182

49. Teare JP, Sherman D, Greenfield SM, et al. Comparison of serum procollagen III peptide concentrations and PGA index for assessment of hepatic fibrosis. Lancet 1993;342:895–898

50. Oberti F, Valsesia E, Pilette C, et al. Noninvasive diagnosis of hepatic fibrosis or cirrhosis. Gastroenterology 1997;113:1609–1616

51. Bonacini M, Hadi G, Govindarajan S, Lindsay KL. Utility of a discriminant score for diagnosing advanced fibrosis or cirrhosis in patients with chronic hepatitis C virus infection. Am J Gastroenterol 1997;92:1302–1304

52. Gaiani S, Gramantieri L, Venturoli N, et al. What is the criterion for differentiating chronic hepatitis from compensated cirrhosis? A prospective study comparing ultrasonography and percutaneous liver biopsy. J Hepatol 1997;27:979–985

53. Aube C, Oberti F, Korali N, et al. Ultrasonographic diagnosis of hepatic fibrosis or cirrhosis. J Hepatol. 1999;30:472–478

54. Mathurin P, Moussalli J, Cadranel JF, et al. Slow progression rate of fibrosis in hepatitis C virus patients with persistently normal alanine transaminase activity. Hepatology 1998;27:868–872

55. Shiffman ML, Hofmann CM, Contos MJ, Luketic VA, Sanyal AJ, Sterling RK, Ferreira-Gonzalez A, Mills AS, Garret C. A randomized, controlled trial of maintenance interferon therapy for patients with chronic hepatitis C virus and persistent viremia. Gastroenterology 1999;117:1164–1172

56. Poynard T, Leroy V, Cohard M, et al. Meta-analysis of interferon randomized trials in the treatment of viral hepatitis: Effects of dose and duration. Hepatology 1996;24:778–789

57. Camma C, Giunta M, Linea C, Pagliaro L. The effect of interferon in chronic hepatitis C: a quantitative evaluation of histology by meta-analysis. J Hepatol 1997;26:1187–1199

58. Capra F, Casaril M, Gabrielli GB, et al. Dolci Alpha-interferon in the treatment of chronic viral hepatitis: effects on fibrogenesis serum markers. J Hepatol 1993;18:112–118

59. Fukuda Y, Nakano I, Katano Y, et al. Assessment and treatment of liver disease in Japanese haemophilia patients. Haemophilia 1998;4:595–600

60. Kaplanski G, Farnarier C, Payan MJ, Bongrand P, Durand JM. Increased levels of soluble adhesion molecules in the serum of patients with hepatitis C. Correlation with cytokine concentrations and liver inflammation and fibrosis. Dig Dis Sci 1997;42:2277–2284

61. Kasahara A, Hayashi N, Mochizuki K, et al. Circulating matrix metalloproteinase-2 and tissue inhibitor of metalloproteinase-1 as serum markers of fibrosis in patients with chronic hepatitis C. Relationship to interferon response. J Hepatol 1997;26:574–583

62. Mazzoran L, Tamaro G, Mangiarotti MA, et al. Effects of interferon therapy on fibrosis serum markers in HCV-positive chronic liver disease. Eur J Gastroenterol Hepatol 1998;10:125–131

63. Napoli J, Bishop GA, McGuinness PH, Painter DM, McCaughan GW. Progressive liver injury in chronic hepatitis C infection correlates with increased intrahepatic expression of Th1-associated cytokines. Hepatology 1996;24:759–765

64. Verbaan H, Bondeson L, Eriksson S. Non-invasive assessment of inflammatory activity and fibrosis (grade and stage) in chronic hepatitis C infection. Scand J Gastroenterol 1997;32:494–499

65. Wong VS, Hughes V, Trull A, Wight DG, Petrik J, Alexander GJ. Serum hyaluronic acid is a useful marker of liver fibrosis in

chronic hepatitis C virus infection. J Viral Hepatol 1998;5: 187–192

66. Yamada M, Fukuda Y, Koyama Y, et al. Serum hyaluronic acid reflects the effect of interferon treatment on hepatic fibrosis in patients with chronic hepatitis C. J Gastroenterol Hepatol 1996;11:646–651

67. Yamada M, Fukuda Y, Nakano I, Katano Y, Takamatsu J, Hayakawa T. Serum hyaluronan as a marker of liver fibrosis in hemophiliacs with hepatitis C virus-associated chronic liver disease. Acta Haematol 1998;99:212–216

Hepatitis C Virus RNA Codes for Proteins and Replicates: Does It also Trigger the Interferon Response?

ANDREA D. BRANCH, Ph.D.

ABSTRACT: *Hepatitis C virus (HCV) is a positive sense virus with a genomic RNA molecule roughly 9,600 nucleotides in length. The single-stranded genomic RNA has a nontranslated region (NTR) at each end and a long open reading frame (coding region) in between. The 5'NTR and portions of the 3'NTR are the most conserved parts of HCV RNA. These conserved regions contain signals for replication and translation. Much of the 5'NTR is folded into a structure that binds ribosomes. This structure, an internal ribosome entry site, promotes the initiation of protein synthesis and is critical for HCV gene expression. The ribosome binding site may extend into the coding region; its exact boundaries are not known. The open reading frame encodes the HCV polyprotein, which is slightly more than 3,000 amino acids in length. The 3'NTR plays a key role in HCV replication and may also influence the rate of HCV protein synthesis. During replication, the genomic RNA is copied by virally encoded enzymes into a complementary antigenomic RNA, which itself is a template for the synthesis of progeny RNAs. At steady state, genomic strands outnumber antigenomic strands about 10 to 1. HCV RNA replication is thought to take place in the cytoplasm and is an error-prone process. It generates a mixed population of RNA sequences (quasispecies), including mutants that may be more fit than the parental type, less fit, or equally fit (but distinct). Natural selection acts upon the progeny RNAs, causing the population to change and drift. Over time, mutation, selection, and population bottlenecks led to the evolution of varied genotypes. The HCV replication complex is a potential source of double-stranded RNA, a powerful inducer of interferon. Thus, HCV-specific double-stranded RNA may trigger the first steps of innate immunity; however, for unknown reasons, the immune system often fails to clear the infection. The plasticity of the HCV genome and the low level of HCV gene expression may counterbalance any immunostimulatory effects of HCV RNA and allow the virus to escape specific immune responses. Antisense drugs and ribozymes directed against HCV RNA are under investigation. Future interventions may include nucleic acid drugs (antisense and ribozymes) and smaller pharmaceuticals that bind to intricate structures in HCV RNA and HCV-specific double-stranded RNA. Infectious clones of HCV RNA are available. These clones and other systems for expressing HCV proteins pave the way for vaccine development.*

KEY WORDS: internal ribosome entry site, double-stranded RNA, interferon, antisense

Objectives

Upon completion of this article, the reader should know the main features of HCV genomic RNA, the relationship between viral replication and interferon induction, and the approaches for developing drugs directed against HCV RNA.

Accreditation

The Indiana University School of Medicine is accredited by the Accreditation Council for Continuing Medical Education to sponsor continuing medical education for physicians. The Indiana University School of Medicine takes responsibility for the contents, quality, and scientific integrity of this activity.

Credit

The Indiana University School of Medicine designates this educational activity for a maximum of 1.0 hours credit toward the AMA Physicians Recognition Award in category one. Each physician should claim only those hours of credit that he/she actually spent in the educational activity.

Disclosure

Statements have been obtained regarding the authors' relationships with financial supporters of this activity. There is no apparent conflict of interest related to the context of participation of the author of this article.

From the Division of Liver Diseases, Department of Medicine, Recanati/Miller Transplantation Institute, Mount Sinai School of Medicine, New York, New York.

Reprint requests: Dr. A. Branch, Division of Liver Diseases, Department of Medicine, Recanati/Miller Transplantation Institute, Mount Sinai School of Medicine, One Gustave L. Levy Place, New York, NY 10029. E-mail: ab8@doc.mssm.edu

Copyright © 2000 by Thieme Medical Publishers, Inc., 333 Seventh Avenue, New York, NY 10001, USA. Tel.: +1(212) 584-4663. 0272–8087,p;2000,20,01,0057,0068,ftx,en;sld00040x

RNA GENOME OF THE HEPATITIS C VIRUS

The blood of patients with hepatitis C virus (HCV) contains infectious virus particles that have an outer envelope with a lipid bilayer and two transmembrane glycoproteins surrounding a nucleocapsid containing the core protein and the HCV genome. The HCV genome is an RNA molecule roughly 9,600 nucleotides in length.[1,2] It contains both RNA structural elements and genetic information encoding the HCV proteins. Upon entry into a susceptible cell, the genomic RNA is released from the particle, binds ribosomes, and is translated.

HCV is classified as a positive sense RNA virus because the virion contains a single-stranded RNA (ssRNA) that is fully equipped to function as a messenger RNA (mRNA). HCV genomic RNA contains a single open reading frame (ORF). The ORF is translated into a polyprotein that is cleaved by cellular and viral proteases to release the structural and nonstructural HCV proteins. Once HCV proteins reach a sufficient level, a switch occurs and a portion of the HCV RNA is diverted from the translational process into the replication pathway. In the first step of HCV RNA replication, viral proteins bind the genomic RNA and copy it into a complementary antigenomic RNA. It is not clear whether the genomic and antigenomic RNAs produce a fully double-stranded RNA (dsRNA) replication intermediate, or remain associated through only a limited number of base pairs.[3] Whatever the exact structure of the replication complex, the antigenomic RNA is copied into positive sense RNA. The steady state ratio of genomic to antigenomic strands is thought to be approximately 10:1 (see Gowans'[4] article in this issue). The progeny positive sense RNAs can feed into three pathways: They can be packaged into infectious particles and released into

the circulation, they can serve as mRNAs for the production of more HCV protein; or they can initiate additional rounds of RNA replication. Replication is thought to occur in the cytoplasm. It is an error-prone process that generates a mixed population of RNA sequences, including mutants that may be more fit than the parental type, less fit, or equally fit (but distinct). Natural selection acts on the progeny RNAs, causing the population to change and drift.[5,6]

This article begins with a description of the structural features of HCV RNAs and a discussion of self-replicating experimental systems. It then examines the possibility that HCV RNA and/or the HCV replication complex triggers the interferon response and concludes with a review of therapeutic interventions designed to interfere with HCV RNA.

LANDMARKS OF HCV GENOMIC RNA

A molecular map of genomic HCV RNA is shown in Figure 1. The genomic RNA has a nontranslated region (NTR) at each end and a coding region in between. The 5′NTR and portions of the 3′NTR are the most conserved parts of the HCV genome. These conserved regions contain signals for replication and translation. The HCV 5′NTR was thought to be 341 nucleotides long in most strains; however, Trowbridge and Gowans[7] recently reported that an additional eight nucleotides are present at the 5′ end. The 5′ terminal moiety of the genomic RNA is not known with certainty; however, the RNA is thought to lack a cap (a structure with an unusual nucleotide linkage that comprises the 5′ terminus of many mRNAs). A short hairpin near the 5′ end may contain signals for replication. The remainder of the 5′NTR forms a structure that binds ribosomes and is im-

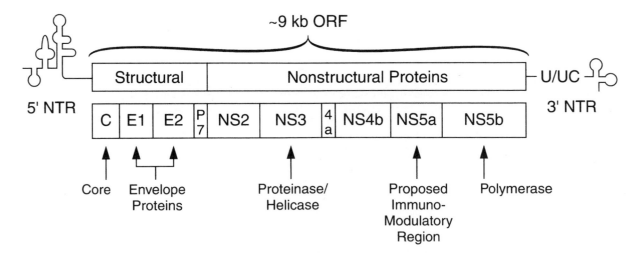

FIG. 1. **Map of the HCV genome.** The HCV genome has a 5′NTR of approximately 340 bases, an ORF of approximately 9,100 bases, and a 3′NTR of approximately 150 bases. The ORF encodes nonstructural proteins and structural proteins.

portant for HCV protein synthesis. This internal ribosome entry site (IRES) may extend into the coding region. The ORF encodes the HCV polyprotein, which is slightly more than 3,000 amino acids in length. The 3'NTR plays an essential role in HCV replication and may also influence the rate of HCV protein synthesis.

STRUCTURAL ELEMENTS IN HCV GENOMIC AND ANTIGENOMIC RNA

5'NTR and the HCV IRES

The highly conserved 5'NTR is a feature of many investigations, whether they are clinical trials or basic research studies. Both quantitative and qualitative polymerase chain reaction diagnostic tests for HCV are directed against this portion of the genomic RNA.[8] The 5'NTR is highly conserved because it forms a major part of a finely honed molecular machine—the IRES—that is essential for viral protein synthesis. In addition, it probably also contains structures required for replication. The IRES binds ribosomes and thereby sets the stage for the initiation of translation at the AUG start codon of the large ORF.

The HCV IRES was originally described by Tsukiyama Kohara et al. in 1992,[9] only a few years after IRES elements were first discovered in members of the *Picornaviridae* family.[10,11] Among viruses in the family *Flaviridae*, members of the genus *Pestivirus* (bovine virus diarrhea virus [BVDV]) have IRES elements with a number of features similar to those of the HCV, whereas members of the genus *Flavivirus* (yellow fever virus) lack IRES elements (Table 1). Lemon and Honda[12] categorize the HCV IRES as a type 3 site and group it with the IRES elements of pestiviruses and GB virus B. (For comparison, enteroviruses [poliovirus] and rhinoviruses have type 1 sites and hepatitis A virus has a type 2 site.[12,13])

TABLE 1.   Various Plus Strand RNA Viruses

Family	Genus	Species	IRES Type
Picornaviridae	Enterovirus	Poliovirus	1
	Rhinovirus		1
	Cardiovirus	EMCV	2
	Hepatovirus	HAV	2
Flaviviridae	Pestivirus	BVDV	3
	Hepacivirus	HCV	3
	Unclassified	GBV-B	3
	Unclassified	GBV-A	4
	Unclassified	GBV-C (HGV)	4
	Flavivirus	YFV	None

HAV, hepatitis A virus; GBV, GB virus; HGV, hepatitis G virus; YFV, yellow fever virus.
From refs. 12 and 13.

Significance of the IRES for HCV Survival and Pathogenesis

Its high degree of sequence conservation indicates that the HCV IRES is essential, and there is no question that this element mediates the initiation of HCV protein synthesis. However, it is not clear what benefit, if any, HCV derives from using an IRES rather than a more conventional structure, such as a cap, to promote initiation. The IRES may be preserved simply because HCV evolved from an IRES-containing virus that lacked capping enzymes and thus is forced to retain a functional IRES to synthesize its proteins. More likely, the HCV IRES has characteristics that confer special benefits, although these characteristics have not yet been defined. Clues can be gleaned from IRES elements of other viruses.

Some IRES-containing viruses, such as poliovirus, achieve a very high rate of production by exploiting differences between IRES-mediated protein synthesis initiation and the conventional cellular pathway. The cap structure present on most cellular mRNAs plays an important role in the conventional pathway. Poliovirus expresses a protein, 2A, that knocks out this pathway by activating a latent cellular proteinase, causing it to cleave a factor, eIF4G, which is required for cap-dependent initiation of protein synthesis.[14,15] Having eliminated competition from capped cellular mRNAs, poliovirus has free access to the cell's protein synthesizing machinery. Poliovirus synthesis proceeds at a brisk pace, producing 400,000 genomes per cell in a matter of hours.[16]

In contrast to poliovirus, HCV has no apparent need to take over the cell's protein synthesizing machinery. In fact, the opposite may be true. On a per-cell basis, the rate of HCV synthesis appears to be very low, at least during chronic infection. As reviewed in the article by Gowans in this issue,[4] calculations of HCV synthesis indicate that each cell needs to produce only 10–100 virions per day to maintain circulating steady state levels. HCV would seem to need a mechanism for *attenuating* viral protein synthesis rather than for maximizing it. A low rate of viral protein synthesis may promote long-term persistence by making it difficult for the immune system to get a fix on the virus.[17] Honda et al.[18] proposed a model in which the IRES downregulates translation. Their model (described below) illustrates how detailed information about IRES structure and function can yield insights into pathogenesis.

Other studies carried out in the Lemon laboratory indicate that the 5'NTRs of different genotypes/strains have distinct translational efficiencies.[19] They compared production of viral capsid and E1 proteins from HCV RNA transcripts that contained almost all of the HCV genome (bases 1–9,454) and no (potentially confounding) foreign reporter protein-coding sequences.

The transcripts included either the 5'NTR of the N2-strain or the H-strain. In both cell-free assays and in transfected cells, RNAs containing the H-strain 5'NTR were translated slightly more efficiently than the N2-strain. Over the years, such small differences could have cumulative clinically significant effects.

Structure and Function of the HCV IRES

A proposed secondary structure of the HCV 5'NTR is shown in Figure 2. It is a modified version of a model originally presented by Brown et al. in 1992[20] and incorporates the results of studies carried out in a number of laboratories (reviewed in reference 12). The current model of the 5'NTR contains four stem-loops and a pseudoknot.[21,22] It is based on phylogenetic analysis of covariant nucleotides in HCV, GBV-B, and pestivirus sequences; physical probing; and mutational studies of IRES function. The nucleotides comprising the stem-loop at the extreme 5'end of the RNA (stem-loop I) are not required for IRES function,[19,23] although they may

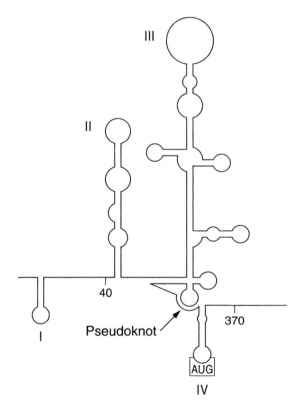

FIG. 2. Structural features of the HCV 5'NTR and IRES.
This model contains several stem-loop elements, a pseudoknot, and an AUG start codon. The stem-loop at the extreme 5'end of the NTR (stem-loop I) is not part of the IRES and may function in replication. The remainder of the model depicts the HCV IRES, which includes nucleotides from about base 40 to base 370. (From refs. 19 and 21 with the kind permission of Dr. Stanley Lemon and the publishers.)

help to regulate this process by reducing the rate of protein synthesis. The heart of the HCV IRES is built out of nucleotides 40–370; however, bases outside this domain may influence IRES function. The AUG start codon is usually at position 342–344.

Remarkably, mutation of the AUG start codon to AUU or CUG only marginally diminishes the efficiency of initiation,[24] revealing that the IRES has a powerful ability to direct the ribosome to the usual initiation site even when the sequence has been altered. This result emphasizes the many differences that exist between the events leading to the placement of the ribosome over the start codon of HCV RNA and those occurring on conventional cellular RNAs. Most cellular mRNAs have a specialized structure at their 5'terminus, an m7G cap. This structure interacts with the cap binding protein complex (eIF4F), initiating a series of reactions that include ribosome binding, ribosome scanning of the mRNA in the 5'to 3'direction, and initiation at the AUG start codon. In contrast, the 40S ribosomal subunit contacts HCV RNA directly at the site of initiation. Any scanning that takes place is restricted to a very limited region of the RNA. One unusual feature of the HCV IRES is its ability to recruit a 40S ribosomal subunit even in the absence of eukaryotic initiation factors and initiator transfer RNA.[25]

18S ribosomal RNA (rRNA) contains a sequence complementary to a 12-base sequence in the IRES of most HCV genotypes. Complementary base pairs may form between these sequence elements. This interaction, if it occurs, is likely to be one of many. Ribosome binding probably involves many contacts—some between accessible sites in rRNA and HCV RNA and others between HCV RNA and ribosomal proteins. Lemon and Honda[12] proposed that the pseudoknot, which is a stable structure located upstream of the AUG initiator codon, helps to position the 40S ribosomal subunit over the initiator codon, acting as a "back-stop." They envision the stem-loop structures upstream of the AUG as a "cradle" for the 40S subunit.[12] Overall, the helical portions of the IRES (the stems of the stem-loop structures) provide a backbone that holds the loop elements in position to bind cellular components such as ribosomal RNA and the anti-codon of the initiator tRNA.

The distal end of the IRES has not yet been fully defined. In 1996, Reynolds et al.[26] reported that the IRES extends into the coding sequence. They found that efficient internal initiation of translation required at least 12–30 nucleotides of the HCV coding sequence. Their observations are supported by studies of other investigators[19,27] but contrast with those of Tsukiyama Kohara et al.[9] and Wang et al.,[28] who demonstrated efficient cap-independent translation of reporter proteins fused directly to the initiator AUG. Zhao et al.[29] used frameshift mutants to show that production of the core peptide is not required for efficient IRES function.

Other studies[18] indicate that the initiator AUG resides in the loop of a stem-loop structure (Fig. 2, stem-loop IV). Engineered mutations that increase the stability of stem-loop IV inhibit translation, evidently by reducing the likelihood that a 40S ribosomal subunit will bind. Collectively, the experiments on this portion of the IRES indicate that the efficiency of HCV protein synthesis is extremely sensitive to sequence and structural changes on either side of the AUG start codon.

Honda et al.[18] speculated that the AUG is housed in a structure with the potential to be switched on and off. It may be switched into the off configuration by interactions with one or more of the proteins expressed during infection, causing protein synthesis to be attenuated. The resulting low level of HCV protein synthesis may make it difficult for the immune system to recognize infected cells.

The actual three-dimensional structure of the 5'NTR is not yet known. However, it is likely to have general features in common with other RNAs. The atomic structures of several small RNAs have been determined by x-ray crystallography and nuclear magnetic resonance spectroscopy. To provide a glimpse of the sort of structure the 5'NTR may have, the crystal structure of a ribozyme (an enzyme composed of RNA) is shown in Figure 3.[30] Knowledge of the atomic structure of the HCV IRES will allow methods of rational drug design to be used to develop pharmaceuticals with an affinity for HCV RNA structural elements (see below).

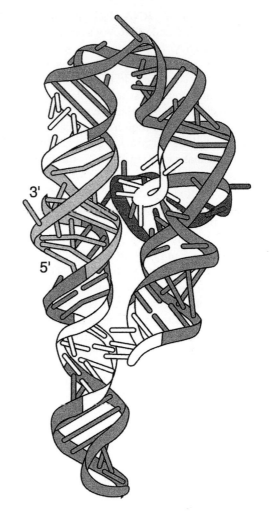

FIG. 3. Crystal structure of a group I ribozyme domain. This structure depicts a 160 nucleotide-long portion of a ribozyme. It illustrates the tendency of RNA molecules fold into compact globular structures rather than to remain as linear chains of nucleotides. (From ref. 30 with permission of Dr. Jennifer Doudna.)

Cellular Proteins that Bind to the IRES

Cellular proteins are likely to help fold the IRES into a functional configuration and may regulate IRES activity. Several proteins bind the HCV IRES. Many of these proteins normally reside primarily in the nucleus but may be present in the cytoplasm in variable amounts or under special circumstances. Ali and Siddiqui[31] reported that La protein, a nucleic acid-dependent ATPase capable of melting RNA helices, enhances IRES activity. The polypyrimidine tract binding protein (PTB, also known as hnRNP I) binds the HCV IRES under some conditions. However, Kaminski et al.[32] found that PTB does not affect IRES activity and concluded that binding is weak. A third nuclear protein, hnRNA L, can be crosslinked to the HCV IRES by exposure to ultraviolet light. Binding of hnRNA L enhances IRES-mediated protein synthesis, possibly through interactions involving PTB. Efficient binding requires the first 33 nucleotides of the ORF and is increased when an additional 28 bases of the ORF are present.[33] Krüger et al.[34,35] recently used a randomized hairpin ribozyme library to seek cellular factors required for HCV IRES-mediated protein synthesis. This approach has the potential to identify a number of additional proteins that mediate HCV IRES function.

Honda et al.[19] searched for downstream sequences influencing IRES-mediated translation by comparing the amount of capsid protein produced from transcripts containing various portions of the ORF. Whether transcripts contained the complete ORF or lacked sequences downstream of nucleotide 1971, no significant differences were found. These experiments provide no indication that the distal portion of the ORF contains RNA signals that affect the rate of initiation of protein synthesis.

Structure and Function of the 3'NTR

A novel structure occurs at the 3' terminus of HCV genomic RNA. Unlike most cellular mRNAs and many viral mRNAs, HCV RNA lacks a polyadenylate [poly(A)] tail. The 3′end of HCV was originally thought to consist of poly(A) or polyuridylate [(poly(U)] tracts but was later found to be a highly conserved 98 nucleotide-long sequence.[2] It is now known that the 3′NTR contains three parts: a variable region that differs extensively between isolates, a poly(U)/polypyrimidine tract (a U/UC-rich region) of variable length, and a 98 nucleotide long terminal sequence. This tail, first described by Tanaka et al. in 1995,[2] is predicted to form three stem-loops.[36,37]

Studies of Ito et al.[38] demonstrated that translation of an IRES-containing transcript was enhanced by the presence of the 3′NTR. The greatest increase was obtained with versions of the 3′NTR that had an intact PTB binding site. Both hnRNP C and PTB interact with the pyrimidine rich region within the 3′NTR.[37,39] Interactions between the 3′and 5′ ends of HCV RNA may create a functional circle. Both RNA–RNA bonds and RNA–protein interactions may help to generate the circular configuration. Oh et al.[40] recently reported that the 3′NTR promotes activity of a recombinant HCV RNA-dependent RNA polymerase. Thus, the 3′NTR is thought to play a role in both HCV translation and replication.

HCV RNA Populations and Strains

Sequence comparisons have provided major insights about HCV. Analysis of HCV RNA from a large number of patients from various geographic locations has revealed several major groups of sequences, called genotypes. Studies of RNAs extracted from individual patients have revealed that the HCV RNAs do not have a single sequence but rather a variety of more or less closely related sequences. This population (swarm) is called a quasispecies,[5,6] and each individual sequence is a "variant." The quasispecies present in a particular individual at a given moment constitutes a specific strain or isolate. Sequence analysis indicates that defective genomes arise during the course of infection and may play a role in persistence and pathogenesis.[6] The clinical significance of genotypes and quasispecies are discussed in the article by Farci and Purcell in this issue.[41]

Clinically significant differences between strains would be missed in many studies of HCV natural history because the standard HCV classification system is based on genotype/subgenotype designations, which are rather broad. Moreover, the designation is typically based on analysis of small portions of the genome, such as the 5′NTR. Current genotyping methods are described by Carithers et al. in the next issue of *Seminars*.[8] In the future, it may be necessary to devise a more fine-grained classification system. Microchip array technology may make detailed global assessments feasible.[42]

Many studies hint that strain-specific viral factors (not distinguishable on the basis of genotype) are important. Two recent studies of liver graft recipients indicate that strain-specific differences can strongly influence HCV pathogenesis. Farci et al.[43] reported that a particular strain of genotype 1a twice induced fulminant hepatitis in a liver graft recipient and caused the most severe hepatitis they had ever observed when inoculated into a chimpanzee. Thus, the extremely severe phenotype of this strain "bred true." Similarly, Vargas et al.[44] found that patients receiving a liver graft from an HCV-infected donor (which presumably carried a mild strain) were more likely to have a favorable outcome if the donor strain prevailed than if the recipient's strain became dominant in the graft.

CHIMERAS, REPLICONS, AND INFECTIOUS CLONED TRANSCRIPTS

HCV replication is inefficient in cell cultures and difficult to study in experimental systems. Fortunately, several aspects of HCV replication and gene expression can be explored through studies of chimeric viruses and replicons. (These replicons are capable of RNA amplification but cannot make mature viruses.) Chimeric viruses are available that contain the HCV IRES and either portions of poliovirus [27,29] or BVDV (a pestivirus).[45] An HCV-poliovirus chimera has been used to test a ribozyme directed against the HCV IRES,[46] illustrating how bioengineered pathogens can be used to develop anti-HCV drugs. Lohmann et al.[47] recently constructed selectable replicons that transduce neomycin resistance and developed HCV-derived RNAs that can be amplified in Huh-7 cells. Genomic sense replicon RNAs reach levels of approximately 1,000–5,000 copies per cell. Antigenomic strands accumulate to 5- to 10-fold lower levels. These replicons do not express HCV structural proteins or NS2, indicting that these proteins are not required for RNA replication. Although the rate of replicon amplification is modest compared with that of many viruses, the replicons will permit important RNA structural elements to be mapped and their drug sensitivities to be tested.

In addition to chimeric viruses and replicons, infectious cloned transcripts provide a third source of novel experimental material for studies of HCV replication. In 1997, Kolykhalov et al.[48] developed plasmids containing full-length copies of HCV RNA. As starting material, they used high titer serum (10^8 HCV RNAs/mL) from a patient in the early phase of infection. Yanagi et al.[49] produced similar transcripts that were also infectious when inoculated into the liver of a chimpanzee. These investigators later demonstrated that the variable region of the 3′NTR is not required for infectivity.[50]

Infectious transcripts allow animals to be inoculated with a nearly pure sequence of HCV RNA. Sequence changes that arise in response to antibodies, inflammatory responses, and other events can then be readily identified. The results obtained thus far shed new light on the connection between HCV persistence and escape variants.[51] Contrary to expectations, one chimpanzee developed persistent infection even though the sequence of the HCV RNA present 60 weeks after inoculation had no changes in hypervariable region 1, a highly variable portion of the E2 protein thought to be a target of neutralizing antibodies. HCV RNA in this chimpanzee and in another inoculated animal developed mutations in other portions of the genome a rate of about 1.5×10^{-3} nucleotide substitutions per site per year. Some of these changes may contribute to persistence.[51] Infectious transcripts facilitate studies of persistence and immune responses and also allow the relationship between HCV strains and pathogenesis to be rigorously examined.

HCV RNA AND IMMUNE RESPONSES

Possible Induction of Interferon by HCV RNA and/or HCV Replication Intermediates

Although the impact of immune responses on HCV RNA evolution is the focus of many studies, the impact of HCV RNA on the state of the immune system has received less attention, although its significance may be as great. Both theoretical considerations and experimental evidence raise the possibility that some form of HCV RNA induces interferon—the human body's first line of immunologic defense against viruses. For example, dsRNA is known to trigger interferon synthesis and viral-specific dsRNA could theoretically be produced in HCV-infected cells because the HCV genome and the antigenome are both composed of RNA. In addition, several lines of evidence indicate that interferon induction occurs during HCV infection. First, HCV-infected Daudi cells produce interferon.[52] Second, livers of HCV-infected chimpanzees contain tubular membrane structures emblematic of interferon exposure.[53] Third, mRNA levels of an interferon response protein, the dsRNA activated protein kinase (PKR), are reported to be elevated in biopsy specimens of patients with chronic HCV;[54] and livers of HCV-infected chimpanzees contain high levels of a second interferon response protein, $2',5'$ oligo(A) synthetase.[55] Because interferon may be induced by HCV RNA, interferon-α treatment is central to the clinical management of chronic infection, and interferon-γ is a Th1 cytokine that may influence the course of disease, knowledge of the interferon system is essential for understanding HCV RNA.

The interferon response is a major form of protection against viruses and thus is of paramount importance to mammalian survival. Transgenic mice deficient in either the type I (α and β) or the type II (γ) interferon receptor rapidly succumb to viral infections. For example, although the median lethal dose of vesicular stomatitis virus is normally in the range of 10^8 plaque forming units, mice lacking the type I interferon receptor die within 3–6 days after receiving 30–50 units.[56] Thus, an intact interferon system raises the lethal dose of this virus 2 million-fold. Cells have an extraordinarily sensitive mechanism for sensing dsRNA and for responding to dsRNA by synthesizing interferons. For example, primary chick embryo cells are capable of responding to a *single molecule* of dsRNA.[57]

Conventional wisdom holds that viral dsRNAs are responsible for interferon induction in most systems. The replication intermediates of RNA viruses, such as HCV, are obvious potential sources of dsRNA. However, the actual trigger of the interferon response can rarely be identified with certainty.[58] For HCV, the situation is particularly cloudy because it is unclear whether the HCV replication complex actually contains dsRNA: dsRNA-enriched fractions are reported to lack detectable levels of antigenomic HCV RNA.[3] Thus, either the antigenomic strands in the replication complex are single stranded throughout most of their length (and thus do not partition into the dsRNA fraction) or they remain affixed to genomic strands and cannot be detected by standard methods. As indicated in Figure 4, viral dsRNA is remarkably resistant to thermal denaturation.[59] Incubation at, or slightly above, 100°C may be required to fully separate the genomic and antigenomic strands. Studies seeking to characterize the HCV replication complex by molecular methods should include dsRNA controls. As an alternative approach, dsRNA-specific antibodies might be used to probe for HCV dsRNA, as has been done for other viruses.[60] Further investigations of HCV dsRNA are needed to define the interplay between HCV and the immune system.

dsRNA-binding Proteins Contribute to the Anti-Viral State in Other Systems and May Interact with HCV RNAs

Several components of the interferon defense system are proteins that bind to dsRNA and certain "highly structured" ssRNAs. It is likely that some form of HCV RNA interacts with one or more of them. These interferon-inducible proteins catalyze reactions that inhibit virus production, and at least one of them, PKR, also alerts the nucleus that a virus has invaded the cell. In response to this PRK-mediated signal, the genes necessary to establish the anti-viral state are transcribed. The three dsRNA-specific enzymes described below—PKR,

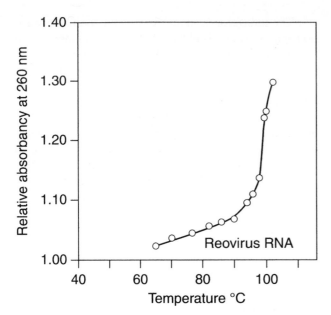

FIG. 4. Thermal denaturation curve of double-stranded viral RNA. Samples of reovirus dsRNA (27 μg/mL) were dissolved in 0.005 M NaCl, 0.001 M phosphate, and 0.0001 M EDTA (pH 7.0); heated for 10 min at temperatures ranging from 64° to 102°C; and absorbancy at 260 nm was measured. The T_m (the temperature at the midpoint of the transition between native RNA and fully denatured RNA) was approximately 99°C. The maximum hyperchromic effect (which occurs when the RNA is maximally disordered) was obtained at 102°C. (From ref. 59.)

2',5'-oligo(A) synthetase, and dsRNA adenosine deaminase—are among the products of the 30 genes induced by interferon.

PKR binds to and is activated by long dsRNA molecules. Binding causes PKR to undergo an autophosphorylation reaction, which activates this kinase. Activated PKR phosphorylates a number of proteins, most notably the translation initiation factor eIF-2. Phosphorylation of eIF-2 blocks its normal functioning and inhibits protein synthesis, thereby diminishing virus production. By phosphorylating certain other proteins, PKR initiates a series of reactions that culminates in the production of interferon and other antiviral proteins. As might be expected given their characteristic adaptability, viruses have developed strategies for protecting themselves against PKR and other components of the interferon response system. For example, an RNA of adenovirus, VAI RNA, causes interferon resistance by binding, but *not* activating, PKR. Adenovirus VAI RNA allows viral synthesis and viral dsRNA production to proceed. It is unlikely that HCV RNA interferes with PKR in a similar manner because VAI RNA is highly abundant and all forms of HCV RNA are relatively scarce. However, it is quite possible that HCV RNA binds to PKR or to another dsRNA binding protein and that this interaction has an effect. Adenovirus VAI RNA demonstrates that

"highly structured" but essentially ssRNA domains (such as the terminal regions of HCV RNA) can have biologically significant interactions with dsRNA binding proteins.

For completeness, it is worth noting that certain viruses produce proteins (rather than RNAs) that block the interferon response. Accordingly, interactions between PKR and the HCV protein NS5a have been explored as a possible cause of interferon resistance.[61,62] However, it is not clear whether HCV-infected cells contain enough NS5a to significantly inhibit PKR, which is a very abundant protein. Human Daudi cells contain about 600,000 molecules. Interferon treatment raises this level three- to fourfold. Interferon-treated cells contain approximately one molecule of PKR per ribosome.[63] Interactions between NS5a and cellular proteins are discussed further by De Francesco et al. in this issue.[64]

The 2',5'-oligo(A) synthetases comprise a group of enzymes that are part of antiviral defenses. The 2',5'-oligo(A) synthetases can be activated by both dsRNA and by highly structured portions of certain ssRNAs. Once activated, the 2',5'-oligo(A) synthetases polymerize ATP into 2',5'-oligo(A), a substance that activates RNase L, a normally latent endonuclease. RNase L degrades ssRNA. Viral RNAs appear to be preferred targets of RNase L. In encephalomyocarditis virus (EMCV)-infected HeLa cells, the 2',5'-oligo(A) synthetases coprecipitating with viral RNAs were only partially activated, suggesting that these enzymes were associated with single-stranded viral RNA rather than dsRNA.[65] Because both adenovirus VAI RNA[66] and heterogeneous nuclear RNA[67] activate 2',5'-oligo(A) synthetases in vitro, extensive regions of perfect duplex structure are clearly not required for activation. If single-stranded EMCV RNAs have structural elements capable of partially activating the synthetases, it is possible that single-stranded HCV RNAs have similar elements, perhaps in the IRES or the 3'NTR. Thus, HCV genomic and antigenomic RNAs, as well as HCV-specific dsRNA, may have the potential to interact with this component of the interferon response system.

The dsRNA adenosine deaminase, dsRAD, is a third enzyme that binds to dsRNA and selected regions of ssRNAs. Like PKR and the 2',5'-oligo(A) synthetases, dsRAD binds to adenovirus VAI RNA in vitro.[68] Deamination by dsRAD reduces the stability of dsRNA because the transformation of adenosine into inosine diminishes Watson-Crick base pairing. In conjunction with a ribonuclease specific for inosine-containing RNA,[69] dsRAD may contribute to the antiviral state. However, its role in anti-viral defense is not as clearly established as that of PKR and the 2',5'-oligo(A) synthetases. dsRAD edits the ssRNA of the delta agent [a.k.a., hepatitis D virus (HDV)] and has been implicated in the production of hypermutated measles virus RNAs during chronic infection. Similar action on HCV dsRNA could introduce mutations, adding to HCV sequence variability and persistence.

PKR and RNase L have been considered to be the principal proteins through which interferons establish the antiviral state. However, interferon retains its ability to confer viral protection in transgenic mice lacking both of these enzymes, although its effects are diminished.[70] This finding indicates profound gaps in knowledge of the innate immune system. As these gaps are filled, the relationship between HCV RNA and interferon-inducible proteins and other components of the innate immune system will become more amenable to study. Given the many interferon-inducible proteins with the potential to bind to HCV RNA, it may seem paradoxical that HCV frequently establishes chronic infection. This paradox points out the need to explore the mechanism that HCV uses to thwart the innate antiviral defenses of the liver.[71] Adaptations that allow HCV to monitor and neutralize innate immune responses may turn out to be as important as those that allow it to escape adaptive immune responses, such as antibodies and cytotoxic T lymphocytes. Adaptive immune responses are discussed by Rehermann in the next issue of *Seminars*.[72]

HCV RNA AS A TARGET FOR PHARMACEUTICALS

A variety of pharmaceuticals directed against HCV RNA are under development. The new drugs that have received the greatest attention thus far are antisense molecules and ribozymes (enzymes composed of RNA). Rapid progress has been made in the investigation of antisense DNA complementary to HCV[73-83] and therapeutic ribozymes for HCV.[46,84-88] Recently, a ribozyme directed against sequences in the HCV IRES was shown to dramatically reduce replication of a chimeric virus containing the HCV IRES and most of the poliovirus genome.[46] This ribozyme has many chemical modifications and is relatively stable compared with ribozymes composed of standard ribonucleotides. Clinical trials are planned for the near future.

Antisense DNAs and chemically modified ribozymes must be delivered as exogenous compounds and then imported into target cells. Alternative interventions use gene therapy vectors to provide a continuous source of unmodified ribozymes and antisense RNAs. Stable expression of therapeutic RNAs from such vectors could create a population of HCV-resistant cells.

Antisense DNAs and ribozymes are designed to bind to HCV RNA through Watson-Crick base pairs and to inhibit the RNA either by sequestering it or by causing it to be degraded. Although antisense drugs and ribozymes hold out the exciting promise of rational drug design, the development of these pharmaceuticals for use against hepatitis viruses has proven to be more challenging than originally anticipated.[89] Antisense molecules often bind to and affect many biologic molecules in addition to their intended target RNAs, giving rise to *nonantisense* effects.[89-94] In 1994, Iizuka et al.[95] performed a well-controlled experiment that demonstrates how potent nonantisense effects can be. They first infected ducks with duck hepatitis B virus (DHBV) and then injected groups of birds either with antisense DNA, control DNA, or saline. At the end of the study, the DHBV DNA in the ducks injected with control DNA was only 0.1% of that in the group injected with saline. A nonantisense effect caused a three-log decline in DHBV DNA. The intensity of nonantisense effects makes it very difficult to obtain pure antisense effects. Furthermore, unless rigorous control studies are carried out, nonantisense effects can easily be mistaken for antisense effects.

One year after the studies of DHBV were published, Krieg et al.[96] discovered that B lymphocytes are activated by DNAs containing a centrally located CG sequence. This activation is thought to occur because the CG sequence element is common in microbial DNA and stimulates the immune system. Immune stimulation may have led to the decline of DHBV DNA that occurred in the ducks treated with control DNA.[95] Valuable guidelines for antisense studies have been published and can also be applied to ribozyme studies.[97]

In addition to antisense drugs for HCV, there is also interest in developing smaller compounds that recognize HCV RNA *structures* (rather than *sequences*). These pharmaceuticals fall into two categories: drugs interacting with three-dimensional structures in HCV (genomic) RNA and drugs binding to the dsRNA helix of the HCV replication complex. The aminoglycoside antibiotics are prototypes of drugs that recognize intricate three-dimensional RNA structural elements. Aminoglycosides bind to elements present in 16S rRNA of bacteria[98,99] and prove that pharmaceuticals that recognize RNA structures can be effective.

FUTURE DIRECTIONS

The availability of HCV RNA-derived replicons and chimeric viruses opens the door to the development of anti-HCV RNA drugs analogous to the aminoglycoside antibiotics. Atomic structural maps of HCV RNA elements will also advance this area of pharmaceutical development and can be expected during the next 5 years. Pharmaceuticals directed against HCV RNAs may act synergistically with existing drugs and with future drugs directed against proteins, such as viral enzymes or cellular factors required for HCV replication and gene expression. Unfortunately, the ability of HCV to bounce back after interferon/ribavirin treatment emphasizes its resilience. HCV will be difficult to eradicate even with long-acting immune modulators and a cocktail of drugs. Thus, HCV vaccine research should be given a high priority—the most effective medical interventions for HCV could turn out to be *derived* from HCV RNA, not directed against it. However, implementation of an HCV vaccine could be problematic in countries with low rates of new infections. Safety requirements will be extraordinarily high for an HCV vaccine if it is to be recommended for administration to the general public. If it is to be aimed at high-risk populations, such as potential drug users, questions will arise about how recipients will be identified. Thus, even as new drugs are sought and vaccines are developed, great efforts should be made to reduce HCV transmission through behavior modification.

Acknowledgments: I thank Dr. Nora Bergasa (Columbia University College of Medicine) for insights; Dr. Robert Carithers (University of Washington) for valuable feedback; Ms. Toby Keller for assistance; Dr. Jose Walewski for helpful comments; and NIDDK grant P01DK50759, project 2, NIDDK grant R01DK52071, the Liver Transplantation Research Fund, and the Artzt Foundation for support.

ABBREVIATIONS

BVDV	bovine viral diarrhea virus
DHBV	duck hepatitis B virus
dsRAD	dsRNA adenosine deaminase
dsRNA	double-stranded RNA
EMCV	encephalomyocarditis virus
HCV	hepatitis C virus
IRES	internal ribosome entry site
mRNA	messenger RNA
NTR	nontranslated region
ORF	open reading frame
PKR	dsRNA activated protein kinase
PTB	polypyrimidine tract-binding protein
rRNA	ribosomal RNA
ssRNA	single-stranded RNA

REFERENCES

1. Choo QL, Kuo G, Weiner AJ, Overby LR, Bradley DW, Houghton M. Isolation of a cDNA clone derived from a blood-borne non-A, non-B viral hepatitis genome. Science 1989;244:359–362

2. Tanaka T, Kato N, Cho MJ, Shimotohno K. A novel sequence found at the 3′terminus of hepatitis C virus genome. Biochem Biophys Res Commun 1995;215:744–749

3. Blight K, Trowbridge R, Gowans EJ. Absence of double-stranded replicative forms of HCV RNA in liver tissue from chronically infected patients. J Viral Hepatitis 1996;3:29–36

4. Gowans EJ. The distribution of markers of hepatitis C virus infection throughout the body. Sem Liver Dis 2000;20:85–102

5. Martell M, Esteban JI, Quer J, et al. Hepatitis C virus (HCV) circulates as a population of different but closely related genomes: quasispecies nature of HCV genome distribution. J Virol 1992;66:3225–3229

6. Higashi Y, Kakumu S, Yoshioka K, et al. Dynamics of genome change in the E2/NS1 region of hepatitis C virus in vivo. Virology 1993;197:659–668

7. Trowbridge R, Gowans EJ. Identification of novel sequences at the 5′terminus of the hepatitis C virus genome. J Viral Hepatitis 1998;5:95–98

8. Carithers RL, Marquardt A, Gretch DR. Diagnostic testing for hepatitis C. Sem Liver Dis 2000;20 (in press)

9. Tsukiyama Kohara K, Iizuka N, Kohara M, Nomoto A. Internal ribosome entry site within hepatitis C virus RNA. J Virol 1992;66:1476–1483

10. Jang SK, Krausslich HG, Nicklin MJH, Duke GM, Palmenberg AC, Wimmer E. A segment of the 5′nontranslated region of encephalomyocarditis virus RNA directs internal entry ribosomes during in vitro translation. J Virol 1988;62:2636–2643

11. Pelletier J, Sonenberg N. Internal initiation of translation of eukaryotic mRNA directed by a sequence derived from poliovirus RNA. Nature 1988;334:320–325

12. Lemon SM, Honda M. Internal ribosome entry sites within the RNA genomes of hepatitis C virus and other flaviviruses. Semin Virol 1997;8:274–288

13. Wimmer E, Hellen CUT, Cao X. Genetics of poliovirus. Annu Rev Genet 1993;27:353–436

14. Etchison D, Milburn SC, Edery I, Sonenberg N, Hershey JWB. Inhibition of HeLa cell protein synthesis following poliovirus infection correlates with the proteolysis of a 220,000-dalton polypeptide associated with eucaryotic initiation factor 3 and a cap binding protein complex. J Biol Chem 1982;257:14806–14810

15. Etchison D, Hansen J, Ehrenfeld E, et al. Demonstration in vitro that eucaryotic initiation factor 3 is active but that a cap-binding protein complex is inactive in poliovirus infected HeLa cells. J Virol 1984;51:832–837

16. Fields BN, Knipe DN. Fundamental Virology. New York: Raven Press,1991, pp.5–1021

17. Branch AD. Replication of hepatitis C virus: Catching it in the act. Hepatology 1996;23:372–375

18. Honda M, Brown EA, Lemon SM. Stability of a stem-loop involving the initiator AUG controls the efficiency of internal initiation of translation on hepatitis C virus RNA. RNA 1996;2:955–968

19. Honda M, Ping LH, Rijnbrand RCA, et al. Structural requirements for initiation of translation by internal ribosome entry within genome length hepatitis C virus RNA. Virology 1996;222:31–42

20. Brown EA, Zhang H, Ping LH, Lemon SM. Secondary structure of the 5′nontranslated regions of hepatitis C virus and pestivirus genomic RNAs. Nucleic Acids Res 1992;20:5041–5045

21. Honda M, Beard MR, Ping LH, Lemon SM. A phylogenetically conserved stem-loop structure at the 5′border of the internal ribosome entry site of hepatitis C virus is required for cap-independent viral translation. J Virol 1999;73:1165–1174

22. Wang C, Le SY, Ali N, Siddiqui A. A pseudoknot is an essential structural element of the internal ribosome entry site located within the hepatitis C virus 5′noncoding region. RNA 1995;1:526–537

23. Rijnbrand R, Bredenbeek P, van der Straaten T, et al. Almost the entire 5′non-translated region of hepatitis C virus is required for cap-independent translation. FEBS Lett 1995;365:115–119

24. Reynolds JE, Kaminski A, Kettinen HJ, et al. Unique features of internal initiation of hepatitis C virus RNA translation. EMBO J 1995;14:6010–6020

25. Pestova TV, Shatsky IN, Fletcher SP, Jackson RJ, Hellen CUT. A prokaryotic-like mode of cytoplasmic eukaryotic ribosome bind-

ing to the initiation codon during internal translation initiation of hepatitis C and classical swine fever virus RNAs. Genes Dev 1998;12:67–83

26. Reynolds JE, Kaminski A, Carroll AR, Clarke BE, Rowlands DJ, Jackson RJ. Internal initiation of translation of hepatitis C virus RNA: The ribosome entry site is at the authentic initiation codon. RNA 1996;2:867–878

27. Lu HH, Wimmer E. Poliovirus chimeras replicating under the translational control of genetic elements of hepatitis C virus reveal unusual properties of the internal ribosomal entry site of hepatitis C virus. Proc Natl Acad Sci USA 1996;93:1412–1417

28. Wang C, Sarnow P, Siddiqui A. Translation of human hepatitis C virus RNA in cultured cells is mediated by an internal ribosome-binding mechanism. J Virol 1993;67:3338–3344

29. Zhao WD, Wimmer E, Lahser FC. Poliovirus/hepatitis C virus (internal ribosomal entry site-core) chimeric viruses: Improved growth properties through modification of a proteolytic cleavage site and requirement for core RNA sequences but not for core-related polypeptides. J Virol 1999;73:1546–1554

30. Cate JH, Gooding AR, Podell E, et al. Crystal structure of a group I ribozyme domain: principles of RNA packing. Science 1996;273:1678–1685

31. Ali N, Siddiqui A. The La antigen binds 5′noncoding region of the hepatitis C virus RNA in context of the initiator AUG codon and stimulates internal ribosome entry site-mediated translation. Proc Natl Acad Sci USA 1997;94:2249–2254

32. Kaminski A, Hunt SL, Patton JG, Jackson RJ. Direct evidence that polypyrimidine tract binding protein (PTB) is essential for internal initiation of translation of encephalomyocarditis virus RNA. RNA 1995;1:924–938

33. Hahm B, Kim YK, Kim JH, Kim TY, Jang SK. Hetergenous nuclear ribonucleoprotein L interacts with the 3′border of the internal ribosomal entry site of hepatitis C virus. J Virol 1998;72:8782–8788

34. Krüger M, Berger C, Welch PJ, Barber J, Wong-Staal F. Identification of cellular regulators of hepatitis C virus internal ribosome entry site (HCV-IRES)-mediated translation using a randomized hairpin ribozyme library. Hepatology 1999;30:355A

35. Krüger M, Beger C, Wong-Staal F. Use of ribozymes to inhibit gene expression. Methods Enzymol 1999;306:207–225

36. Blight KJ, Rice CM. Secondary structure determination of the conserved 98-base sequence at the 3′terminus of hepatitis C virus genome RNA. J Virol 1997;71:7345–7352

37. Ito T, Lai MMC. Determination of the secondary structure of and cellular protein binding to the 3′-untranslated region of the hepatitis C virus. J Virol 1997;71:8698–8706

38. Ito T, Tahara SM, Lai MMC. The 3′-untranslated region of hepatitis C virus RNA enhances translation from an internal ribosomal entry site. J Virol 1998;72:8789–8796

39. Gontarek RR, Gutshall LL, Herold KM, et al. hnRNP C and polypyrimidine tract-binding protein specifically interact with the pyrimidine-rich region within the 3′NTR of the HCV RNA genome. Nucleic Acids Res 1999;27:1457–1463

40. Oh JW, Ito T, Lai MMC. A recombinant hepatitis C virus RNA-dependent RNA polymerase capable of copying the full-length viral RNA. J Virol 1999;73:7694–7702

41. Farci P, Purcell RH. Clinical significance of hepatitis C genotypes and quasispecies. Semin Liver Dis 2000;20:103–126

42. Service RF. Microchip arrays put DNA on the spot. Science 1998;282:396–399

43. Farci P, Munoz SJ, Shimoda A, et al. Experimental transmission of hepatitis C virus-associated fulminant hepatitis to a chimpanzee. J Infect Dis 1999;179:1007–1011

44. Vargas HE, Laskus T, Wang LF, et al. Outcome of liver transplantation in hepatitis C virus-infected patients who received hepatitis C virus-infected grafts. Gastroenterology 1999;117:149–153

45. Frolov I, McBride S, Rice CM. cis-Acting RNA elements required for replication of bovine viral diarrhea virus-hepatitis C virus 5′nontranslated region chimeras. RNA 1998;4:1418–1435

46. Macejak DJ, Jensen KL, Bellon L, Pavco PA, Blatt LM. Inhibition of viral replication by nuclease resistant hammerhead ribozyme directed against hepatitis C virus RNA. Hepatology 1999;30:409A

47. Lohmann V, Korner F, Koch JO, Herian U, Theilmann L, Bartenschlager R. Replication of subgenomic hepatitis C virus RNAs in a hepatoma cell line. Science 1999;285:110–113

48. Kolykhalov AA, Agapov EV, Blight KJ, Mihalik K, Feinstone SM, Rice CM. Transmission of hepatitis C by intrahepatic inoculation with transcribed RNA. Science 1997;277:570–574

49. Yanagi M, Purcell RH, Emerson SU, Bukh J. Transcripts from a single full-length cDNA clone of hepatitis C virus are infectious when directly transfected into the liver of a chimpanzee. Proc Natl Acad Sci USA 1997;94:8738–8743

50. Yanagi M, St. Claire M, Emerson SU, Purcell RH, Buhk J. In vivo analysis of the 3′untranslated region of the haptitis C virus after in vitro mutagenesis of an infectious cDNA clone. Proc Natl Acad Sci USA 1999;96:2291–2295

51. Major ME, Mihalik K, Fernandez J, et al. Long-term follow-up of chimpanzees inoculated with the first infectious clone for hepatitis C virus. J Virol 1999;73:3317–3325

52. Shimizu YK Feinstone SM, Kohara M, Purcell RH, Yoshikura H. Hepatitis C virus: Detection by electron microscopy of intracellular virus particles. Hepatology 1996;23:205–209

53. Kamimura T, Bonino F, Ponzetto A, Feinstone SM, Gerin J, Purcell RH. Cytoplasmic tubular structures in liver of HBsAg carrier chimpanzees infected with delta agent and comparison with cytoplasmic structures in non-A, non-B hepatitis. Hepatology 1983;3:631–637

54. Yu SH, Enomoto N, Nagayama K, Kurosaki M, Sato C. Overexpression of dsRNA-activated protein kinase (PKR) in the liver with chronic hepatitis C. Hepatology 1999;30:359A

55. Thimme RL, Guidotti G, Bukh J, Koch R, Pemberton J, Purcell RH, Chisari FV. Different intrahepatic cytokine profiles during acute HBV and HCV infection in the same chimpanzees. Hepatology 1999;30:411A

56. Muller U, Steinhoff U, Reis LF, et al. Functional role of type I and type II interferons in antiviral defense. Science 1994;264:1918–1921

57. Marcus PI, Sekellick MJ. Defective interfering particles with covalently linked [±/−]RNA induce interferon. Nature 1977;266:815–819

58. Jacobs BL, Langland JO. When two strands are better than one: the mediators and modulators of the cellular responses to double-stranded RNA. Virology 1996;219:339–349

59. Gomatos PJ, Tamm I. The secondary structure of reovirus RNA. Proc Natl Acad Sci USA 1963;49:707–714

60. Magliano D, Marshall JA, Bowden DS, Vardaxis N, Meanger J, Lee JY. Rubella virus replication complexes are virus-modified lysosomes. Virology 1998;240:57–63

61. Enomoto N, Sakuma I, Asahina Y, et al. Mutations in the nonstructural protein 5A gene and response to interferon in patients with chronic hepatitis C virus 1B infection. N Engl J Med 1996;334:77–81

62. Gale M, Blakely CM, Kwieciszewski B, et al. Control of PKR protein kinase by hepatitis C virus nonstructural 5A protein: molecular mechanisms of kinase regulation. Mol Cell Biol 1998;18:5208–5218

63. Jeffrey IW, Kadereit S, Meurs EF, et al. Nuclear localization of the interferon-inducible protein kinase PKR in human cells and transfected mouse cells. Exp Cell Res 1995;218:17–27

64. De Francesco R, Neddermann P, Tomei L, Steinkühler C, Gallinari P, Folgori A. Biochemical and immunological properties of

the nonstructural proteins of the hepatitis C virus: implications for development of antiviral agents and vaccines. Semin Liver Dis 2000;20:69–84

65. Gribaudo G, Lembo D, Cavallo G, Landolfo S, Lengyel P. Interferon action: binding of viral RNA to the 40-kilodalton 2'-5'-oligoadenylate synthetase in interferon-treated HeLa cells infected with encephalomyocarditis virus. J Virol 1991;65:1748–1757

66. Desai SY, Patel RC, Sen GC, Malhotra P, Ghadge GD, Thimmapaya B. Activation of interferon-inducible 2'-5'oligoadenylate synthetase by adenoviral VAI RNA. J Biol Chem 1995;270:3454–3461

67. Nilsen TW, Maroney PA, Robertson HD, Baglioni C. Heterogeneous nuclear RNA promotes synthesis of (2',5')oligoadenylate and is cleaved by the (2',5')oligoadenylate-activated endoribonuclease. Mol Cell Biol 1982;2:154–160

68. Lei M, Liu Y, Samuel CE. Adenovirus VAI RNA antagonizes the RNA-editing activity of the ADAR adenosine deaminase. Virology 1998;245:188–196

69. Scadden AD, Smith CW. A ribonuclease specific for inosine-containing RNA: A potential role in antiviral defence? EMBO J 1997;16:2140–2149

70. Zhou A, Paranjape JM, Der SD, Williams BR, Silverman RH. Interferon action in triply deficient mice reveals the existence of alternative antiviral pathways. Virology 1999;258:435–440

71. O'Farrelly C, Crispe IN. Prometheus through the looking glass: Reflections on the hepatic immune system. Immunol Today 1999;20:394–398

72. Rehermann B. Interaction between HCV and the immune system. Semin Liver Dis 2000;20:137

73. Wakita T, Wands JR. Specific inhibition of hepatitis C virus expression by antisense oligodeoxynucleotides. In vitro model for selection of target sequence. J Biol Chem 1994;269:14205–14210

74. Mizutani T, Kato N, Hirota M, Sugiyama K, Murakami A, Shimotohno K. Inhibition of hepatitis C virus replication by antisense oligonucleotide in culture cells. Biochem Biophys Res Commun 1995;212:906–911

75. Alt M, Renz R, Hofschneider PH, Paumgartner G, Caselmann WH. Specific inhibition of hepatitis C viral gene expression by antisense phosphorothioate oligodeoxynucleotides. Hepatology 1995;22:707–717

76. Hanecak R, Brown Driver V, Fox MC, et al. Antisense oligonucleotide inhibition of hepatitis C virus gene expression in transformed hepatocytes. J Virol 1996;70:5203–5212

77. Mizutani T, Kato N, Saito S, Ikeda M, Sugiyama K, Shimotohno K. Characterization of hepatitis C virus replication in cloned cells obtained from a human T-cell leukcmia virus Type 1-infected cell line. J Virol 1996;70:7219–7223

78. Eisenhardt S, Samstag W, Jahn-Homann K, et al. Comparison of the inhibitory effect of different chemically modified *antisense* oligodeoxynucleotides on hepatitis C viral gene expression. Hepatology 1996;24:396A

79. Lima WF, Brown Driver V, Fox M, Hanecak R, Bruice TW. Combinatorial screening and rational optimization for hybridization to folded hepatitis C virus RNA of oligonucleotides with biological antisense activity. J Biol Chem 1997;272:626–638

80. Alt M, Renz R, Hofschneider PH, Caselmann WH. Core specific antisense phosphorothioate oligodeoxynucleotides as potent and specific inhibitors of hepatitis C viral translation. Arch Virol 1997;142:589–599

81. Wu CH, GY Wu. Targeted inhibition of hepatitis C virus-directed gene expression in human hepatoma cell lines. Gastroenterology 1998;114:1304–1312

82. Zhang H, Hanecak R, Brown-Driver V, et al. Antisense oligonucleotide inhibition of hepatitis C virus (HCV) gene expression in livers of mice infected with and HCV-vaccinia virus recombinant. Antimicrob Agents Chemother 1999;43:347–353

83. Brown-Driver V, Eto T, Lesnik E, Anderson KP, Hanecak RC. Inhibition of translation of hepatitis C virus RNA by 2'-modified antisense oligonucleotides. Antisense Nucleic Acid Drug Dev 1999;9:145–154

84. Lieber A, He CY, Polyak SJ, Gretch DR, Barr D, Kay MA. Elimination of hepatitis C virus RNA in infected human hepatocytes by adenovirus-mediated expression of ribozymes. J Virol 1996;70:8782–8791

85. Sakamoto N, Wu CH, Wu, GY. Intracellular inhibition of HCV protein synthesis by hammerhead ribozyme expression vectors. Hepatology 1996;24:357A

86. Ohkawa K, Yuki N, Kanazawa K, et al. Comparison of three different hammerhead ribozymes for cleavage efficiency of hepatitis C virus RNA in vitro. Hepatology 1996;24:396A

87. Alt M, Schussler S, Steigerwald R, Hofschneider PH, Caselmann WH. Hepatitis C virus-specific *hammerhead* ribozymes cleave target RNA efficiently and inhibit viral gene expression. J Hepatol 1996;25(Suppl 1):73

88. Sakamoto N, Wu CH, Wu GY. Intracellular cleavage of hepatitis C virus RNA and inhibition of viral protein translation by hammerhead ribozymes. J Clin Invest 1996;98:2720–2728

89. Branch AD. Instructive surprises from antisense treatments for viral hepatitis and other diseases. Proc VIII Intl Symp Viral Hepatitis 1998;(Suppl 1):33–39

90. Gura T. Anti sense has growing pains. Science 1995;270:575–577

91. Stein CA. Phosphorothioate antisense oligodeoxynucleotides: Questions of specificity. TIBTECH 1996;14:147–149

92. Crooke ST, Bennett CF. Progress in antisense oligonucleotide therapeutics. Annu Rev Pharmacol Toxicol 1996;36:107–129

93. Branch AD. A hitchhiker's guide to antisense and nonantisense biochemical pathways. Hepatology 1996;24:1517–1529

94. Branch AD. A good antisense molecule is hard to find. Trends Biochem Sci 1998;23:45–50

95. Iizuka A, Watanabe T, Kubo T, et al. M13 bacteriophage DNA inhibits duck hepatitis B virus during acute infection. Hepatology 1994;19:1079–1087

96. Krieg AM, Yi AK, Matson S, et al. CpG motifs in bacterial DNA trigger direct B-cell activation. Nature 1995;374:546–549

97. Stein CA, Krieg AM. Problems in interpretation of data derived from in vitro and in vivo use of antisense oligodeoxynucleotides. Antisense Res Dev 1994;4:67–69

98. Moazed D, Noller HF. Interaction of antibiotics with functional sites in 16S ribosomal RNA. Nature 1987;327:389–394

99. Gravel M, Melancon P, Brakier Gingras L. Cross-linking of streptomycin to the 16S ribosomal RNA of *Escherichia coli*. Biochemistry 1987;26:6227–6232

SEMINARS IN LIVER DISEASE—VOL. 20, NO. 1, 2000

Biochemical and Immunologic Properties of the Nonstructural Proteins of the Hepatitis C Virus: Implications for Development of Antiviral Agents and Vaccines

RAFFAELE DE FRANCESCO, Ph.D., PETRA NEDDERMANN, Ph.D., LICIA TOMEI, Ph.D., CHRISTIAN STEINKüHLER, PAOLA GALLINARI, Ph.D., and ANTONELLA FOLGORI, Ph.D.

ABSTRACT: *Infection with the hepatitis C virus (HCV) is the major cause of non-A, non-B hepatitis worldwide. The viral genome, a positive-sense, single-stranded, 9.6-kb long RNA molecule, is translated into a single polyprotein of about 3,000 amino acids. The viral polyprotein is proteoytically processed to yield all the mature viral gene products. The genomic order of HCV has been determined to be C → E1 → E2 → p7 → NS2 → NS3 → NS4A → NS4B → NS5A → NS5B. C, E1, and E2 are the virion structural proteins. Whereas the function of p7 is currently unknown, NS2 to NS5B are thought to be the nonstructural proteins. Generation of the mature nonstructural proteins relies on the activity of viral proteinases. Cleavage at the NS2–NS3 junction is accomplished by a metal-dependent autocatalytic proteinase encoded within NS2 and the N-terminus of NS3. The remaining downstream cleavages are effected by a serine proteinase contained also within the N-terminal region of NS3. NS3, in addition, contains an RNA helicase domain at its C-terminus. NS3 forms a heterodimeric complex with NS4A. The latter is a membrane protein that acts as a cofactor of the proteinase. Although no function has yet been attributed to NS4B, NS5A has been recently suggested to be involved in mediating the resistance of the HCV to the action of interferon. Finally, the NS5B protein has been shown to be the viral RNA-dependent RNA polymerase. This article reviews the current understanding of the structure and the function of the various HCV nonstructural proteins with particular emphasis on their potential as targets for the development of novel antiviral agents and vaccines.*

KEY WORDS: hepatitis, virus, replication

Infection with the hepatitis C virus (HCV) is the major cause of non-A, non-B hepatitis worldwide. As of today there is no effective therapy to cure chronic hepa-titis caused by persistent infection with HCV. Similarly, a vaccine to prevent infection by this virus has yet to be discovered. There is thus an obvious need to develop ef-

Objectives

Upon completion of this article, the reader should be able to 1) summarize the role of the HCV nonstructural proteins with respect to viral replication and host immune response and 2) understand the implication of HCV nonstructural proteins as targets for the development of antiviral agents and vaccines.

Accreditation

The Indiana University School of Medicine is accredited by the Accreditation Council for Continuing Medical Education to sponsor continuing medical education for physicians. The Indiana University School of Medicine takes responsibility for the contents, quality, and scientific integrity of this activity.

Credit

The Indiana University School of Medicine designates this educational activity for a maximum of 1.0 hours credit toward the AMA Physicians Recognition Award in category one. Each physician should claim only those hours of credit that he/she actually spent in the educational activity.

Disclosure

Statements have been obtained regarding the authors' relationships with financial supporters of this activity. There is no apparent conflict of interest related to the context of participation of the author of this article.

From the Istituto di Ricerche di Biologia Molecolare, "P. Angeletti," Pomezia, Rome, Italy.

Reprint requests: Dr. Raffaele De Francesco, Istituto di Ricerche di Biologia, Molecolare, "P. Angeletti," Pomezia, Rome, Italy.

fective therapeutic strategies to cure HCV-associated hepatitis, and it is likely that improvements in the clinical treatment of this disease will only be possible if we acquire detailed knowledge of the HCV biology. This review summarizes the current understanding of the biochemical and immunologic properties of the various viral nonstructural proteins.

HCV POLYPROTEIN PROCESSING

The HCV genome is a positive-sense, single-stranded, 9.6-kb-long RNA molecule. The viral genome contains a single open reading frame encoding a polyprotein of about 3,000 amino acids. The HCV polyprotein undergoes co- and posttranslational proteolytic processing in the cytoplasm or in the endoplasmic reticulum (ER) of the infected cell to give rise to at least 10 mature proteins.[1] Three different proteolytic activities that are involved in this process have been identified so far. The polypeptides liberated from the amino terminus of the polyprotein are the structural proteins and include the nucleocapsid C protein (p19/21); two envelope glycoproteins, E1 (gp31–35) and E2 (gp70); and p7, a 7-kDa protein generated by limited processing of an E2–p7 precursor. These polypeptides arise from cleavages catalyzed by cellular signal peptidases associated with the lumen of the ER.[1] The region of the polyprotein downstream of E2–p7 harbors the nonstructural proteins and is processed by two HCV-encoded proteolytic enzymes (Fig. 1). The NS2–NS3 junction is cleaved by a zinc-dependent proteinase associated with NS2 (p23) and the N-terminus of NS3. The C-terminal remainder of the HCV polyprotein is further processed to give rise to mature NS3 (p70), NS4A (p8), NS4B (p27), NS5A (p56/p58), and NS5B (p68) proteins by a virus-encoded serine proteinase contained within the NS3 protein.[2–6] The latter enzyme functions as a heterodimeric proteinase, requiring the noncovalent association with the viral protein NS4A for optimal catalytic activity.[7]

A distinct temporal hierarchy of cleavage events was observed that is initiated by an intramolecular cut between NS3 and NS4A, giving rise to the activated heterodimeric NS3/4A proteinase. This enzyme in turn processes the NS5A–5B site first, giving rise to the mature viral polymerase, NS5B, followed by cleavage between NS4A and NS4B, and finally by processing of the NS4B–NS5A junction. The role of the temporal order of processing events is not understood, but in analogy to what is known from other RNA viruses, one can speculate that it may be an important requirement to ensure the successful replicative cycle of HCV. Hence, tampering with the processing kinetics, or even abolishing certain cleavage events, is likely to severely impair viral replication. In line with this hypothesis, it has been re-

cently shown that knocking out either of the two viral proteinases by introducing appropriate mutations in cDNAs encoding the HCV genome abolishes their infectivity in chimpanzees.[8]

THE NS2/3 PROTEINASE

The mature N-terminus of NS3 is generated by the intramolecular cleavage performed by a viral proteinase encoded within the NS2 and NS3 regions of the HCV polyprotein. Mutagenesis experiments showed that the NS3 serine proteinase domain, but not its catalytic activity, were required for processing at this junction.[9,10] A deletion mutagenesis analysis made to map the minimum domain required for efficient processing at the NS2–NS3 site indicated an N-terminal boundary between residues 898 and 923 within NS2, whereas a sharp drop in cleavage efficiency was observed upon C-terminal truncations beyond residue 1,207 within NS3.[9–12] Radiosequencing of the mature cleavage products showed that processing at the NS2–NS3 junction occurs between Leu1026 and Ala1027, within the amino acid sequence Gly-Trp-Arg-Leu-Leu-↓-Ala-Pro-Ile[9] (where the arrow indicates the scissile bond). Membranes were shown to enhance cleavage efficiency at the NS2–NS3 junction,[12] and membrane-activation could be mimicked by detergent micelles.[13]

Thiol-reactive agents such as iodacetamide or N-ethylmaleimide or the chloromethylketone tosyl-phenyl-chloromethylketone were shown to inhibit the enzyme.[13] Also, metal chelators such as EDTA or phenanthroline abolished cleavage, and subsequent addition of zinc or cadmium was able to restore activity.[10,13] The metal dependence of the NS2/3 proteinase activity led Hijikata et al.[10] to propose that NS2/3 might be a zinc-dependent metalloproteinase. Thus, these authors mutagenized all conserved histidine, cysteine, and glutamic acid residues within NS2/3 with the goal of identifying possible metal ligands. After this procedure, residues His-952 and Cys-993, located within NS2, were identified as essential for proteolytic activity. However, the finding of a structural zinc binding site in the NS3 proteinase domain[14–17] has shed some doubt on the involvement of these residues as metal ligands. In fact, zinc could possibly be required for the NS2–NS3 proteinase activity because it stabilizes the structure of the NS3 component of the NS2/3 proteinase. Wu et al.[18] have recently discussed the possible mechanisms by which the cleavage between NS2 and NS3 might occur. Those authors came to the conclusion that the existing data are compatible with either a cysteine proteinase or a zinc-dependent metalloproteinase being responsible for the processing event. According to the former hypothesis, a cysteine proteinase having His-952 and Cys-993 as a catalytic dyad may be invoked as responsible

AMINO ACIDS	PROTEIN	FUNCTION
·810-1026	NS2	Component of Zn-dependent auto-proteinase
·1027-1657	NS3	Ser proteinase domain RNA/DNA Helicase domain
·1658-1711	NS4A	NS3 Ser proteinase cofactor
·1712-1972	NS4B	?
·1973-2420	NS5A	Interferon-α resistance
·2421-3010	NS5B	RNA-dependent RNA polymerase

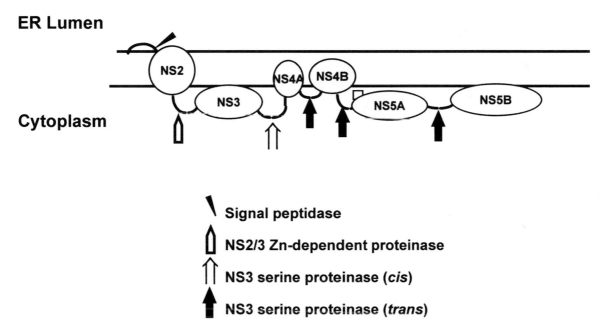

FIG. 1. Schematic representation of the polyprotein proteolytic processing and hypothetical membrane topology of the HCV nonstructural proteins.

for the cleavage event. According to this hypothesis, zinc would merely serve the purpose of stabilizing the structure of the NS3 proteinase domain without playing any role in catalysis. This view is also shared by Gorbalenya and Snijder,[19] who classified NS2/3 as a cysteine proteinase.

An alternative mechanism may be envisaged, invoking a zinc-dependent metalloproteinase as catalyst in the scission of the NS2–NS3 junction. In favor of this hypothesis is the observation that in the crystal structure of the NS3 proteinase domain,[15,17] the bound zinc of NS3 is in close proximity to the N-terminus of the enzyme and hence to the NS2–NS3 junction.[18] In addition, both x-ray crystallography[16] and nuclear magnetic reso-

nance (NMR) studies[20] have shown that the coordinating histidine residue is endowed with a considerable flexibility, compatible with a switch of the metal binding site between an "open" and a "close" conformation. It could be speculated that the open conformation, with the histidine moving away to leave a waterbound zinc ion located in the proximity of the NS2–NS3 junction, may play a role in hydrolysis.

In summary, the exact details about the mechanism adopted by the NS2/3 proteinase remains elusive primarily because of the autocatalytic nature of the proteolytic cleavage it catalyzes and the inherent difficulty associated with expressing and purifying an active protein. An in vitro assay, based on biochemically defined or purified components, is still lacking. This in turn has made the design of potent and selective and antiviral agents targeting the NS2/3 proteinase extremely difficult. Despite these difficulties, several groups have characterized many interesting properties of the NS2/3 proteinase, thus opening the avenue to the discovery of compounds capable of interfering with its activity.

NS3/4A PROTEINASE

The serine proteinase contained within the viral protein NS3 catalyzes four of five processing events that take place during the maturation of the nonstructural portion of the HCV polyprotein (Fig. 1). The NS3 proteinase displays its catalytic activity as a noncovalent heterodimeric complex with the viral protein NS4A.[21] The NS3 minimal proteinase domain has been mapped by deletion mutagenesis to the N-terminal 180 amino acids of NS3.[21–25] Within this region, the conserved residues that form the enzyme catalytic triad, namely His-1083, Asp-1107, and Ser-1165, are found. The remainder of the NS3 protein, namely its ~450 C-terminal residues, harbor an RNA helicase (see below). The artificially truncated serine proteinase and helicase domains retain their respective catalytic activities, and the relative ease of purification of the truncated forms in comparison with the full-length construct have led many workers in the field to primarily focus on the truncated enzymes. Recent findings, however, suggest that binding of the NS4A proteinase cofactor to the full-length enzyme besides activating the proteinase also downregulates the helicase activity, pointing to a significant cross talk between the two functional domains of the NS3 protein.[26]

In transfected cells, NS3 and NS4A were shown to form a stable complex.[21] A region of about 30 amino acids at the N-terminus of NS3 is necessary for both complex formation and modulation of the proteolytic activity by NS4A.[21,27,28] In addition to activating the serine proteinase, NS4A targets the NS3 protein to the membranes of the ER.[29] Deletion mutagenesis experiments have shown that a 14-amino acid central hydrophobic region of NS4A (amino acids 1,678–1,691) is sufficient for the activation of the NS3 proteinase.[28,30–32] This region is preceded by a very hydrophobic N-terminal portion, possibly forming a *trans*-membrane α-helix involved in membrane targeting, and is followed by a more hydrophilic portion that appears not to be required for the cofactor activity. Interestingly, the effect of NS4A on the proteolytic activity of NS3 can be efficiently mimicked in vitro by synthetic peptides encompassing the 14-amino acid central region of NS4A.[30–32]

Both x-ray crystallography[15–17] and NMR spectroscopy[33] have been used to determine the three-dimensional structure of the isolated NS3 proteinase domain, either in its free form or complexed to NS4A-derived peptides. These studies revealed that the NS3 proteinase folds in a canonical chymotrypsin-like fold, consisting of two ß-barrel-like domains (Fig. 2A). The residues of the catalytic triad are located in a groove at the interface of the two domains. The NS4A peptide is embedded into the core of the NS3 proteinase domain and stabilized by the N-terminus of NS3, which literally forms a molecular clamp around the NS4A cofactor. In the structure without NS4A, the N-terminal region of NS3 is essentially unfolded.[16–33] The activation mechanism of NS4A thus appears to be linked to its capacity of conferring structural stability to the N-terminal ß-barrel in the complexed enzyme.

A distinguishing structural feature of the NS3 proteinase is the presence of a tetrahedral zinc binding site formed by residues Cys-1123, Cys-1125, Cys-1171, and His-1175 (Fig. 2A). The zinc binding site lies on the opposite side of the molecule from the active site and was shown to have a structural rather than a catalytic role.[14] Substitution of any of the cysteine residues involved in metal coordination by alanine greatly reduces the proteinase activity in vitro, whereas mutation of His-1175 has a minor effect on enzymatic activity.[10,34] In line with these experimental findings, the side chain of His-1175 was shown not to participate directly to metal coordination but rather to bind the metal indirectly through a water molecule. This may have implication for the zinc-dependent cleavage at the NS2–NS3 cleavage site by the NS2/3 proteinase (see above). A similar binding motif for a structural metal ion is found in 2A proteinase of picornavirus.[35] Picornavirus 2A is a cysteine proteinase with a chymotrypsin fold. Remarkably, in these highly variable viral RNA genomes, the metal-binding site is even more conserved than the catalytic residues.

The NS3 cleavage sites have the consensus sequence Asp/Glu-Xaa$_4$-Cys-↓-Thr-Ser/Ala (were Xaa indicates any amino acid and the arrow indicates the scissile bond) with cleavage occurring after cysteine in all-*trans* cleavage sites (i.e., NS4A–NS4B, NS4B–NS5A, and NS5A–NS5B) or after threonine in the intramolecular cleavage site between NS3 and NS4A. The primary specificity of a proteinase is defined by the side chain of the amino acid that precedes the scissile bond (i.e., the P1 position). (We follow the nomenclature of Schechter and Berger[36] in designating the cleavage sites as P6-P5-P4-P3-P2-P1 . . . P1'-P2'-P3'-P4'-, with the scissile bond between P1 and P1' and the C-terminus of the substrate on the prime site.) The specificity for the P1 amino acid is imposed by the shape of the S1 pocket on the enzyme (often referred to as the proteinase specificity pocket). The specificity pocket of the enzyme is shallow and closed at its bottom by Phe-1180, as previously predicted by homology modeling.[37] The nature of this pocket explains the preference of the NS3 proteinase for cysteine in the substrate P1 position (Fig.

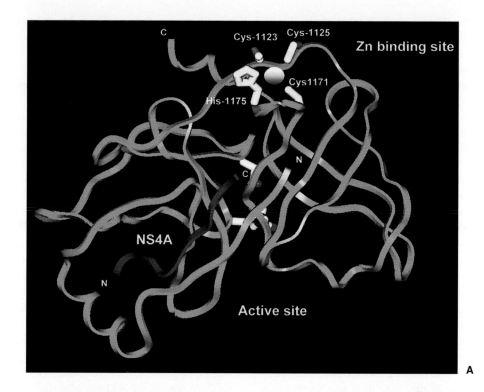

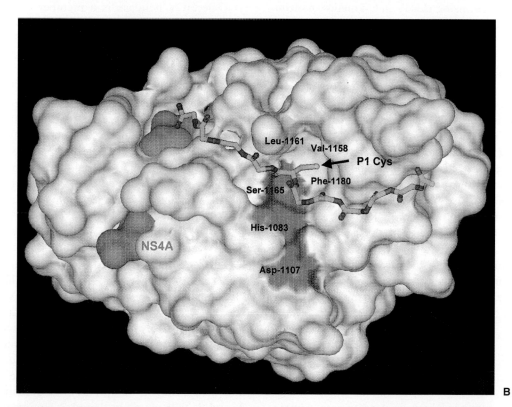

FIG. 2.   **(A) Ribbon representation of three-dimensional crystal structure of the NS3 serine proteinase domain (green) complexed with an NS4A$_{21-34}$ cofactor peptide (red).** The side chains of the catalytic triad amino acids are indicated in white and are visible in the back of the molecule. The side chains of Cys-1123, Cys-1125, Cys-1171, and His-1175 (yellow) were modeled to form a tetrahedral metal binding site. The structural zinc ion is indicated in magenta. N and C indicate the N-terminus and the C-terminus of the NS3 protein (white) and of the NS4A peptide (yellow). **(B)** Surface representation of the of three-dimensional crystal structure of the NS3 serine proteinase domain (white) complexed with an NS4A$_{21-34}$ cofactor peptide (magenta) and with a decapeptide substrate. The residues of the catalytic triad are shown in red. The amino acid that define the proteinase S1 specificity pocket are shown in yellow. The side chain of the substrate P1 Cys is shown bound in the S1 pocket.

2B). Apart from the P1 specificity pocket, the surface of the enzyme involved in substrate recognition is rather flat and solvent exposed (Fig. 2B). This finding accounts for the apparent lack of substrate specificity between P1 and P6. A cluster of positively charged residues is present on the surface of NS3 at a distance that allows their interaction with the acidic residue found in the substrate P6 position.

This rather featureless substrate-binding site provides a rationale for the enzyme's requirement of at least decamer peptide substrates spanning from P6 to P4'.[38–40] These substrate peptides derive their binding energy from a series of weak interactions distributed along the recognition surface. Clearly, this peculiar mechanism of substrate recognition is a difficult starting point for the development of small molecule inhibitors of the enzyme.

Analysis of the interaction of the NS3 proteinase with its peptide substrates led to the discovery that the enzyme is competitively inhibited by its N-terminal cleavage products.[41–43] The extent of product inhibition experienced by the NS3 proteinase is uncommon in this family of enzymes. The binding mode of cleavage products to the active site of the proteinase was therefore investigated in detail using steady state kinetics, molecular modeling, site directed mutagenesis, and NMR spectroscopy as tools[41,44,45] and was more recently confirmed by the x-ray structure of the full-length NS3 protein.[46] According to those studies, the hexapeptide products bind to the enzyme's active site in a ß-strand conformation via two electrostatic anchoring points involving an acidic residue in the P6 position and the P1 α carboxylate. The former residue binds to a cluster of positively charged residues that also form the P6 binding site for the substrate. Conversely, the P1 α carboxylate was shown to engage in hydrogen bond interactions with the catalytic histidine, the amide protons of the residues that form the oxyanion hole of the enzyme—Ser-1165 and Gly-1163—and with the side chain amino group of the conserved Lys-1162. The discovery of product inhibition lead to the development of several hexapeptide inhibitors with nanomolar potencies[42,43,47] that may be regarded as promising starting points for the development of more druglike molecules.

NS3 RNA HELICASE

In addition to the N-terminal proteinase domain, the HCV NS3 has conserved sequence motifs that are the hallmark of RNA helicases.[48] RNA helicases are enzymes capable of unwinding duplex RNA. This is accomplished in a reaction that is coupled with the hydrolysis of nucleoside triphosphate (NTP). In fact, all RNA helicases characterized to date possess RNA-stimulated NTPase activity. Most likely, hydrolysis of NTP is required to generate the energy necessary to disrupt the hydrogen bonds that keep the two RNA strands annealed.

Various forms of recombinant proteins containing the C-terminal domain of NS3 have been shown to possess polynucleotide-stimulated NTPase activity,[49–52] duplex unwinding activity,[51,53–57] and single-stranded (ss) polynucleotide binding activity.[55,56,58] The minimal requirement for these activities lies within the C-terminal 465 amino acids of NS3 that represent a functionally and structurally separate domain.[53] Interestingly, the HCV NS3 helicase has some very unique properties: it can unwind double-stranded dsRNA and dsDNA and RNA/DNA heteroduplexes in the 3' to 5' direction (this convention implies that the enzyme required a 3'-overhang to start the unwinding reaction) using any NTP or (deoxy)NTP as energy source.[55] Recently, studies on the full-length enzyme have shown that the N-terminal proteinase domain has little if any effect on the NTPase and helicase activities associated with the C-terminal domain.[59] However, NS4A-mediated stabilization of NS3 in the active proteinase conformation appears to downregulate its capacity to unwind dsRNA, but not the NTPase activity.[26]

The HCV helicase is a member of the so-called DEXH helicase family.[60,61] The name "DEXH" is due to the fact that an invariant sequence, namely Asp-Glu-Xaa-His, is found in correspondence of the active site of the enzymes belonging to these family (see also below). Like the other members of the DEXH family, the HCV helicase contains six conserved sequence motifs (numbered I to VI). Several mutational studies[62–64] related to recently acquired structural information[65,66] have now demonstrated a defined function for four of these six motifs in the NS3 helicase. Motif I (Gly-Ser-Gly-Lys-Thr, or Walker motif A) is involved in binding the terminal phosphate groups of the nucleotide cofactor, whereas the acidic residues of motif II (the actual DEXH motif, Asp-Glu-Cys-His, or Walker motif B) are responsible for chelating the Mg^{++} of the Mg–NTP complex. The histidine residue of motif II together with motif III (Thr-Ala-Thr) and the conserved glutamine and arginine residues of motif VI (Glu-Arg-Xaa-Gly-Arg-Xaa-Gly-Arg) are implicated in coupling NTP hydrolysis to nucleic acid unwinding. The three-dimensional structures of the isolated NS3 helicase domain[65–67] and that of the helicase domain within the full-length NS3 protein[46] have been determined. The enzyme comprises three domains termed 1, 2, and 3, with domains 1 and 2 having very similar fold. The ATP-binding site is situated in a cleft between domains 1 and 2. This cleft that is lined with conserved motifs I through VI. On the basis of these studies, NS3 can be considered part of a large class of helicases that have a 3' to 5' directionality and share a number of structural features, despite the very limited

As a result, the range of probes, labels, tissue preparation protocols, and, not least, samples reported in the literature is daunting and makes direct comparisons of data very difficult. It is important to note that all reported studies appeared to satisfy the controls that were performed. However, none of the studies performed a posthybridization melt curve, recognized as a highly stringent control.[18] Furthermore, the use of cold probes to compete with labeled probes is circular and fails to control for nonspecific hybridization.

In addition, several studies report the detection of negative sense HCV RNA by ISH despite the fact that this is 10- to 100-fold less abundant in the naturally infected liver than positive sense (genomic) RNA. In experiments designed to determine the nature of negative sense vRNA in Kunjin virus (a member of the *Flaviviridae*)-infected cells, it was determined that the negative strand was not found as free ssRNA but was only detected after denaturation of the dsRF.[19] Because HCV can be expected to replicate in a similar manner to the flaviviruses, it can be predicted that the detection of negative sense HCV RNA by ISH will require prior denaturation of the tissue section. Indeed, the detection of positive sense vRNA can also be predicted to benefit from such a denaturation step, as a proportion of positive sense RNA is likely to be present as a component of the RF. In addition, although the 5' untranslated region (UTR), which is the most highly conserved region of the HCV genome, is often chosen as the target for ISH studies, this region contains a high degree of secondary structure (Fig. 1) composed of base-paired stems and loops.[20] This structure is essential for the function of the internal ribosome entry site (IRES) necessary for viral protein synthesis,[21] and consequently, it is most likely that detection of HCV RNA by ISH to the 5' UTR target will also require prior denaturation of the tissue sample.

Detection of HCV RNA in Individual Liver Cells

I have chosen to present the data related to the detection of HCV RNA by ISH by reviewing the early data (before 1995) that suggest that the proportion of infected cells is low and then to review more recent data that suggest the opposite. Consequently, as many of the interim studies simply confirmed the earlier studies, these publications are not reviewed.

Several early studies with probes representing the 5'UTR or the equally highly conserved core gene regions were performed that reported the detection of HCV RNA in some hepatocytes and in monocytes.[22–25] These studies all remarked on the difficulties in the detection of the vRNA; all studies reported a cytoplasmic distribution of HCV RNA, although the study from Lamas et al.[23] also reported a nuclear distribution. The

patients in this study were also HIV positive. Negative and positive sense vRNA was also detected in two studies,[23,25] whereas the others[22,24] used dsDNA probes, which were unable to identify the polarity of the target. The latter study [24] used dsDNA probes to the core gene region, because this was considered a more suitable target than the 5'UTR, which it was recognized may need prior denaturation for detection. A later study[26] also detected positive and negative sense vRNA, but in a majority of hepatocytes in contrast to the above studies, with a probe to the 5'UTR, and only detected positive sense vRNA in mononuclear cells. This study used a four-layer system to detect the hybridized digoxygenin (DIG)-labeled RNA probe, and this may account for the detection of an increased proportion of HCV-infected hepatocytes. However none of the studies that claimed to detect the 5'UTR or negative sense vRNA subjected the tissue sections to a denaturation step. In view of the possibility that negative sense RNA may only be present as a component of the dsRF, then it is possible that these signals were nonspecific. Alternatively, HCV may replicate in a manner consistent with the production of negative sense vRNA that is not a component of the dsRF. The study from Yamada et al.[25] was unusual in the choice of probes; three pairs of oligodeoxynucleotides (sense and antisense) were used that were tailed with ATT repeats at the 5'and 3'ends. The oligodeoxynucleotides were then ultraviolet irradiated to form T-T dimers, which formed haptens, and the bound probes were detected with a horseradish peroxidase (HRPO)-conjugated antibody to the T-T dimer. No details have been reported on the relative sensitivity of this protocol compared with the use of more conventional probes.

Similar contemporary studies were unable to detect any vRNA in hepatocytes,[27,28] but one of these studies demonstrated that mononuclear cells were positive for vRNA.[27] In this study, it was considered likely that hepatocytes were also infected with HCV, but this was beyond the level of sensitivity of the assay. On the other hand, a study[29] using a dsDNA probe from the NS5 region (mainly NS5B) claimed that HCV RNA was detected in mononuclear cells, biliary epithelial cells, and sinusoidal cells in addition to hepatocytes. It was found that 1–5% of hepatocytes were positive for vRNA. Furthermore, the authors noted a correlation between the presence of HCV RNA and cell injury in the biliary epithelium. Using strand-specific probes to the 5'UTR, positive and negative sense vRNA was also detected in the same cell populations, although negative strand was not detected in the biliary epithelium. The significance of this is unclear but may relate to the levels of virus in the different cell populations. More recently, primary biliary epithelial cells were shown to support the replication of HCV in vitro.[30] However, HCV RNA was detected in the nucleus and cytoplasm of the positive cells,[29] a surprising finding, which raises some concerns over the specificity of the data. Although the tissue sections used to detect the positive and negative sense vRNA were denatured before hybridization, additional confirmation of the specificity of these signals (generated by RNA probes to the 5'UTR) would have been possible had this step been omitted on some sections, but this was not performed.

Because an earlier study suggested that formalin-fixed, paraffin embedded HCV-positive liver samples, as used by Nouri Aria et al.,[29] were prone to produce nonspecific signals in hepatocyte nuclei,[31] it is possible that the nuclear signals were nonspecific. However, a study[32] using oligodeoxynucleotide probes from the 5'UTR and core regions of the genome on paraformaldehyde-fixed frozen sections also showed that the bulk of the signal was localized to the nucleus of infected hepatocytes. Nevertheless, because there are no data (see below) to support a nuclear phase in the replication cycle of flaviviruses, this is a puzzling finding. The signal detected in the mononuclear cells with a radioactive probe[27] has been interpreted as a nuclear signal in recent reviews,[13–15] but this claim was not made in the original publication, and it is likely that the signal originated from the small cytoplasm of these cells.

A useful approach to resolve the apparent difficulties in the detection of HCV RNA was to examine liver biopsy samples from experimentally infected chimpanzees. One study used an ss oligodeoxynucleotide probe (50 nt) complementary to a region in the 5'UTR.[33] The results showed that most hepatocytes were positive for positive sense (genomic) vRNA 2 days after experimental infection with 0.5 mL of undiluted plasma from a patient with persistent HCV infection, before the appearance of the vRNA in the blood 1–2 days later, as determined by RT-PCR. In this study, the tissue sections were subjected to a heating step to denature the 5'UTR before hybridization, and it was suggested that this step was necessary for detection of the vRNA. This latter point is consistent with the proposed structure of the 5'UTR. No attempt was made to detect the negative strand. The hepatocytes remained positive, sometimes intermittently, for 11–20 weeks. It is unfortunate that the study did not attempt to detect vRNA by RT-PCR in RNA samples extracted from the liver, to complement the ISH data, or attempt to detect vRNA by Northern blot hybridization, and one is left to ponder the point raised by the authors themselves on the discrepancy between the number and intensity of putative HCV RNA-positive hepatocytes on the one hand and the absence of viremia on the other.

A recent study using RNA probes directed to the 5'UTR also claimed to detect vRNA in most hepatocytes in liver biopsy samples from HCV carrier patients and chimpanzees.[1] Both positive and negative sense vRNA appeared to be detected in this study. In common with the studies reported above,[29,33] the tissue sections were subjected to a denaturation step to ensure that the 5'UTR target was denatured, but no evidence was presented to indicate that this step was necessary nor was the use of undenatured sections considered as a negative control.[1] The limit of detection of HCV RNA by ISH in cultured Daudi cells infected with the virus was claimed to be 14 genome equivalents per cell.[1] However, no details were presented on the methodology to detect the vRNA in the cells, in contrast to the method to detect the vRNA in the liver sections. A number of control steps including pretreatment of the sections with RNase, followed by RNasin to protect the probe from digestion were performed. However, as only a small residue of RNase is required to digest the probe, it is unfortunate that the RNase digestion of the tissue was not followed by a proteinase digestion step to eliminate any residual RNase. In these circumstances, it is difficult to determine if the loss of signal was attributed to RNase digestion of the target or the probe. An additional control to compete the labeled probe with unlabeled probe was also performed, but as discussed above this control is not stringent.

Nevertheless, the results of the study[1] look convincing; 15–81% of the hepatocytes in the human liver samples were positive for positive strand HCV RNA and 64–84% were positive in the chimpanzee samples, whereas no signals were generated in a range of liver samples from patients with non-HCV hepatitis and from individuals with normal liver. It was calculated that each hepatocyte in two representative human samples contained 6.5 and 4.5 genome copies (positive sense) of HCV RNA, respectively. If these results are correct, then this represents a highly sensitive ISH assay. However, the data begin to lose credibility if one considers that this level of vRNA in such a high proportion of hepatocytes is likely to be detectable by Northern blot hybridization. Furthermore, RT-PCR analysis of RNA extracted from the samples showed that negative strand vRNA was 10- to 50-fold less abundant than positive strand vRNA, and this is totally inconsistent with the apparent detection of the negative strand in a similar proportion of hepatocytes that contained 6.5 copies of positive sense RNA.[1] Consequently, it is difficult to conclude that the signals were specific.

Recently, vRNA was detected in a proportion of hepatocytes but not other cell types in liver biopsy samples from 10 patients who were infected with genotype 1b, using a dsDNA probe to the 5'UTR hybridized in the presence of dextran sulfate.[34] The distribution of the positive hepatocytes was assessed by digital image analysis, which showed that the infected hepatocytes appeared to be distributed randomly, suggesting that cell–cell spread of the virus did not occur. The mean viral load in individual hepatocytes was shown to be similar in the 10 samples and the viral load in blood was shown to correlate with the proportion of infected hepatocytes in the respective liver samples, although it was conceded in a follow-up study that this correlation was not strong.[35] The initial study represents an attempt to correlate the results of the ISH analysis with the RT-PCR data and is to be commended. However, as 87% of hepatocytes in case 10 in this study were scored as HCV RNA positive and this correlated with a high viral load $(1.2 \times 10^6/mL)$ in the blood, it could be expected that this and similar samples would be positive by Northern blot hybridization, and consequently this can be considered to be a discrepancy. In addition, a nuclear signal was detected in a proportion of the hepatocytes, and the tissue sections were not subjected to a denaturation step before hybridization, again raising some concerns over specificity.

Because it is clear that the level of HCV RNA in the infected liver is exceedingly low, the use of in situ PCR has been explored to detect the vRNA. In situ PCR to detect HCV RNA is performed after an initial RT step, either by direct incorporation of labeled nucleotides during the PCR (direct in situ PCR) or indirectly using ISH to detect the amplicons after the PCR (indirect in situ PCR). From first principles and to follow the procedures (Southern blot hybridization, nested PCR) used to ensure that amplicons produced in conventional RT-PCR are specific, it is preferable to use indirect in situ -PCR, but this is more technically demanding. An initial study[36] that compared the sensitivity of detection of HCV RNA by ISH and in situ PCR found that although ISH only detected HCV RNA-positive cells in one of six liver samples, both direct and indirect in situ PCR detected positive cells in all six samples. The study also highlighted the importance of a "hot start" PCR after the RT step to ensure specificity and the need to pretreat the sections with DNase; failure to perform this latter step resulted in endogenous DNA repair by the *Taq* polymerase and the appearance of a strong nonspecific nuclear signal. Indeed, a later study was unable to remove the source of this nonspecific signal even with prior DNase digestion.[28] The Nuovo et al. study[36] showed that a high proportion of hepatocytes in some liver lobules were HCV RNA positive, whereas only a few cells in other lobules were positive. The signal was reported to be perinuclear and was not restricted to hepatocytes, as Kupffer cells and bile duct epithelia were also positive.

A similar study that also used direct in situ PCR to target the core gene region[37] also detected vRNA in the cytoplasm of 5–25% of hepatocytes and a few mononuclear cells in four of six liver samples that were examined. A follow-up study from the same group[38] confirmed the detection of HCV RNA in approximately 5% of hepatocytes, showed a correlation between hepatic vRNA and viral load, but failed to show any correlation between hepatic vRNA and the histologic activity index (HAI) or serum alanine aminotransferase (ALT). More-over, the proportion of HCV RNA-positive hepatocytes was reduced in patients who were treated with interferon, providing additional proof of the specificity of the signal. On the other hand, a recent study using both direct and indirect in situ -PCR suggested that the vRNA was detected in the nucleus of hepatocytes, bile duct cells, and lymphocytes.[39] Aside from the intracellular localization, the signal in the hepatocytes remained constant even in responders to interferon treatment, and consequently it is difficult to accept that the signal was specific.

The above reports to detect HCV RNA by in situ PCR highlight the difficulties in using this technique to detect HCV RNA. Two recent reviews emphasize the care required for successful detection of HCV RNA in this manner.[13,40] The most realistic interpretation is that around 5–25% of hepatocytes are infected with the virus, the virus RNA is localised to the perinuclear region or the cytoplasm of the infected cell, and that the level of intracellular virus is very low indeed.

Detection of HCV RNA in Tumor Cells

Persistent infection with HCV often results in chronic liver disease and hepatocellular carcinoma (HCC) in a proportion of individuals. The mechanism for the development of the HCC is quite unclear, and a number of studies have examined tumor tissue for the presence of HCV RNA by ISH in an attempt to determine if these cells are infected.

A high proportion of hepatocytes was positive for viral antigens and vRNA using a protocol to examine the distribution of these markers simultaneously.[41] The study noted that infected cells generally contained viral antigens and RNA; hepatocytes were the major infected cell, although occasional mononuclear cells were also infected; the intracellular distribution of the viral products was cytoplasmic; and denaturation of the samples was required for efficient and reproducible detection of the vRNA. Although it was noted that cells in tumorous regions of the liver were also positive for HCV markers, no correlation was noted between viral antigens/RNA and histologic features. It was suggested that negative strand vRNA constituted a high proportion of the vRNA in the infected cells. The results and arguments to support this statement were not well developed, and one is left once again to ponder the specificity, if the levels of positive- and negative-strand vRNA, as detected by ISH, fail to agree with the generally accepted findings that positive strands are 10- to 100-fold more abundant, as determined by RT-PCR.

A second study to examine the distribution of HCV in tumor and nontumor tissue also detected positive- and negative-strand vRNA in both areas of the liver.[42] A mixture of three antisense and sense oligonucleotide probes, respectively, with T-T dimers described previously[25] were used that were detected with an HRPO-conjugated antibody to the T-T dimer. The probes were directed to the 5'UTR and to the NS4B gene region; the tissue sections were not denatured in this study, but the use of the NS4B probe may not require this step. A comparison with the individual probes was not performed. The positive strand was detected in the nontumor tissue in 10 of 15 patients studied and the minus strand in 7 of 15. The proportion of vRNA-positive hepatocytes varied between a few cells to >50%. The distribution of cells containing the positive and negative strands was similar, and only hepatocytes were shown to be positive. Examination of the tumor tissue showed that 9 of 15 patients had detectable positive strand whereas only 4 of 15 had detectable negative strand. This was interpreted to mean that hepatoma cells showed reduced permissiveness for HCV replication compared with normal hepatocytes. The study also suggested that there was no correlation between HCV RNA and histology or tumor differentation, no correlation between vRNA in the tumor compared with nontumorous tissue, and no correlation between intracellular HCV RNA and viral load/ALT. The high quality of the figures was particularly noteworthy. This resulted from the use of resected liver samples, which were treated specifically for ISH, rather than the use of samples that were formalin fixed for routine histologic analysis before examination by ISH. A previous study that used dsDNA probes from the core region in the presence of dextran sulfate also detected vRNA in tumor cells and normal hepatocytes in tissues that were treated in a similar manner.[43]

Positive sense vRNA was detected in the nucleus and cytoplasm of lymphoma cells in a primary hepatic lymphoma but not in the hepatocytes of one case, whereas hepatocytes but not the lymphoma cells were considered to be positive in two other cases.[44] This study used an RNA probe against the 5'UTR, but the sections were not denatured and no attempt was made to detect negative sense RNA. Although the results are consistent with the previous detection of HCV RNA in the nucleus of infected cells, the data lack conviction and no details of the proportion of HCV-positive cells were presented.

Commentary

Despite the large number of studies (or perhaps due to the large number), there is no consensus on the cellular or intracellular distribution of HCV RNA in the naturally infected liver. Conflicting data on the proportion of infected hepatocytes are common, and because this may differ among different patients, it is possible that a consensus will never be reached. Differences between samples may also account for the detection of HCV RNA in

cells other than hepatocytes, although this appears to be less likely and more a feature of the methods used.

Current understanding of the HCV replication process suggests that the ratio of positive-to-negative sense RNA is >10:1 and that the vRNA may need denaturation to permit successful hybridization and detection in situ. This is particularly true of the 5'UTR, which is a common target for ISH studies as a result of the high degree of nucleotide conservation in this region and the negative strand. The proportion of 5'UTR molecules that forms an authentic IRES within the infected cell at any one time is unknown. Moreover, the proportion of positive sense vRNA that is engaged in transcription as opposed to translation is a component of the dsRF and ss genomic RNA can be expected to be rapidly exported from the cell.

It is surprising that more emphasis has not been placed on studies with BVDV, which can be cultured in vitro. Studies of tissue samples of naturally infected cattle demonstrated quite clearly that vRNA was restricted to the cytoplasm of infected cells.[45,46] Indeed, the distribution as detected with an RNA probe from the highly conserved p125 gene region of a noncytopathic strain of virus (analogous to the 3'region of HCV NS3) was identical to the distribution of viral proteins. No attempt was made to detect negative-strand vRNA. However, the lack of nuclear localization of the positive-strand vRNA was viewed as additional evidence for the specificity of the ISH reaction.

Although the core protein of different members of the Flaviviridae can be found in the nucleus of the infected cell, it has not been proved that this contributes to replication, and in an example that readers of this review may be more familiar with, nuclear HBcAg is unrelated to the HBV replication process.[47] An explanation for the apparent appearance and detection of HCV RNA in the nucleus of infected cells has been to suggest that HCV has a nuclear phase of replication like the flaviviruses.[14] However, there are no data to support such a phase. Close attention to the details of flavivirus replication shows that replication is perinuclear,[48] and although viral replicase activity is associated with the nuclear fraction after cell fractionation studies, it is extremely difficult to remove all traces of extranuclear membranes from the nuclei. Consequently, residual replicase activity is thought to be associated with these adherent membranes (Westaway EG, 1999 personal communication). Furthermore, BrU-labeled nascent RNA was found only the cytoplasm of actinomycin D-treated Kunjin virus-infected cells,[49] and replication complexes were detected by immunogold labeling only in the cytoplasm of infected cells.[50] It is possible that HCV replication is also perinuclear, as the core protein expressed in eukaryotic cells has also been detected in this location.[51]

Thus, although much of the ISH data presented in the above studies appears to be authentic, inconsistencies are common, although it is clear that the probes generated a signal. Many individuals are suspicious of data generated by ISH, and as a result the data will only be widely accepted if it is consistent with other data. Several studies described a nuclear distribution of vRNA; although one cannot be certain that this may be part of the pathogenetic process, the likelihood is higher that this is nonspecific. Several other studies reported the detection of negative strand vRNA in a ratio that differed to the ratio that is accepted from RT-PCR and from Northern blot analysis of BVDV-infected cells.[5] Other studies reported negative strand detection without a prior denaturation step, whereas still others reported intrahepatic HCV RNA in the absence of viremia. As a result, the data lose credibility. Despite the complex nature of the method, the studies that used in situ -PCR appear credible, and one study reported a loss of signal as a result of interferon treatment.

HCV REPLICATION IN LIVER CELLS AS DETERMINED BY THE DETECTION OF VIRAL PROTEINS IN SITU

The in situ detection of viral antigens in liver cells has the potential to clarify aspects of pathogenesis and help in the histologic diagnosis. Although theoretic considerations dictate that the detection of viral structural proteins may represent contamination (as defined above) or phagocytosis, especially in monocytes/macrophages, this is seldom the case in practice. Consequently, the intracellular detection of viral structural proteins is usually accepted as evidence of ongoing active virus replication. This is particularly so for viruses that produce low levels of nonstructural proteins, which are often enzymes required for the replication and processing of the viral–genome and –protein products. HBV is a good example of this, as the detection of the polymerase and X proteins has proved problematic and confusing, in contrast to the detection of the core and surface antigens.

However, as discussed above, an unknown proportion of the structural proteins expressed in HCV-infected cells will be exported as nascent virions. As a result, because the HCV proteins are synthesized as a polyprotein, which is co- and posttranslationally processed to produce equimolar concentrations of the mature viral polypeptides, the nonstructural proteins that are retained in the infected cell can be assumed to represent more suitable targets. Nevertheless, the detection of the nonstructural proteins will be dependent on their half-life in the infected cell, and little information is available on this.

The in situ detection of viral antigens in tissue samples by immunohistochemistry depends on two major factors: the quality of the antiserum and whether the tis-

sue sample is fixed or unfixed. A discussion on procedures to successfully raise hyperimmune antisera is out of the scope of this review but can be found elsewhere.[52] However, many workers choose to use commercially available antisera and consequently are unable to influence this component. Nevertheless, a number of studies have been performed with human polyclonal antibodies. Although these antibodies are by definition largely uncharacterized, they can prove useful because they are directed to epitopes that are expressed during natural infection. It has been possible to adsorb such antibodies with purified recombinant viral proteins to determine which major antigenic targets are recognized and to confirm the specificity of the reaction.

Laboratory staff may be unable to influence whether the tissue sample is fixed for routine histologic processing or examined as fresh frozen sections. Although formalin-fixed paraffin-embedded tissue is still most convenient, the loss of antigenicity of many viral proteins makes frozen sections the optimum sample. Many aspects of the detection of HCV proteins by immunohistochemistry, including the appropriate controls, were discussed recently,[12] and consequently the following discussion concentrates on the data generated. I have divided this part of the review into different sections, based on the detection of the viral proteins with human antibodies or with antibodies raised in other species to the structural proteins and nonstructural proteins, although these sections are not rigid due to an overlap in some studies.

Detection of HCV Antigens with Human Antisera

The detection of HCV antigens was first described with a direct fluorescein isothiocyanate (FITC)-conjugated human or chimpanzee polyclonal antibody.[53] This conjugate detected the antigens in the cytoplasm of hepatocytes in frozen sections from chimpanzees with acute or persistent HCV infection and patients with persistent infection. Careful adsorption studies with recombinant HCV proteins determined that the major target of the FITC conjugate was the NS3 protein, with some activity against the NS4 protein. It was determined that 50–70% of hepatocytes in the chimpanzee liver samples were HCV antigen positive, whereas only 5–20% of hepatocytes in the human carriers were positive. This was followed by a similar study[54] using the same FITC-conjugated antibody. This study showed that HCV antigen was detected in 30 of 35 liver biopsy samples taken from HCV carriers before treatment with interferon and suggested no correlation between expression of viral antigen and viral load. However, low levels of HCV antigen expression were predictive of a good response to interferon. Furthermore, patients who responded to the interferon treatment showed a reduction in the intensity of staining and in the number of antigen-positive hepatocytes. These results helped to confirm the specificity of the antigen detection system. A recent study[55] using the same conjugate to examine the expression of the nonstructural proteins in liver transplant recipients with recurrent HCV infection showed that the level of expression of the viral antigens and the proportion of the infected hepatocytes correlated with the viral load, in contrast to the above study.[54] The Vargas et al. study[55] detected viral antigen in the cytoplasm of only 30% of recipients within the first month of transplant, whereas antigen was detected in all recipients 1 month or later after transplantation. The proportion of infected cells varied but many samples showed >20% of positive cells.

HCV antigens were also detected in hepatocytes, mononuclear cells, and bile duct epithelial cells in patients with end-stage liver disease.[56] Approximately 1–5% of hepatocytes were shown to be positive in frozen sections using a biotin-labeled human polyclonal IgG preparation, whereas only a small proportion of the mononuclear and bile duct cells in some patients were positive. The HCV antigens recognized by the human conjugate in this study were not defined but included the core and NS5 proteins, as shown by the detection of these proteins in recombinant baculovirus-infected cells. The conjugate detected the HCV antigens in 13 of 14 frozen sections from resected liver samples taken from patients with end-stage liver disease but only in 1 of 3 similar samples that were formalin fixed and paraffin embedded. The same report[56] described the detection of the core protein in formalin-fixed paraffin-embedded tissues, in 1–2% of hepatocytes, and in isolated mononuclear cells but not the bile duct epithelia using a mixture of monoclonal antibodies to the core protein.

An elegant study that used a pool of human polyclonal IgG conjugated with FITC described a correlation between a response to interferon therapy and a low number of HCV antigen-positive hepatocytes,[57] as suggested previously.[54] However, the patients who were most resistant to interferon therapy were infected with genotype 1b, and consequently it was unclear if the genotype or the number of HCV-positive hepatocytes was responsible for the nonresponse. In an effort to increase the sensitivity of the direct immunofluorescence assay used in this study, the authors used multilayers; the initial FITC-conjugated human antibody was followed by a mouse monoclonal antibody to FITC and then by HRPO-conjugated rabbit anti-mouse and HRPO-conjugated swine anti-rabbit that were detected with diaminobenzidine. This strategy resulted in positive hepatocytes in 31 of 38 patients; there was a great variation in the number and intensity of positive cells that were often focal with no preferred lobular distribution. In a series of colocalization experiments, it was

demonstrated clearly that CD8+ lymphocytes were often found in contact with HCV antigen-positive hepatocytes, and an increase in the number of these CD8+ cells correlated with increased levels of ALT. The HCV-positive hepatocytes were also shown to express detectable levels of human leukocyte antigen A, B, and C and intracellular adhesion molecule-molecules, suggesting that they represented suitable targets for cytotoxic T lymphocytes. Moreover, there was no correlation between the number of positive hepatocytes and the HAI, a finding that is compatible with an immune-mediated mechanism for hepatocyte injury in HCV infection.[57]

In a refinement of the method used in that study, the authors used antigen-specific antibodies selected and affinity purified by binding to the HCV antigens contained in the bands of a recombinant immunoblast 3 test kit.[58] The rationale behind this, to use naturally derived antibodies to recognize the native form of the proteins, seems flawed, as the antibodies were selected by recombinant proteins bound to nitrocellulose, but the approach showed that the individual viral proteins were detected in the same hepatocyte populations, as might be expected.

A study of 10 patients after liver transplantation using human monoclonal antibodies to core and NS4[59] failed to detect viral antigen within 2 weeks of the transplant, whereas 2 weeks later, both antigens were detected in the cytoplasm of individual hepatocytes in 3 patients. Six months posttransplantation, both antigens were detected in samples from all 10 recipients. The design of this study provides additional evidence for the specificity of the HCV antigen detection.

Detection of HCV Structural Proteins in the Infected Liver Using Nonhuman Antibodies

Although the above studies provided useful novel data, previous experience with human polyclonal antisera showed that the use of hyperimmune antisera to individual specific viral antigens raised in another species was likely to increase sensitivity and provide additional information.[47] Nevertheless, two studies that did use hyperimmune antisera on frozen sections were unable to detect the core protein or detected negligible levels in samples from chronic carriers or a carrier chimpanzee.[14,60] Thus, it is possible that the antisera failed to recognize the intracellular form of the protein or that the concentration of the protein was below the level of detection, perhaps as a result of the rapid secretion of the protein in mature virus particles.

However, these reports are in contrast to several others, which report the successful detection of the core protein, and this highlights some of the difficulties in working with HCV. In a study of 48 biopsy samples, which were fixed in Zamboni's solution before the examination of frozen sections, core, E1, and NS3 proteins were detected in approximately one quarter, but overall 19 of 48 were positive for any of the proteins using monoclonal antibodies raised in mice.[61] The proportion of positive cells differed in different patients, but samples that were antigen positive showed a higher HAI. A later study using the same monoclonal antibodies on acetone-fixed frozen sections reported the detection of core, E1, NS3, and NS5 in tumor tissue from three of nine patients with HCC.[62] A higher proportion (6/14) of samples were core antigen positive when frozen sections were examined with a mouse monoclonal antibody to the second hydrophilic region of the core protein (ca. amino acids 100–120) followed by an HRPO-conjugated anti-mouse.[25] On the other hand, a study of snap-frozen tissue from which frozen sections were fixed in cold acetone showed that E2 (and NS3— see below) were detected in eight of eight samples examined.[63] The antigens were present as distinct punctate foci in the cytoplasm of hepatocytes and infiltrating mononuclear cells and resembled the staining pattern reported by others who expressed recombinant HCV proteins in mammmalian cells.[64] A mouse monoclonal antibody to amino acids 5–19 of the core protein also detected core antigen in frozen sections, in the form of specific cytoplasmic granules in a proportion of hepatocytes in 21 of 28 carriers.[65] One percent formalin fixation of the frozen sections was optimal for detection of the HCV antigens in one study,[60] whereas an acetone/chloroform fixation protocol was determined to be optimal in another study.[66]

The study described above[60] showed that the immunogenicity of HCV proteins in hepatocytes but not lymphocytes was reduced by fixation with organic solvents, and although no clear explanation was forthcoming, it was suggested that this may be related to differences in the cell types. However, a recent review[13] outlined some apparent discrepancies in the data, based on a similar study using the same anti-peptide antisera reported only nonspecific staining.[66] It is most important to note that the antisera used in the former study[60] were adsorbed against a normal human liver homogenate before use, and this step did not appear to have been performed in the second study.[66] In addition, preadsorption of the antisera with the specific peptide eliminated the signal.[60] Although the detection system also differed in these two studies (immunofluorescence vs. immunoperoxidase, respectively), the lack of the vital liver homogenate adsorption step is sufficient to explain the contrasting results.

Nevertheless, the second study[66] showed that the core antigen was detected in the cytoplasm of 1–10% of hepatocytes in 75% of viremic individuals with a number of mouse monoclonal antibodies to an epitope contained within aa 26–45 of the core protein, whereas

monoclonal antibodies to aa 39–74 failed to react. Core antigen was also detected in anti-HCV-positive individuals who were not viremic as determined by RT-PCR (see below). Using this protocol, a second study from the same group[67] showed that core antigen, detected with the above monoclonal antibodies, and NS4, detected with a human monoclonal antibody, were detected in 38 of 46 individuals with chronic hepatitis, whereas this figure rose to 40 of 46 when either core or NS4 was detected. In contrast to the study reported above,[61] there was no correlation between levels of antigen expression and the HAI, although a correlation between antigen expression and viral load was noted. In agreement with the study reported above,[54] patients with lower levels of antigen expression before interferon therapy were more likely to respond to therapy, and viral antigens became undetectable in patients who showed a good response to the therapy. This study[67] also showed an unusual twist that reinforced the specificity of the immunohistochemistry, because the anti-NS4 monoclonal antibody that was raised to a genotype 1-specific sequence was unable to detect NS4 expression in patients who were infected with other genotypes.

Thus, although many of the anti-peptide antibodies described above were tested against and reacted with the peptide in ELISA, the antibodies often failed in immunohistochemistry. These studies highlight the need to screen antibodies, particularly monoclonal antibodies, by immunohistochemistry, if this is the intended use. The above data also highlighted that it is often impossible to detect HCV proteins in formalin-fixed paraffin-embedded tissue,[60,66] probably due to reduced immunoreactivity resulting from the fixation process. More recent data suggest that it may be possible to detect HCV antigens if the tissues are subjected to a microwave antigen-retrieval system.[68] In this study, E1, E2, and NS5 were detected in isolated hepatocytes or in groups of hepatocytes. It was concluded that HCV antigens may persist in liver tissue from nonviremic anti-HCV-positive individuals. The same study also reported the detection of HCV RNA by RT-PCR in RNA purified from the same formalin-fixed paraffin-embedded tissue despite the clearance of viremia.[68] Nevertheless, the above data indicate quite clearly that fresh frozen tissue is preferable for the detection of HCV antigens by immunohistochemistry.

Detection of HCV Nonstructural Proteins in the Liver with Nonhuman Antibodies

An early study reported the detection of the HCV antigen encoded by the c100 clone (mainly NS4 and a small region of the carboxy terminus of NS3) using a combination of mouse monoclonal antibodies in unfixed frozen sections from patients with acute and chronic hepatitis C.[69] It was reported that 50–70% of hepatocytes showed cytoplasmic staining in the acute phase, whereas less than 20% were positive in individuals with chronic hepatitis. There was no correlation with cell necrosis or inflammation. Attempts to detect the core and NS3 proteins failed, perhaps due to problems with the monoclonal antibodies, discussed above. In contrast, in another study using frozen sections,[60] NS3 was detected in hepatocytes and B and T lymphocytes with a rabbit anti-peptide (amino acids 1192–1240). The distribution mirrored the detection of E2 described above,[60] and the intracellular staining pattern was similar to the discrete punctate cytoplasmic pattern described above for E2.

The apparent detection of NS4 in formalin-fixed paraffin-embedded samples using a rabbit polyclonal antibody raised to peptide aa 1694–1735 was also reported. A four-layer detection system was developed that appeared to detect the protein in the cytoplasm of 60–90% of hepatocytes in 10 patients with severe chronic hepatitis.[70] In this case, a correlation between the levels of intrahepatic antigen and viral load was noted. However, the protein was virtually undetectable in frozen sections using the same antibody.[60] The same rabbit anti-NS4 peptide was used to examine the distribution of NS4 in formalin-fixed paraffin-embedded samples from liver transplant recipients; 5–20% of the hepatocytes were positive in the cytoplasm of 50% of the patients.[71]

In contrast, a recent study using formalin-fixed paraffin-embedded tissue was only able to detect the occasional NS4-positive cell using a mouse monoclonal antibody (TORDJI-22); in addition to positive hepatocytes, it was noted that endothelial and bile duct epithelial cells were also positive.[72] However, a previous report suggested that this monoclonal antibody generated false-positive reactions,[28] and this has been confirmed subsequently.[73] This latter report suggested that the antibody reacted with hepatocytes that showed ballooning, irrespective of the etiology. Thus, particularly in view of the high proportion of NS4-positive hepatocytes noted in the above reports,[69,70] that contrast with the proportion positive for HCV structural proteins and the nonreproducible nature of NS4 detection in frozen sections, reports on the detection of NS4 in formalin-fixed paraffin-embedded tissue samples should be viewed with some caution.

A rabbit antibody raised to NS5B (aa 2636–2828) detected the protein in 19 of 34 individuals with chronic hepatitis C.[11] The antigen was reputed to show a similar distribution to HCV RNA detected by ISH with a cDNA probe to the core gene region and was localized in the endoplasmic reticulum in a varying proportion of hepatocytes ranging from a diffuse to patchy distribution. Immunoblot analysis of a lysate from a HCV-positive biopsy sample was also positive for NS5B (see below).

The paucity of information related to the detection of the NSP by specific polyclonal or monoclonal antibodies is surprising in view of the success of the human polyclonal antisera that appear to recognize NS3 selectively. This may be related to a lack of cross-reactivity across the genotypes, because the nonstructural proteins are not so highly conserved as the core protein.

Detection of HCV Proteins by Immunoblot

There are two reports of the detection of HCV proteins in lysates prepared from samples of HCV-infected livers; the first reported the detection of a 44-kDa protein using a rabbit antibody to E2.[10] Deglycosylation of the protein with N-glycanase converted the protein to 38-kDa, close to the predicted molecular weight for E2. Because the fully glycosylated form of E2 is reported to be around 70-kDa, it is unclear why a polypeptide of this size was not detected, but this may be related to the antibody that was raised to an unglycosylated form of the protein expressed in *Escherichia coli*.

The second report detected an 84-kDa protein using a rabbit antibody to NS5B.[11] This polypeptide was detected in whole cell lysates and in the microsomal fraction but not the mitochondrial or nuclear fractions of the lysates. Although the electrophoretic mobility of this polypeptide differs to that predicted for NS5B, there are numerous examples of proteins that migrate in an anomalous manner, and this should not be viewed as evidence of nonspecificity, particularly because nothing is known of the expression profiles of HCV proteins in natural infection.

If these reports can be confirmed, then this would suggest that the levels of HCV proteins in the naturally infected liver may be higher than suspected from data generated by RT-PCR analysis to detect the virus genome.

Commentary

In contrast to the detection of the vRNA, the detection of the viral proteins appears to be more reproducible. Surprisingly, the detection of the viral proteins was most successful with human antibodies, and consensus data were accumulated. It is possible that the human antibodies are more successful because they recognize the native forms of the viral proteins more efficiently than hyperimmune antisera raised to recombinant proteins. Nevertheless, antisera to specific proteins, raised in other species, also detected viral proteins.

The specificity of antigen detection was proved beyond a doubt by a combination of controls, including adsorption studies, by the use of serotype-specific antibodies and by the studies that documented the disappearance or appearance of the antigens in patients who were treated with interferon and in those who received a transplanted liver, respectively. In all cases, the viral antigens were detected in the cytoplasm of a proportion of hepatocytes that ranged from ~1% to >20% and in a smaller proportion of lymphocytes and bile duct cells. However, there is only one report[56] on the detection of viral antigen in bile duct cells, and this should be confirmed by others.

It is clear that frozen sections are necessary for the detection of viral antigens by immunohistochemistry. The use of formalin-fixed paraffin-embedded tissue leads to loss of immunoreactivity and appears to result in the nonspecific detection of NS4 through a mechanism that is not clear. The intracellular distribution of the antigens appeared to be in the form of discrete granular staining, as determined by the use of fluorescein-labeled conjugates, whereas enzyme-labeled conjugates showed a lower resolution, and the products were localized within the cytoplasm. Two viral proteins were detected by immunoblot in lysates from HCV-infected liver samples.

These studies agreed that low levels of antigen positive hepatocytes before treatment with interferon correlated with a good response, and in turn this response resulted in a reduced intensity and proportion of HCV antigen-positive hepatocytes. In addition, although it was not unanimous, there was a suggestion that the proportion of infected hepatocytes correlated with the viral load. In contrast, there was no correlation with the degree of hepatocyte injury. This is consistent with immune-mediated injury, and one study demonstrated CD8+ cells in contact with hepatocytes that displayed plasma membrane glycoproteins that are necessary for clearance by the cellular immune response.

EXTRAHEPATIC SITES OF HCV REPLICATION

Studies to examine the distribution of HCV in different tissues and cells have proved extraordinarily difficult due to the low levels of vRNA in the infected carrier and problems with the specific amplification of negative sense HCV RNA by RT-PCR from nucleic acids purified from cell lysates. The strand-specific detection of HCV RNA is fraught with technical difficulties, which were not recognized for some time after the widespread introduction and use of RT-PCR to detect HCV RNA.[74–76] These studies showed that false priming, random priming, or self-priming by cellular RNA resulted in the apparent amplification of negative strands even from in vitro synthesized RNA that contained no negative sense vRNA. Many of these problems have been overcome by the use of RT enzymes that

work at elevated temperatures, coupled with the use of tagged primers.[77] Consequently, early reports of the detection of negative sense HCV RNA as a marker of HCV replication, before the introduction of these innovations, should be viewed with extreme caution. It is vital for individual research workers to validate the negative strand-specific nature of the RT-PCR in their own laboratories, and when this is accomplished, it is possible to achieve a discrimination of around 1×10^4 between the correct and incorrect strands. Equally important, given our newfound understanding of strand-specific RT-PCR, is the need for manuscript reviewers and journal editors to ensure that the methods used to generate data are appropriate. It is clear that this is not happening at present, and this simply confuses the issues for those readers who are unaware of the subtleties of strand-specific RT-PCR and poses an unacceptable burden on readers who do, as they have to read the fine print to ensure that the technology is appropriate. In the following paragraph of this review, I have generally restricted the discussion to manuscripts that addressed these problems and that appear to have used a genuine strand-specific RT-PCR.

Sites Determined by RT-PCR

Some workers have chosen to exhaustively wash the cell population under study (e.g., peripheral blood mononuclear cells [PBMC]) and, having demonstrated that the last wash was negative for HCV RNA by RT-PCR, have concluded that vRNA detected in RNA purified from the cells must have originated from an intracellular site.[78] Although a positive result is suggestive of HCV infection of the cells, this is not conclusive.

Using a strand-specific RT-PCR, it has been documented that negative-strand HCV RNA was detected in the liver, lymph node, bone marrow, pancreas, thyroid, adrenal, and spleen of autopsy samples from individuals who were co-infected with HIV and HCV.[79] The vRNA was most commonly detected in the liver, lymph nodes, and pancreas. A similar study of co-infected individuals from the same authors[80] determined that PBMC were also infected with HCV; this conclusion was based on the detection of negative-strand vRNA in the cells and on the fact that the nucleotide sequence of the 5'UTR, amplified from the PBMC by RT-PCR differed to that amplified from serum, suggesting that the virus in the two sites had evolved independently. It is likely that the widespread extrahepatic distribution of HCV RNA resulted from HIV-associated immunosuppression. Data that are consistent with the detection and replication of HCV RNA resulting from immunosuppression were presented[81] that described the detection of negative sense vRNA in PBMC in immunosuppressed liver transplant recipients. In contrast, vRNA could not be detected in PBMC harvested from HCV patients who were not co-infected with human immunodeficiency virus (HIV) or otherwise immunosuppressed.[82] Similar data were reported by others.[2,83] The latter study[83] suggested that circulating dendritic cells may have been infected.

On the other hand, other studies support the concept that circulating PBMC are infected in the typical HCV carrier.[84,85] The latter study[85] targeted the core gene region for the detection of negative-strand vRNA, as this region was considered to be less structured than the 5′UTR, leading to an increase in specificity of negative-strand detection and highlighted a contrast between the detection of negative-strand vRNA in 75% of liver samples but only in 8% of PBMC samples. Genetic diversity between vRNA nucleotide sequences amplified from serum, PBMC, and liver was also interpreted to mean that HCV could infect PBMC[86]; although this study did not use negative strand-specific RT-PCR, the PBMC were thoroughly washed and then digested with trypsin, before extraction and purification of the total RNA from the cells, to ensure that any blood-derived virus particles, which were nonspecifically bound to the plasma membrane, were removed.

A study to compare HCV RNA in PBMC in acute and chronic hepatitis C determined that vRNA was undetected during acute infection[87]; on the other hand, 12 of 48 patients with chronic hepatitis C infection were positive for vRNA in PBMC, and although 6 of 12 were reported to contain negative sense vRNA, the assay was not strand specific. However, 5 of 12 patients who had detectable levels of vRNA in the PBMC were reported to be negative for vRNA in the serum, and as a result it is difficult to argue that the PBMC were simply contaminated with blood-derived virus. There may be technical reasons to explain this dichotomy, but the phenomenon (serum negative, PBMC positive) has been reported previously.[88,89] One of these studies[88] also reported that the core protein was detected in the cytoplasm rather than the plasma membrane of monocytes but was undetected in lymphocytes of 3 of 11 patients as determined by fluorescein activated cell sorter (FACS) analysis of permeabilized PBMC.

These conflicting data make it difficult to determine if HCV truly infects PBMC. In an effort to resolve this issue, SCID mice were inoculated with PBMC derived from HCV carriers and the serum and blood cell fraction examined for HCV RNA over several weeks.[90] There was concordance between the detection of positive sense vRNA in the serum and positive and negative sense vRNA in the cells of those mice that were HCV RNA-positive 8 weeks after inoculation, leading to the conclusion that the virus was able to replicate in the PBMC during this time.

In conclusion, the conflicting data may result from true differences in PBMC infection by different geno-types, samples taken from patients at different stages in the disease process, and differences in the sensitivity of the RT-PCR, particularly for the detection of negative sense vRNA. The data suggest at least that the virus can infect PBMC, but the level of replication is extremely low.

Extrahepatic Replication as Detected by Examination In Situ

An alternative explanation for the above conflicting results is that the proportion of PBMC infected is low. Several groups have attempted to address this point by ISH or in situ -PCR examination of PBMC from carriers. One study,[91] which used ISH with RNA probes to detect positive or negative sense vRNA in the 5′UTR, appeared to detect vRNA in 0.01–0.03% of cells, a figure that rose to 0.3% after the cells were stimulated with phytohaemaglutinin (PHA). However, the cells were not subjected to a denaturation step before hybridization, which may be necessary to melt the highly structured nature of the 5′UTR (see above). In a similar study in which the cells were subjected to a denaturation step, PBMC from 6 of 11 viremic patients were reported to be positive for either HCV antigens or HCV RNA.[92] Approximately 0.15–1% of the cells derived from bone marrow or PBMC were positive in the macrophage/mononuclear B- and T-cell populations. Positive and negative sense vRNA were detected in the cells using two pairs of DIG-labeled oligodeoxynucleotide probes (45nt) representing the 5′UTR and the 5′UTR/core region, respectively. Denaturation of the cells was necessary for detection of the vRNA, but in an unusual finding, it was reported that the negative strand signal was stronger than that of the positive strand. This is unusual and leads to some concern over the specificity that was discussed more fully above. A study using in situ PCR to examine the prevalence of HCV RNA in PBMC reported that 0.2–0.8% of cells in 14 of 28 HCV patients were positive; incorporation of the fluorescein-labeled primers into amplicons within the cells was determined by immunofluoresence microscopy or FACS.[93] A conventional strand-specific RT-PCR using tagged primers on RNA extracted from the cells detected negative sense vRNA in 12 of 14 samples that were shown to contain HCV RNA by in situ PCR.[93] Collectively, the data suggest PBMC infection by HCV, but the level and proportion of infected cells is likely to be very low.

Localization of HCV Antigens in Cryoglobulinemia

Persistent infection with HCV is often associated with nonhepatic diseases,[94] including HCV-related mixed cryoglobulinemia. The HCV core NS3 and NS4 antigens were detected in small blood vessels in the skin (and in the cytoplasm of hepatocytes) in patients with mixed cryoglobulinemia using a range of monoclonal antibodies.[95] The detection of these proteins in the skin was not thought to represent virus replication in this site but rather immune deposits. The source of the nonstructural proteins that are necessary for virus replication and are normally intracellular is unknown, but it is possible that HCV-infected lysed cells were the source. This report awaits confirmation. An additional report from the same authors, which examined lymph nodes in HCV carriers with type II mixed cryoglobulinemia, also detected the core NS3 and NS4 proteins in lymphoid cells of the interfollicular areas and in circulating mononuclear cells of capsular blood vessels. It was suggested that HCV infection precedes neoplastic transformation, and consequently HCV may have a role in the development of lymphoma.[96]

A similar study of patients with cryoglobulinemia using ISH detected vRNA in association with inflamed blood vessels and in the epidermis of six patients who were HCV RNA positive in the serum but not in patients with cryoglobulinemia who were HCV RNA negative.[97] However, although it was reported that negative strand vRNA was detected in two patients with the highest level of viremia, it was suggested that the detection of the vRNA did not represent replication in this site but complexes formed in situ. Thus, these data can only be regarded as preliminary and also require confirmation. A recent study[98] was unable to detect negative sense HCV RNA by RT-PCR in skin samples from carriers with lichen ruber planus or cutaneous vasculitis, and consequently it is most unlikely that the virus replicates in any skin cells.

Commentary

Technical problems related to the detection of negative-strand HCV RNA have hindered progress to determine extrahepatic sites of replication. However, these problems have now been overcome, and recent data, generated using recognized strand-specific protocols, can now be regarded as reliable. Negative-strand RNA was detected in a range of tissue samples from HCV carriers who were co-infected with HIV and most commonly in liver, PBMC, lymph nodes, and pancreas, and it is likely that these sites support HCV replication. Whether the same tissues are infected in patients who are not HIV co-infected is still unclear.

Considerable effort has been expended to determine if PBMC are infected with HCV. A number of studies have simply washed the cells, shown that the last wash was negative for HCV RNA, and then concluded that the cells were infected on the basis of the detection of vRNA in the cell lysate. This is suggestive but

not ideal. Similarly, trypsin treatment of the cells to remove virus attached to the cell surface in a nonspecific manner is also not conclusive, unless proof is available that the tryspin has removed cell surface molecules (e.g., CD4, CD19, etc).

Nevertheless, RT-PCR analysis from several studies suggests that PBMC are infected, and reports of HCV RNA-positive PBMC in the absence of HCV viremia are intriguing. Although a corollary of these data are to assume problems with PCR contamination, several reports support this concept, and because there is acceptance that both HBV and HCV can persist in the liver in individuals who have apparently recovered from infection, it is possible that virus persistence is equally possible in other cell types.

However, the data pertaining to HCV infection of PBMC derived by ISH are still equivocal, and consequently the proportion of infected cells cannot be estimated accurately at this stage. A study using in situ PCR followed by microscopy or FACS analysis suggested that less than 1% of cells were infected, but this study needs to be confirmed. This is also true of the data related to the detection of viral antigens and RNA in lymph nodes and skin. However, given the cumulative viral load over the years in HCV carriers, most of whom respond immunologically to the virus proteins, it would not be unusual to find viral antigens in the lymph nodes.

Acknowledgments: I thank Professor E. G. Westaway and Dr. David Warrilow for helpful discussions and critical reading of the manuscript. The figure was prepared by Sandra Goodwin and Dr. W. B. Lott, and I am grateful for this contribution. Sandra Goodwin also collated the references.

ABBREVIATIONS

ALT	alanine aminotransferase
BVDV	bovine viral diarrhea virus
DIG	digoxygenin
FACS	fluorescence activated cell sorter
FITC	fluorescein isothiocyanate
HAI	histologic activity index
HBV	hepatitis B virus
HCC	hepatocellular carcinoma
HCV	hepatitis C virus
HRPO	horseradish peroxidase
IRES	internal ribosome entry site
ISH	in situ hybridization
PBMC	peripheral blood mononuclear cells
RF	replicative form
RI	replicative intermediate
RT-PCR	reverse transcriptase polymerase chain reaction
UTR	untranslated region
vRNA	viral RNA

REFERENCES

1. Agnello V, Abel G, Knight GB, Muchmore E. Detection of widespread hepatocyte infection in chronic hepatitis C. Hepatology 1998;28:573–584

2. Lanford RE, Cahvez D, Chisari FV, Sureau C. Lack of detection of negative-strand hepatitis C virus RNA in peripheral blood mononuclear cells and other extrahepatic tissues by the highly strand-specific rTth reverse transcriptase PCR. J Virol 1995;69: 8079–8083

3. Burleson FG, Chambers TM, Wiedbrauk DL. Virology: A Laboratory Manual. San Diego: Academic Press:

4. White DO, Fenner FJ. Viral Replication in Medical Virology, 4th ed. San Diego: Academic Press, 1994

5. Gong Y, Trowbridge R, Macnaughton TB, Westaway EG, Shannon AD, Gowans EJ. Characterisation of RNA synthesis during a one-step growth curve and of the replication mechanism of bovine viral diarrhea virus. J Gen Virol 1996;77:2729–2236

6. Neumann AU, Lam NP, Dahari H, Gretch DR, Wiley TE, Layden TJ, Perelson AS. Hepatitis C viral dyanamics in vivo and the antiviral effect of interferon-alfa therapy. Science 1998;282: 103–107

7. Choo Q-L, Kuo G, Weiner AJ, Overby LR, Bradley DW, Houghton M. Isolation of a cDNA clone derived from a bloodborne non-A, non-B viral hepatitis genome. Science 1989;244: 359–362

8. Kolykhalov AA, Agapov EV, Blight KJ, Mihalik K, Feinstone SM, Rice CM. Transmission of hepatitis C by intrahepatic inoculation with transcribed RNA. Science 1997;277:570–574

9. Negro F, Krawczynski K, Quadri R, Rubbia-Brandt L, Mondelli M, Zarski J-P, Hadengue A. Detection of genomic- and minus-strand of hepatitis C virus RNA in the liver of chronic hepatitis C patients by strand-specific semiquantitative reverse-transcriptase polymerase chain reaction. Hepatology 1999;29:536–542

10. Nakamoto Y, Kaneko S, Honda M, Unoura M, Cheong J, Harada A, Matsushima K, Kobayashi K, Murakami S. Detection of the putative E2 protein of hepatitis C virus in human liver. J Med Virol 1994;42:374–379

11. Tsutsumi M, Urashima S, Takada A, Date T, Tanaka Y. Detection of antigens related to hepatitis C virus RNA encoding the NS5 region in the livers of patients with chronic type C hepatitis. Hepatology 1994;19:265–272

12. Blight KJ, Gowans EJ. In situ hybridization and immunohistochemical staining of hepatitis C virus products. Viral Hepat Rev 1995;1:143–155

13. Lau JYN, Krawczynski K, Negro F, Gonzalez-Peralta RP. In situ detection of hepatitis C virus—a critical review. J Hepatol 1996; 24(Suppl 2):43–51

14. Scheuer PJ, Krawczynski K, Dhillon AP. Histopathology and detection of hepatitis C virus in liver. Semin Immunopathol 1997;19:27–45

15. Negro F. Detection of hepatitis C virus RNA in liver tissue: an overview. Ital J Gastroenterol Hepatol 1998;30:205–210

16. Brahic M, Haase AT. Detection of viral sequences of low reiteration frequency by in situ hybridization. Proc Natl Acad Sci USA 1978;75:6125–6129

17. Gerhardt GS, Kawasaki ES, Bancroft FC, Szabo P. Localization of a unique gene by direct hybridization in situ. Proc Natl Acad Sci USA 1981;78:3755–3759

18. Gowans EJ, Jilbert AR, Burrell CJ. Detection of specific DNA and RNA sequences in tissues and cells by in situ hybridization. In: RH Symons, ed. Nucleic Acid Probes. Boca Raton, FL: CRC Press, 1989; pp. 139–158

19. Khromykh AA, Westaway EG. Subgenomic replicons of the Flavivirus Kunjin: construction and applications. J Virol 1997;71: 1497–1505

20. Honda M, Rijnbrand R, Abell G, Kim D, Lemon SM. Natural variation in translational activities of the 5′nontranslated RNAs of hepatitis C virus genotypes 1a and 1b: evidence for a long-range RNA-RNA interaction outside of the internal ribosome entry site. J Virol 1999;73:4941–4951

21. Wang C, Le SY, Ali N, Siddiqui A. An RNA pseudoknot is an essential structural element of the internal ribosome entry site located with the hepatitis C virus 5′noncoding region. RNA 1995;1:526–537

22. Lau JYN, Davis GL. Detection of hepatitis C virus RNA genome in liver tissue by non-isotopic in situ hybridization. J Med Virol 1994;42: 268–271

23. Lamas E, Baccarini P, Housset C, Kremsdorf D, Brechot C. Detection of hepatitis C virus (HCV) RNA sequences in liver tissue by in situ hybridization. J Hepatol 1992;16:219–223

24. Tanaka Y, Enomoto N, Kojima S, Tang L, Goto M, Marumo F, Sato C. Detection of hepatitis C virus RNA in the liver by in situ hybridization. Liver 1993;13:203–208

25. Yamada G, Nishimoto H, Endou H, et al. Localization of hepatitis C viral RNA and capsid protein in human liver. Dig Dis Sci 1993;38:882–887

26. Gastaldi M, Massacrier A, Planells R, et al. Detection by in situ hybridization of hepatitis C virus positive and negative RNA strands using digoxigenin-labeled cRNA probes in human liver cells. J Hepatol 1995;23:509–518

27. Blight K, Trowbridge R, Rowland R, Gowans E. Detection of hepatitis C virus RNA by in situ hybridization. Liver 1992;12: 286–289

28. Komminoth P, Adams V, Long AA, Roth J, Saremaslani P, Flury R, Schmid M, Heitz PhU. Evaluation of methods for hepatitis C virus detection in archival liver biopsies. Path Res Pract 1994; 190:1017–1025

29. Nouri Aria KT, Sallie R, Sangar D, Alexander GJM, Smith H, Byrne J, Portmann B, Eddleston ALWF, Williams R. Detection of genomic and intermediate replicative strands of hepatitis C virus in liver tissue by in situ hybridization. J Clin Invest 1993; 91:2226–2234

30. Loriot M-A, Bronowicki J-P, Lagorce D, et al. Permissiveness of human biliary epithelial cells to infection by hepatitis C virus. Hepatology 1999;29:1587–1595

31. Endo H, Yamada G, Nakane PK, Tsuji T. Localization of hepatitis C virus RNA in human liver biopsies by in situ hybridization using thymine-thymine dimerized oligo DNA probes: improved method. Acta Med Okayama 1992;46:355–364

32. Haruna Y, Hayashi N, Hiramatsu N, Takehara T, Hagiwara H, Sasaki Y, Kasahara A, Fusamoto H, Kamada T. Detection of hepatitis C virus RNA in liver tissues by an in situ hybridization technique. J Hepatol 1993;18:96–100

33. Negro F, Pacchioni D, Shimizu Y, Miller RH, Bussolati G, Purcell RH, Bonino F. Detection of intrahepatic replication of hepatitis C virus RNA by in situ hybridization and comparison with histopathology. Proc Natl Acad Sci USA 1992;89:2247–2251

34. Gosvalez J, Rodriguez-Inigo E, Ramiro-Diaz JL, Bartolome J, Tomas JF , Oliva H, Carreno V. Relative quantitation and mapping of hepatitis C virus by in situ hybridization and digital image analysis. Hepatology 1998;27:1428–1434

35. Rodriguez-Inigo E, Bartolome J, deLucas S, Manzarbeitia F, Pardo M, Arocena C, Gosalvez J, Oliva H, Carreno V. Histological damage in chronic hepatitis C is not related to the extent of infection in the liver. Am J Pathol 1999;154:1877–1881

36. Nuovo GJ, Kidonnici K, MacConnell P, Lane B. Intracellular localization of polymerase chain reaction (PCR)-amplified hepatitis C cDNA. Am J Surg Pathol 1993;17:683–690

37. Lau GKK, Fang JWS, Wu PC, Davis GL, Lau JYN. Detection of hepatitis C virus genome in formalin-fixed paraffin-embedded liver tissue by in situ reverse transcription polymerase chain reaction. J Med Virol 1994;44:406–409

38. Lau GKK, Davis GL, Wu SPC, Gish RG, Balart LA, Lau JYN. Hepatitic expression of hepatitis C virus RNA in chronic hepatitis C: a study by in situ reverse-transcription polymerase chain reaction. Hepatol 1996;23:1318–1323

39. Walker FM, Dazza M-C, Dauge M-C, Boucher O, Bedel OC, Henin D, Lehy T. Detection and localization by in situ molecular biology techniques and immunohistochemistry of hepatitis C virus in livers of chronically infected patients. J Histochem Cytochem 1998;46:653–660

40. Muratori L. in situ reverse transcriptase-polymerase chain reaction: an innovative tool for hepatitis C virus RNA detection and localization, and for quantification of infected cells. Eur J Histochem 1998;42:133–136

41. Sansonno D, Cornacchiulo V, Racanelli V, Dammacco F. in situ simultaneous detection of hepatitis C virus RNA and hepatitis C virus-related antigens in hepatocellular carcinoma. Cancer 1997;80:22–33

42. Ohishi M, Sakisaka S, Harada M, et al. Detection of hepatitis-C virus and hepatitis-C virus replication in hepatocellular carcinoma by in situ hybridization. Scand J Gastroenterol 1999; 34:432–438

43. Tang L, Tanaka Y, Enomoto N, Marumo F, Sato C. Detection of hepatitis C virus RNA in hepatocellular carcinoma by in situ hybridization. Cancer 1995;76:2211–2216

44. Ohsawa M, Itomita Y, Hashimoto M, Kanno H, Aozasa K. Hepatitis C viral genome in a subset of primary hepatitic lymphomas. Mod Pathol 1998;11:471–478

45. Booth PJ, Stevens DA, Collins ME, Brownlie J. Detection of bovine viral diarrhea virus antigen and RNA in oviduct and granulosa cells of persistently infected cattle. J Reprod Fertil 1995;105:17–24

46. Desport M, Collins ME, Brownlie J. Detection of bovine virus diarrhea virus RNA by in situ hybridization with digoxigenin-labelled riboprobes. Intervirology 1994;37:269–276

47. Gowans EJ, Burrell CJ, Jilbert AR, Marmion BP. Cytoplasmic (but not nuclear) hepatitis B virus (HBV) core antigen reflects HBV DNA synthesis at the level of the infected hepatocyte. Intervirology 1996;24:220–225

48. Westaway EG. Flavivirus replication strategy. Adv Virus Res 1987;33:45–90

49. Westaway EG, Khromykh AA, Mackenzie JM. Nascent flavivirus RNA colocalized in situ with double-stranded RNA in stable replication complexes. Virology 1999;258:108–117

50. Westaway EG, Mackenzie JM, Kenney MT, Jones MK, Khromykh AA. Ultrastructure of Kunjin virus-infected cells: colocalization of NS1 and NS3 with double-stranded RNA, and of NS2B with NS3, in virus-induced membrane structures. J Virol 1997;71:6650–6661

51. Barba G, Harper F, Harada T, et al. Hepatitis C virus core protein shows a cytoplasmic localization and associates to cellular lipid storage droplets. Proc Natl Acad Sci USA 1997;94:1200–1205

52. Harlow E, Lane D. Antibodies: A Laboratory Manual. New York: Cold Spring Harbor Laboratory, 1988

53. Krawczynski K, Beach MJ, Bradley DW, et al. Hepatitis C virus antigens in hepatocytes: Immunomorphologic detection and identification. Gastroenterology 1992;103:622–629

54. Di Bisceglie AM, Hoofnagle JH, Krawczynski K. Changes in hepatitis C virus antigen in liver with antiviral therapy. Gastroenterology 1993;105:858–862

55. Vargas V, Krawczynski K, Castells L, Martinez N, Esteban J, Allende H, Esteban R, Guardia J. Recurrent hepatitis C virus infection after liver transplantation: immunohistochemical assessment of the viral antigen. Liver Transplant Surg 1998;4: 320–327

56. Nouri-Aria KT, Sallie R, Mizokami M, Portmann BC, Williams R. Intrahepatic expression of hepatitis C virus antigens in chronic liver disease. J Pathol 1995;175:77–83

57. Ballardini G, Groff P, Pontisso P, Giostra F, Francesconi R, Lenzi M, Zauli D, Alberti A, Bianchi FB. Hepatitis C virus (HCV) genotype, tissue HCV antigens, hepatocellular expression of HLA-A, B, C, and intercellular adhesion-1 molecules. J Clin Invest 1995;95:2067–2075

58. Ballardini G, Groff P, Giostra F, Francesconi R, Miniero R, Ghetti S, Zauli D, Bianchi FB. Hepatocellular codistribution of c100, c33, c22 and NS5 hepatitis C virus antigens detected by using immunopurified polyclonal spontaneous human antibodies. Hepatol 1995;21:730–734

59. Gane EJ, Naoumov MB, Qian K-P, Mondelli MU, Maertens G, Portmann BC, Lau JYN, Williams R. A longitudinal analysis of hepatitis C virus replication following liver transplantation. Gastroenterology 1996;110:167–177

60. Blight K, Lesniewski RR, LaBrooy JT, Gowans EJ. Detection and distribution of hepatitis C-specific antigens in naturally infected liver. Hepatology 1994;20:553–557

61. Hiramatsu N, Hayashi N, Haruna Y, Kasahara A, Fusamoto H, Mori C, Fuke I, Okayama H, Kamada T. Immunohistochemical detection of hepatitis C virus-infected hepatocytes in chronic liver disease with monoclonal antibodies to core, envelope and NS3 regions of the hepatitis C virus genome. Hepatology 1992;16:306–311

62. Haruna Y, Hayashi N, Kamada T, Hytiroglou P, Thung SN, Gerber MA. Expression of hepatitis C virus in hepatocellular carcinoma. Cancer 1994;73:2253–2258

63. Blight K, Lesniewski R, LaBrooy J, Trowbridge R, Gowans EJ. Localization of hepatitis C virus proteins in infected liver tissue by immunofluorescence. Gastroenterol Japon 1993;28(Suppl 5): 55–58

64. Selby MJ, Choo Q-L, Berger K, et al. Expression, identification and subcellular localization of the proteins encoded by the hepatitis C viral genome. J Gen Virol 1993;74:1103–1113

65. Yap S-H, Willems M, Van den Oord J, et al. Detection of hepatitis C virus antigen by immuno-histochemical staining: a histological marker of hepatitis C virus infection. J Hepatol 1994;20: 275–281

66. Gonzalez-Peralta RP, Fang JWS, Davis GL, et al. Optimization for the detection of hepatitis C virus antigens in the liver. J Hepatol 1994;20:143–147

67. Gonzalez-Peralta RP, Fang JWS, Davis GL, et al. Significance of hepatic expression of hepatitis C viral antigens in chronic hepatitis C. Dig Dis Sci 1995;40:2595–2601

68. Dries V, Von Both I, Muller M, et al. Detection of hepatitis C virus in paraffin-embedded liver biopsies of patients negative for viral RNA in serum. Hepatology 1999;29:223–229

69. Sansonno D, Dammacco F. Hepatitis C virus c100 antigen in liver tissue from patients with acute and chronic infection. Hepatol 1993;18:240–245

70. Blight K, Rowland R, Hall PM, Lesniewski RR, Trowbridge R, LaBrooy JT, Gowans EJ. Immunohistochemical detection of the NS4 antigen of hepatitis C virus and its relation to histopathology. Am J Pathol 1993;143:1568–1573

71. Gretch DR, Bacchi CE, Corey L, et al. Persistent hepatitis C virus infection after liver transplantation: clinical and virological features. Hepatol 1995;22:1–9

72. Brody RI, Eng S, Melamed J, et al. Immunohistochemical detection of hepatitis C antigen by monoclonal antibody TORDJI-22 compared with PCR viral detection. Anat Pathol 1998;110: 32–37

73. Doughty AL, Painter DM, McCaughan GW. Nonspecificity of monoclonal antibody Tordji-22 for the detection of hepatitis C virus in liver transplant recipients with cholestatic hepatitis. Liver Transplant Surg 1999;5:40–45

74. Willems M, Moshage H, Yap SH. PCR and detection of negative HCV RNA strands. Hepatol 1993;17:526

75. McGuinness P, Bishop GA, McCaughan GW, Trowbridge R,

Gowans EJ. False detection of negative strand hepatitis C RNA. Lancet 1994;343:551–552

76. Lanford RE, Sureau C, Jacob JR, White R, Fuerst T. Demonstration of in vitro infection of chimpanzee hepatocytes with hepatitis C virus using strand specific RT-PCR. Virology 1994; 202:606–614

77. Sangar DV, Carroll AR. A tale of two strands:reverse transcriptase polymerase chain reaction detection of hepatitis C virus replication. Hepatology 1998;28:1173–1176

78. Zehender G, Meroni L, De Maddalena C, Varchetta S, Monti G, Galli MK. Detection of hepatitis C virus RNA in CD19 peripheral blood mononuclear cells of chronically infected individuals. J Infect Dis 1997;176:1209–1214

79. Laskus T, Radkowski M, Wang L-F, Vargas H, Rakela J. Search for hepatitis C virus extrahepatic replication sites in patients with acquired immune deficiency syndrome: specific detection of negative-strand viral RNA in various tissues. Hepatol 1998;28:1398–1401

80. Laskus T, Radkowski M, Wang L-F, Jang SJ, Vargas H, Rakela J. Hepatitis C virus quasispecies in patients infected with HIV-1: correlation with extrahepatic viral replication. Virology 1998; 248:164–171

81. Radkowski M, Wang L-F, Vargas HE, Rakela J, Laskus T. Detection of hepatitis C virus replication in peripheral blood mononuclear cells after orthotopic liver transplantation. Transplantation 1998;66:664–666

82. Laskus T, Radkowski M, Wang L-F, Cianciara J, Vargas H, Rakela J. Hepatitis C virus negative strand RNA is not detected in peripheral blood mononuclear cells and viral sequences are identical to those in serum: a case against extrahepatic replication. J Gen Virol 1997;78:2747–2750

83. Mellor J, Haydon G, Blair C, Livingstone W, Simmonds P. Low level or absent in vivo replication of hepatitis C virus and hepatitis G virus/GB virus C in peripheral blood mononuclear cells. J Gen Virol 1998;79:705–714

84. Maggi F, Fornai C, Vatteroni ML, et al. Differences in hepatitis C virus quasispecies composition between liver, peripheral blood mononuclear cells and plasma. J Gen Virol 1997;79: 1521–1525

85. Lerat H, Berby F, Trabaud MA, Vidalin O, Major M, Trepo C, and Inchauspe G. Specific detection of hepatitis C virus minus-strand RNA in hematopoietic cells. J Clin Invest 1996;97: 845–851

86. Navas S, Martin JH, Quiroga JA, Catillo I, Carreno V. Genetic diverstiy and tissue compartmentalization of the hepatitis C virus genome in blood mononuclear cells, liver, and serum from chronic hepatitis C patients. J Virol 1998;72:1640–1646

87. Chang T-T, Young K-C, Yang Y-J, Lei H-Y, Wu H-L. Hepatitis C virus RNA in peripheral blood mononuclear cells: comparing acute and chronic hepatitis C virus infection. Hepatol 1996;23: 977–981

88. Bouffard P, Hayashi PH, Acevedo R, Levy N, Zeldis JB. Hepatitis C virus is detected in a monocyte/macrophage subpopulation of peripheral blood mononuclear cells of infected patients. J Infect Dis 1992;166:1276–1280

89. Muratori L, Giostra F, Cataleta M, et al. Testing for hepatitis C virus sequences in peripheral blood mononuclear cells of patients with chronic hepatitis C in the absence of serum hepatitis C virus RNA. Liver 1994;14:124–128

90. Bronowicki J-P, Loriot M-A, Thiers V, Grignon Y, Zignego AL and Brechot C. Hepatitis C virus persistence in human hematopoietic cells injected into SCID mice. Hepatology 1998; 28:211–218

91. Moldvay J, Deny P, Pol S, Brechot C, Lamas E. Detection of hepatitis C virus RNA in peripheral blood mononuclear cells of infected patients by in situ hybridization. Blood 1994;83:2 69–273

92. Sansonno D, Iacobelli AR, Cornacchiulo V, Iodice G, Dammacco F. Detection of hepatitis C virus (HCV) proteins by immunofluorescence and HCV RNA genomic sequences by non-isotopic in situ hybridization in bone marrow and peripheral blood mononuclear cells of chronically HCV-infected patients. Clin Exp Immunol 1996;103:414–421

93. Muratori L, Gibellini D, Lenzi M, Cataleta M, Muratori P, Morelli MC, Bianchi FB. Quantification of hepatitis C virus-infected peripheral blood mononuclear cells by in situ reverse transcriptase-polymerase chain reaction. Blood 1996;7: 2768–2774

94. Hadziyannis S. Nonhepatic manifestations and combined diseases in HCV infection. Dig Dis Sci 1996;41(Suppl):63S–74S

95. Sansonno D, Cornacchiulo V, Iacobelli AR, De Stefano R, Lospalluti M, Dammacco F. Localization of hepatitis C virus antigens in liver and skin tissues of chronic hepatitis C virus-infected patients with mixed cryoglobulinemia. Hepatol 1995;21: 305–312

96. Sansonno D, De Vita S, Cornacchiulo V, Carbone A, Boiocchi M, Dammacco F. Detection and distribution of hepatitis C virus-related proteins in lymph nodes of patients with type II mixed cryoglobulinemia and neoplasia or non-neoplastic lymphoproliferation. Blood 1996;88:4638–4645

97. Agnello V, Abel G. Localization of hepatitis C virus in cutaneous vasculitic lesions in patients with type II cryoglobulinemia. Arthritis Rheum 1997;40:2007–2015

98. Mangra A, Andriulli A, Zenarola P, Lomuto M, Cascavilla I, Quadri R, Negro F. Lack of hepatitis C virus replication intermediate RNA in diseased skin tissue of chronic hepatitis C patients. J Med Virol 1999;59:277–280

Clinical Significance of Hepatitis C Virus Genotypes and Quasispecies

PATRIZIA FARCI, M.D.[1] and ROBERT H. PURCELL, M.D.[2]

ABSTRACT: *Hepatitis C virus (HCV) is a major cause of morbidity and mortality worldwide. The infection becomes chronic in about 85% of infected individuals, in the face of a strong humoral and cellular immune response. One of the most important features of HCV is its high degree of genetic variability, which is due to the inherent low fidelity of the viral replication machinery. As a consequence, HCV circulates in vivo as a population of divergent, albeit closely related, genomes exhibiting a distribution that follows the model referred to as a quasispecies. The genetic variability of HCV is complex and has been classified into four hierarchical strata: genotypes, subgenotypes, isolates, and quasispecies. Over the past few years, an extraordinary interest has been focused on the biologic and clinical implications of the genetic variability of HCV. Although there is consensus that the genotypes may influence the out come of antiviral therapy, their clinical significance in the natural history of the disease, as well as in transmission, infectivity, and pathogenesis of HCV infection, remains elusive. Conversely, evidence has accumulated that the quasispecies nature of HCV provides a large reservoir of biologically different viral variants that may have important clinical implications for viral persistence by immune escape mechanisms, for the generation of antiviral drug resistance, and for the development of an effective vaccine. This article reviews the state of the art on the biologic and clinical implications of the genetic variability of HCV.*

KEY WORDS: hepatitis C virus, genetic variability, genotypes, quasispecies, clinical implications

Hepatitis C virus (HCV) is an important public health problem because it is a major cause of chronic hepatitis, cirrhosis, and hepatocellular carcinoma (HCC) worldwide.[1-3] Currently, HCV-related end-stage liver disease is the leading indication for orthotopic liver transplantation.[4] The most striking feature of this virus is its ability to induce chronic infection in at least 85% of infected individuals.[5-7] Prospective studies of posttransfusion and community-acquired hepatitis C have provided unique cohorts of patients with long-term follow-up, which have been instrumental in unraveling the natural history of the disease, and in elucidating the

---

Objectives
Upon completion of this article, the reader will understand: 1) the mechanisms behind the genetic variability of the HCV genome; 2) the difference between viral genotypes and HCV quasispecies; and 3) the clinical implications of genotypes and HCV quasispecies.

Accreditation
The Indiana University School of Medicine is accredited by the Accreditation Council for Continuing Medical Education to sponsor continuing medical education for physicians. The Indiana University School of Medicine takes responsibility for the contents, quality, and scientific integrity of this activity.

Credit
The Indiana University School of Medicine designates this educational activity for a maximum of 1.0 hours credit toward the AMA Physicians Recognition Award in category one. Each physician should claim only those hours of credit that he/she actually spent in the educational activity.

Disclosure
Statements have been obtained regarding the authors' relationships with financial supporters of this activity. There is no apparent conflict of interest related to the context of participation of the author of this article.

From the [1]Department of Medical Sciences, University of Cagliari, Italy, and [2]Hepatitis Viruses Section, Laboratory of Infectious Diseases, National Institute of Allergy and Infectious Diseases, National Institutes of Health, Bethesda, Maryland.

Reprint requests: Dr. P. Farci, Department of Medical Sciences, University of Cagliari, Via S. Giorgio 12, 09124 Cagliari, Italy. E-mail: farcip@pacs.unica.it

molecular events associated with acute and chronic HCV infection. Chronic hepatitis C is associated with continuous viral replication in vivo, as documented in some cases for more than 20 years.[8] The clinical course of chronic hepatitis C is usually indolent and subclinical.[9,10] In some patients, however, the disease may be rapidly progressive, leading to liver-related death within 6 years after primary infection.[6] Prospective studies failed to identify any clinical, serologic, or virologic features that predict the outcome of the disease.[11,12] Although HCV infection progresses to chronicity in most cases, about 15% of patients experience an acute self-limited hepatitis associated with viral clearance and recovery.[2,5,6] The immunologic correlates of HCV clearance are still undefined.

Clinical and experimental studies conducted both before and after the discovery of HCV suggested that natural HCV infection does not induce protective immunity in the host. Cross-challenge studies demonstrated that convalescent chimpanzees could be reinfected several times with either homologous or heterologous HCV strains, each time showing histopathologic evidence of acute hepatitis.[13–15] The risk of developing chronic HCV infection was in this setting similar to that observed after primary infection. Evidence that HCV may cause more than one episode of acute hepatitis C in the same individual came from the analysis of multiply transfused β-thalassemic children.[16] The second episodes of acute hepatitis were clinically indistinguishable from the first and, as seen in the chimpanzee model, were associated in most cases with the development of chronic hepatitis. Superinfection with heterologous HCV strains, documented both in humans[17] and in chimpanzees[18] chronically infected with HCV, provided additional evidence that HCV is unable to induce protective immunity.

The mechanisms responsible for the lack of protective immunity elicited by natural or experimental HCV infection are at present unknown. The study of the role of host factors, such as inefficient cellular or humoral immune responses, or viral factors, such as the ability of the virus to use effective mechanisms of immune evasion, has been an area of intensive investigation over the past few years. However, the observation of vigorous humoral and cellular immune responses during the acute and chronic phases of HCV infection, including specific anti-envelope antibodies[19] and multispecific cytotoxic T lymphocytes (CTL),[20,21] suggests that viral factors may play a key role in HCV persistence. Similar to other RNA viruses, HCV is characterized by a high degree of genetic variability. Over the past few years, evidence has accumulated that the genetic variation of HCV may be implicated as a mechanism of viral persistence. This review explores the biologic implications of the viral antigenic variation, with particular emphasis on the quasispecies nature of HCV and its clinical relevance in the pathogenesis, therapy, and prevention of HCV infection.

GENETIC VARIABILITY OF THE HCV GENOME

HCV is a spherical enveloped virus, approximately 50 nm in diameter,[22] which has been classified within a third genus (*Hepacivirus*) of the *Flaviviridae* family.[23] The viral genome is a single-stranded linear RNA of positive sense. It is approximately 9.6 kb in size and contains a single open reading frame (ORF) bracketed by 5′and 3′ noncoding (NC) regions.[24] The 5′ NC region consists of approximately 340 nucleotides, forms a stem-loop structure, and contains an internal ribosomal entry site.[25] Immediately downstream of the 5′ NC region is the single large ORF of approximately 9,000 nucleotides encoding a polyprotein precursor of 3,010–3,033 amino acids that is cotranslationally or posttranslationally cleaved into separate proteins by a combination of host and viral proteases. The structural proteins, which include the capsid protein (core), two envelope proteins (E1 and E2), and possibly a small protein of unknown function (P7) are at the 5′ end, followed by at least six nonstructural (NS) proteins (NS2, NS3, NS4A, NS4B, NS5A, and NS5B). The 3′ NC region consists of approximately 50 nucleotides, a polypyrimidine tract, and a recently discovered highly conserved terminal sequence of approximately 100 nucleotides.[26] Like the 5′ NC region, the 3′ NC region is thought to have considerable secondary structure.

Similar to other RNA viruses, HCV is characterized by a high degree of genetic heterogeneity,[27] resulting from the fact that the viral RNA polymerase lacks a proof-reading 3′–5′ exonuclease activity,[28] which is an important repair mechanism. For HCV, the rate of nucleotide misincorporation by the viral RNA polymerase has been calculated to be approximately 10^{-3} to 10^{-4} base substitutions per genome site per year[29,30] (Fig. 1). Thus, HCV shares with other RNA viruses a high mutation rate, which is often 1,000 to 1,000,000-fold greater than the mutation rate of DNA viruses.[28] For some RNA viruses, the mutation rate appears to be near the maximum that can be tolerated without catastrophic loss of genetic information.[31] Furthermore, many RNA virus genomes appear to tolerate the replacement of more than half of their nucleotides without loss of viability. Thus, the small size of many RNA genomes, their high mutation rate, and their tolerance to genetic diversity all favor the establishment of complex mixtures of related viruses in the same patient. As a consequence of the low fidelity of the viral replication machinery, HCV is never present in vivo as a homogeneous population of identical RNA genomes but rather as a mixture of divergent, albeit closely related, genomes, exhibiting a dis-

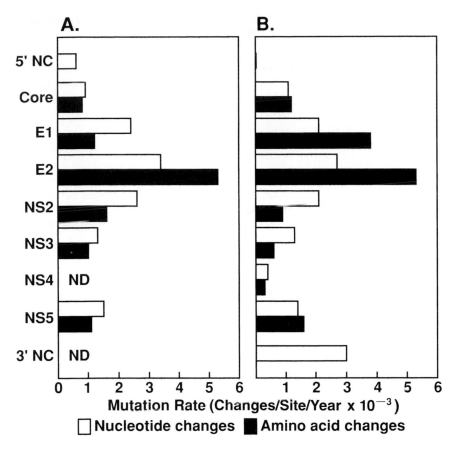

FIG. 1. Mutation rate in different regions of the HCV genome. (A) Strain H77, derived at two time points, 13 years apart, from a chronically infected individual.[29] **(B)** Strain HC-J4, derived at two time points, 8.2 years apart, from a chronically infected chimpanzee.[30]

tribution that follows the model referred to as a quasispecies.[32]

Genetic variability is one of the most important features of the HCV genome. In this respect, it resembles the human immunodeficiency virus (HIV), a member of the virus family *Retroviridae*.[33] Like HIV, the genetic heterogeneity of HCV is not uniform throughout the genome[24,27] (Fig. 1). The most highly conserved regions were identified in parts of the 5′ NC region and the terminal 3′ NC region. The capsid protein is the most highly conserved region of the ORF, followed by conserved sequences in the NS3 and NS5B proteins. The most heterogeneous regions of the genome are the genes encoding the two envelope proteins, E1 and E2. The N terminus of the E2 gene contains a domain of 31 amino acids, which is the most variable region of the entire HCV genome and has been called the first hypervariable region (HVR1).[34,35] A second hypervariable region located just 3′ of HVR1 has been described and named HVR2, but it seems to be limited only to strains of genotype 1b.[35] The HVR2 is only approximately seven amino acids in length and its significance is not well un-

derstood. Thus, the genetic heterogeneity of HCV is complex. It has been classified into four hierarchical strata: genotypes, subgenotypes, isolates, and quaispecies. A description of these follows.

HCV GENOTYPES

Definition

Studies of HCV isolates collected worldwide have documented significant genetic variation.[36–38] The genomic sequences of the most distantly related HCV isolates vary by as much as 35%. Thus, the genetic distance between HCV isolates is comparable with that found between the genera of enteroviruses and rhino viruses within the *Picornaviridae* family and to that between different serotypes of other *Flaviviridae* (i.e., dengue virus types 1–4). Based on their genetic heterogeneity, it is now generally accepted that HCV has evolved into major genetic groups (genotypes) that are further divided into subgroups (subgenotypes or subtypes).[38–40] A total of six major genotypes, designated in order of discovery as 1 through 6, has been identified; more than 50 subtypes have been described, designated by lower case letters in order of discovery for each genotype. An increasing number of novel subtypes is emerging within all genotypes except 5 as the analysis of geographic areas worldwide widens.[41,42] Difficulties were recently encountered in the classification of HCV isolates obtained from southeast Asia. These isolates were proposed as new major genotypes designated as 7 through 11.[43,44] However, more detailed phylogenetic analysis of such variants suggests that these isolates, with the exception of genotype 10, should instead be classified as divergent subtypes of type 6, whereas isolates designated as genotype 10 should instead be classified as divergent subtypes of genotype 3.[45,46] These genetically diverse subtypes are evidence that HCV heterogeneity in reality may be a continuum. Nevertheless, the tiered hierarchical classification of HCV[40] remains of practical use for studies of the molecular epidemiology and transmission of HCV worldwide.

The detection of distinct signature motifs within the HCV genome has permitted genotype analysis based on partial HCV sequences.[37] Several studies have demonstrated that analysis of the E1[47] or NS5b[48] genes of HCV leads to a reliable and more practical classification of the different HCV isolates. Moreover, although sequencing of the entire E1 and NS5b genes is essential for a definitive determination of the HCV genotypes, analysis of a fragment of about 100 nucleotides within E1 was found to be sufficient to predict the genotype of 51 isolates collected worldwide, representing all 6 genotypes and 12 subtypes.[47]

Over the past few years, with the development of commercial assays for the identification of HCV genotypes,[42] an impressive number of studies have investigated the molecular epidemiology of HCV infection worldwide and possible interactive effects between HCV genotypes and the pathogenesis or therapy of hepatitis C. However, the different methods used for genotyping and the different criteria for patient inclusion have made comparison of results obtained in different studies difficult.[37] In particular, several confounding variables related to the clinical and virologic characteristics of the patients, including the quasispecies nature of individual isolates, the viral titer, the stage of the disease, the history of alcohol consumption, and the local epidemiology, were not always taken into consideration, which may explain the opposite results obtained in different studies.[49] Indeed, although there is consensus that the HCV genotype may influence the outcome of antiviral therapy, no consensus has been reached on other important issues, such as the effects of genotype on transmission, infectivity, pathogenesis, and natural history of the disease.

Distribution

The evidence so far accumulated indicates that the major genotypes of HCV differ in their global distribution.[37,41,42] Isolates of genotypes 1, 2, and 3 are widely distributed throughout the world, but significant differences emerge when the geographic distribution of the subtypes is examined. The most common genotypes present in America, Europe, and Japan are genotypes 1, 2, and 3. Within genotype 1, the most frequent worldwide, subtype 1a is predominant in Western Europe and North America, whereas subtype 1b is the most common in Japan and in Southern and Eastern Europe; subtype 1c was detected only in Indonesia where it represents more than 20% of genotype 1 isolates. Among genotypes 2 and 3, also widely distributed throughout the world, subtype 2c is confined to a restricted region of Northern Italy; subtype 3b to Japan, Nepal, Thailand, and Indonesia; and subtypes 3c–3f to Nepal. Genotype 3a has been commonly detected in younger populations in Western countries, particularly among intravenous drug users. Genotype 4 appears to be a Pan-African type (4a is the principal genotype in Egypt, with four other subtypes in Gabon and Zaire). Genotype 5 represents the main genotype in South Africa and has only sporadically been detected outside of Africa. Genotype 6 and its many variants have been found in Asia.

Although the data obtained from several studies on the overall geographic distribution of the HCV genotypes worldwide are generally consistent, it is important to point out that some factors may introduce a selection bias, such as the groups of individuals studied.[50] In hemophiliacs and dialysis patients, the HCV genotype may reflect either the genotype found in blood products[51,52] or transmission of specific genotypes within a dialysis unit.[53] The genotype distribution also differs between intravenous drug users and other groups of HCV-infected individuals.[54] Recent epidemiologic surveys conducted in Italy have demonstrated that genotype 2 is prevalent in the general population with asymptomatic infection even in areas where type 1b was reported to be the most prevalent, suggesting that the reported prevalence of the different HCV genotypes was population based and either included mostly asymptomatic carriers or was from a tertiary referral center and included mostly symptomatic patients.[55–57] This bias may also explain why, overall, genotype 2 is less frequently detected than type 1.

The analysis of HCV genotypes can also provide evidence of changes in HCV epidemiology. Recent European studies have documented the emergence of subtypes 1a and 3a and a decline of subtypes 2a/c and 1b in younger patients,[58] most likely reflecting the high prevalence of the former genotypes in intravenous drug users and their recent extension from this reservoir to the general population. Although studies reporting the segregation of HCV genotypes within specific groups of patients are potentially interesting, it has to be emphasized that some of the proposed associations are premature and require further studies before any conclusions can be drawn.

CLINICAL IMPLICATIONS OF THE HCV GENOTYPES

HCV Genotype and Natural History of Hepatitis

Studies conducted both in humans and in chimpanzees have clearly demonstrated that various HCV genotypes are not associated with major biologic differences: To date, all the genotypes and subtypes have been found to be both hepatotropic and pathogenic. Importantly, all the HCV genotypes can induce chronic infection. Studies in hemophiliacs also have provided evidence of no difference in the infectivity, transmissibility, and pathogenicity among HCV genotypes.[59] Analysis of the levels of viremia, which should accurately reflect viral replicative capacity, did not show any significant differences among HCV genotypes collected from different clinical settings and geographic areas, including blood donors from around the world,[60] patients with chronic liver disease from the United States,[61] and patients undergoing orthotopic liver transplantation.[62] However, several studies of Japanese patients with chronic liver disease, with few exceptions, showed that the levels of viremia were significantly higher with genotype 1b than with genotypes 2a or 2b.[37]

The critical question of the significance of the HCV genotypes and subtypes for pathogenesis is still controversial. After the interesting observation of Pozzato et al.[63] that genotype 1b was associated with more severe liver disease than infection with other genotypes in Japan and Italy, evidence both for and against such an association was provided. The evidence in favor was based on the findings that liver cirrhosis and HCC were detected significantly more frequently in patients infected with genotype 1b than in patients infected with other genotypes.[64–70] A series of other studies, however, failed to confirm such an association.[71–79] Although the reasons for these contradictory results are still unknown, several confounding factors may have contributed. Among them, the fact that patients infected with genotype 1b were significantly older than those infected with other genotypes strongly supports the hypothesis that a cohort effect could explain the association between genotype 1b and cirrhosis or HCC.[80] Similarly, and related to this, another confounding factor might be incorrect estimates of the duration of dis-

ease, because in a high proportion of sporadic cases no precise estimate of the time of infection is possible; thus, a longer duration of the disease might explain the association between genotype 1b and progression of the disease,[81] especially in areas where genotype 1b may have been present for a longer time.

Although all of the above-mentioned studies were cross-sectional and thus liable to potential statistical biases, conflicting results have also emerged from a limited number of recent prospective cohort studies.[82–84] In a large prospective study of cirrhotic patients conducted in Italy, Bruno et al.[82] demonstrated that genotype 1b was a highly significant independent risk factor for the development of HCC. However, two other prospective studies failed to confirm an association between genotype 1b and severity or progression of the disease.[83,84] The influence of the viral genotype on the outcome of the disease was also assessed in three case-control studies.[85–87] The results of these studies did show a relationship between genotype 1b and the development of HCC in cirrhotic patients.

Conflicting results have also emerged from analyses of the association between HCV genotype and outcome of HCV infection after liver transplantation. Although some studies showed that patients infected with genotype 1b developed more severe liver disease after transplantation,[88–92] others failed to detect such an association.[93,94] The effect of HCV genotypes on superinfection in patients who underwent orthotopic liver transplantation was also investigated.[95] In a study of 14 HCV-infected patients who underwent orthotopic liver transplantation and received a liver graft from an HCV-infected donor, the strain of the recipient was found to prevail in six patients, whereas the donor's strain replaced the recipient's strain in eight patients. In five donor–recipient pairs in which one patient was infected by genotype 1 (either 1a or 1b) and the other by a different genotype (i.e., 2c, 3a, 5b), the former invariably became predominant after transplantation. Similarly, genotype 1b consistently replaced genotype 1a. This study confirmed that HCV superinfection does occur in humans and provided evidence that genotype 1 (1b or 1a) may have biologic advantages over the other HCV genotypes. Patients retaining their own strain after transplantation had more severe disease than those who acquired the donor strain, suggesting that, at least in some patients, viral factors might play an important role in the pathogenesis of HCV-related liver disease. In light of the evidence so far accumulated both in humans and chimpanzees, HCV-infected patients may not be protected against superinfection by heterologous HCV strains. Because of the general shortage of graft donors and the steadily increasing need for liver tranplantation in end-stage HCV-related liver disease worldwide, it will be important to understand better the impact of

HCV superinfection on the natural history of the disease in transplanted patients.

Based on the studies discussed above, an answer to the question of whether genotypes play a role in the pathogenesis of HCV infection remains unresolved. In light of the conflicting findings, it is important to emphasize that several confounding factors may hamper the interpretation of different clinical studies. Variations in patient characteristics at the time of enrollment, especially age, duration of the infection, histologic stage of the disease, and specific cofactors, such as alcohol consumption, make it difficult to compare the results reported in the literature. For example, in a recent study aimed at evaluating the risk factors associated with the progression of liver fibrosis in patients with chronic hepatitis C, Poynard et al.[96] found a significant association between the rate of fibrosis progression and age at infection, alcohol consumption, and male sex; by contrast, no association was seen between progression of the fibrosis and genotypes. Another important question is the lack of uniform criteria in evaluating the risk factors associated with the progression of the disease. Only rarely were multiple parameters simultaneously studied, including the HCV genotypes, the level of viremia, the histologic findings, the duration of the infection, alcohol consumption, and age at infection. Furthermore, the recent observation that occult hepatitis B virus infection in HCV-infected patients accelerates the evolution to cirrhosis, the most important risk factor for the development of HCC,[97] further emphasizes that a wide spectrum of factors may modify the natural history of chronic hepatitis C.

HCV Genotype and Response to Antiviral Therapy

Alpha-interferon (IFN) is the only therapy of proven benefit for patients with chronic hepatitis C. Such treatment, however, is effective in only 10–20% of cases. More recently, a combination of alpha-IFN and ribavirin, an oral nucleoside analogue, was shown to increase the rate of sustained response to 30–40% in naive patients[98] and in relapsed patients,[99] but the rate did not differ significantly in prior nonresponders to IFN alone. Thus, most patients with chronic hepatitis C are resistant to antiviral therapy. Several attempts have been made to identify factors predictive of the response to IFN therapy.[100] Among them, increasing interest has been focused on virologic factors, such as the role of the HCV genotypes, in determining the outcome of antiviral therapy. In contrast to the conflicting results obtained in studies of the interactive effects of the HCV genotypes on the natural history of HCV infection, more consistent data have been accumulated

on the association between genotype and response to therapy. Patients infected with genotype 1 (in particular 1b) and genotype 4 respond poorly to IFN treatment compared with patients infected with genotypes 2 and 3. In an extensive review of 15 studies, sustained response after short courses of IFN treatment was achieved in only 18.1% of 536 patients with genotype 1 but in 54.9% of the 288 patients with other genotypes.[100] An association between HCV genotype and response to treatment also emerged when IFN was given in combination with ribavirin to naive patients[98] and to those who relapsed after an initial response to therapy with IFN alone.[99]

The mechanisms by which most of the HCV isolates are resistant to IFN therapy are still not fully defined. The mechanism of action of IFN includes transcriptional induction of several antiviral genes, such as the double-stranded RNA-activated protein kinase (PKR), which inhibits protein synthesis by phosphorylation of eIF2α, a translation initiation factor. Recently, Taylor et al.[101] demonstrated a remarkable homology between a 12 amino acid sequence in the E2 envelope protein of HCV and phosphorylation sites in PKR and eIF2α. Of importance, the genotype most resistant to IFN therapy (1a and 1b) contains a sequence with greater homology to PKR and eIF2α than do the most IFN-sensitive genotypes (2a, 2b, and 3a). These results suggest that a possible mechanism of HCV genotype 1's IFN-resistance resides in the ability of its E2 protein to bind and inhibit the activity of PKR, thereby abrogating the inhibitory effect that this kinase exerts on protein synthesis and cell growth. Another interferon sensitivity-determining region has been found in NS5A; this is discussed elsewhere in this review.

QUASISPECIES NATURE OF HCV

The concept of quasispecies was introduced for the first time by Manfred Eigen.[102] He proposed this concept to describe the diverse and rapidly evolving populations of related but different RNA clones arising as a result of Darwinian evolution during the early phases of life on earth.[103,104] These principles have been applied in modern virology to describe RNA virus populations with a common origin but encompassing distinct viral genomes as a result of stochastic variations, inherent ability to replicate, and selective pressure exerted by the host environment.[105] The rapid evolution of RNA viruses may represent a fundamental strategy of adaptation for survival. It is due to the low fidelity of the viral replicase, which leads to the continuous generation of mutants among progeny RNA genomes.[28] It is important to emphasize that the variants present within the quasispecies do not reflect the spectrum of mutants generated during the error prone replication process but rather the result of a competitive selection among such mutants based on their replicative ability in a given environment.[106] Thus, genomes displaying a higher ability to produce progeny (fitness), relative to the other components of the quasispecies, will tend to be more represented.[107] Generally, the viral quasispecies encompasses a "master" genome, which is quantitatively predominant, and a multitude of minor genomes, representing variable proportions of the total population. It is assumed that at any given moment during the natural history of the infection, the quasispecies distribution re presents the best fitting population that has established a status of equilibrium, transient though it may be, with the host.[105] This equilibrium can be lost suddenly as a consequence of changes in the host environment, with rapid quasispecies evolution (i.e., loss of dominance by previous master sequences and rise to dominance of new master sequences), leading to the generation of virus population disequilibrium.[107,108] Conversely, relative long-term stasis of the viral population can be observed when a virus of greater fitness replicates in a defined relatively constant host environment. Probably the most effective selective constraint within the environment is represented by the specific host immune responses, whether cellular (i.e., CTL) or humoral (i.e., neutralizing antibodies). As pointed out by Eigen and Schuster,[103] it is the quasispecies population in its complex, not the individual genomes, that constitutes the actual target of selection by the immune system. Thus, at any given moment the selective pressure of the host results in a precise, albeit transient, homeostatic quasispecies distribution.

Methods for the Analysis of the HCV Quasispecies

The study of the HCV quasispecies is complex, and several parameters can be used for its characterization.[107] The development of refined molecular techniques for nucleic acid amplification, such as the polymerase chain reaction (PCR), has provided the tools for a dramatic advancement in our knowledge of the HCV quasispecies. In the pre-PCR era, direct RNA fingerprinting was used for analyzing the quasispecies of viruses that were present in sufficient titer in biologic samples or that could be amplified by the use ex vivo culture systems.[109,110] However, the relatively low viral load of HCV in patient samples and the lack of ex vivo amplification systems prevented a reliable approach to the study of HCV. The introduction of reverse transcriptase (RT)-PCR has overcome these limitations by allowing the in vitro exponential amplification by thermostable polymerase (Taq-polymerase) of minute

amounts of the HCV genome, extracted from biologic samples, after RT of the viral RNA into cDNA. By this method, sufficient amounts of cDNA are produced to be analysed by a wide array of techniques.

The degree of heterogeneity within the HCV quasispecies can be evaluated at two different levels: the genetic complexity, defined as the total number of viral variants identified in a single sample, and the genetic diversity, defined as the average genetic distance among the different variants.[111] Molecular cloning of the RT-PCR products, followed by sequencing of individual clones, is the most accurate method currently available for defining HCV quasispecies. A sufficient number of molecular clones must be included in the analysis for an adequate representation of the viral population. Indeed, sequencing of fewer than 20 molecular clones almost invariably results in an artifactual simplification of the HCV quasispecies, accounting only for the major viral variants.[112] The predominant master sequence may or may not coincide with the consensus sequence of the quasispecies, which is defined as the sequence containing the nucleotide most frequently detected at each position of the sequence analyzed. Furthermore, the consensus sequence might not represent any of the individual genomes present in the quasispecies and is subject to changes as the sequences of additional clones are added to the alignment; however, it may be useful as an overall reference sequence for identifying changes that affect the global population[107] (Fig. 2).

Although molecular cloning of RT-PCR amplicons followed by sequencing is the methodology of choice for a complete characterization of the HCV quasispecies, it is highly labor intensive. Thus, the widespread application of HCV quasispecies studies in different clinical settings has prompted investigators to develop alternative techniques that are simpler and faster; however, these methods fail to identify specific nucleotide residues and therefore do not permit precise analysis of the genetic diversity of individual viral variants. The most common of these techniques are single-stranded conformation polymorphism (SSCP),[113,114] temperature-gradient gel electrophoresis,[115] and gel-shift analysis.[116] All these methods are based on the differential gel mobility of amplified DNA products containing nucleotide mutations and thus they provide a general representation of the quasispecies complexity (number of variants). The major limitation of these techniques is that they do not permit investigation of the correlations between specific residues within a genomic region and phenotypic or clinical traits of interest.[107] Similarly, these techniques do not allow a precise tracking of individual viral variants during longitudinal analysis of quasispecies evolution. Nevertheless, it must be recognized that even analysis by molecular cloning and sequencing has potential drawbacks because selec-

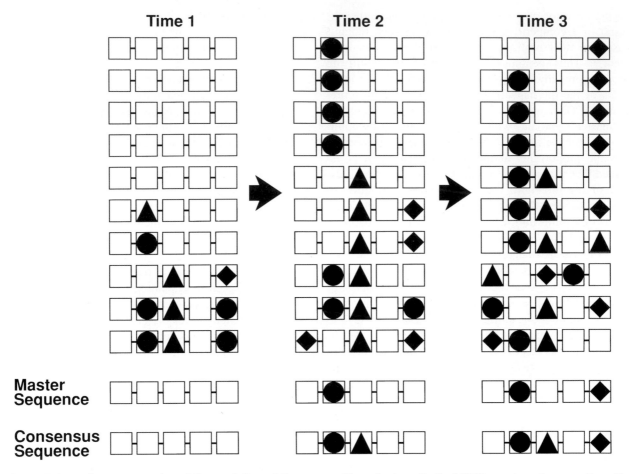

FIG. 2.   Schematic representation of the evolution of the composition of a hypothetical HCV quasispecies over time. For each time point, 10 different viral genomes, and the consensus and the master sequences are shown. The consensus sequence is defined as the sequence containing the nucleotides most frequently detected at each position. The master sequence is the predominant sequence found in the viral population at each time point; it may (time point 1) or may not (time points 2 and 3) be identical to the consensus sequence. The solid symbols denote different nucleotide substitutions with respect to the initial dominant sequence.

tion during amplification and cloning procedures may result in a biased quasispecies representation.[117]

Genetic Complexity and Diversity of the HCV Quasispecies

Evidence of a quasispecies distribution of the HCV genome within single infected individuals was initially obtained from studies in which HCV was either molecularly or biologically cloned. The first description that HCV circulates in vivo as a quasispecies was provided by Martell et al.,[32] who studied an individual coinfected with HCV and HIV. By sequence analysis of 27 molecular clones, they demonstrated that about half of the circulating RNA molecules were identical (master sequence), whereas the remaining consisted of a spectrum of mutants differing from each other at one to four nucleotide sites. Several studies have subsequently expanded on these observations and confirmed that HCV circulates in vivo as a complex population of closely re-

lated viral variants.[118-122] Other important evidence of the quasispecies nature of HCV was obtained from studies of experimental transmission in chimpanzees. Comparative sequence analysis between the well-characterized strain H77 used for inoculation and the viruses recovered from the chimpanzees demonstrated that none of the sequences recovered was identical to the consensus sequence of strain H77.[123] Sequence analysis of nine near full-length clones recovered from pooled plasma of an acutely infected chimpanzee demonstrated that all sequences differed from each other.[124]

The fact that the HVR1 shows the highest degree of variability has been instrumental both for the identification of individual viral strains and for investigation of the degree of the genetic complexity and diversity of the HCV quasispecies. An extensive sequence analysis of the HVR1 from 104 molecular clones derived from the H77 inoculum demonstrated that at least 19 different viral strains were present simultaneously within the inoculum (Fig. 3, left). The predominant sequence (master) was represented by 70 of 104 clones.[125] The

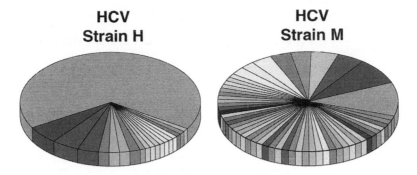

FIG. 3. Genetic complexity of two HCV strains derived from the NIH prospective study of posttransfusion non-A, non-B hepatitis[126] during the acute phase of hepatitis. The analysis was based on 31 amino acids representing the HVR1 of the E2 gene, spanning map positions 384–414 of the HCV genome. **(Left)** Strain H77 (104 molecular clones). A total of 19 different viral variants was detected.[125] **(Right)** Strain M77 (81 molecular clones). A total of 53 different viral variants was detected. See text for details.

remaining 34 consisted of a multitude of different variants, represented by 6, 5, 4, 2, or 1 clone, respectively. Four variants were represented by two clones each and 11 by a single clone. However, the degree of genetic complexity can be dramatically higher, as shown by the analysis of another strain of HCV (strain M), also derived from a patient included in the NIH prospective study of posttransfusion hepatitis C.[126] Sequence analysis of the HVR1 (31 amino acids) from 81 molecular clones showed that 53 different variants were simultaneously present within a single sample (Fig. 3, right). In this case, the dominant strain was represented by only 11% of the entire viral population; other variants were represented by only 9%, 5%, 4%, and 3%; and most 44 variants, were represented by a single clone each (P. Farci, H. J. Alter, unpublished observations 1999). The genetic distance among the different variants within a single sample differed from each other (at the amino acid level; clones of 31 amino acids) at 1–8 sites in strain H77 (Fig. 4A) and at 1–10 sites within strain M (Fig. 4B).

CLINICAL IMPLICATIONS OF THE HCV QUASISPECIES

In recent years, the gap between basic science and clinical research increasingly has been altered by the rise of molecular medicine, a new area of investigation that has shifted the focus to the mechanisms of disease at the molecular level. The wide application of these novel techniques to human virology has dramatically advanced our knowledge of viral pathogenesis and of the complex interactions between viruses and their host. A paradigm of the collision between molecular biology and clinical medicine has been the study of the HCV quasispecies and of its biologic implications, particularly for viral persistence, for drug resistance and for vaccine failure.[127,128] Nevertheless, this extraordinary

progress has also posed a new series of unresolved questions.

Immune Escape as a Mechanism of Viral Persistence

Humoral Immunity

As stated above, extensive clinical and experimental studies, performed both before and after the discovery of HCV, raised concerns about the degree of protective immunity elicited by HCV in the host. The observations that convalescent chimpanzees are not protected against reinfection with either homologous or heterologous HCV strains, the occurrence of multiple episodes of acute hepatitis C in polytransfused β-thalassemic children, and the evidence of superinfection of chronically infected HCV carriers with heterologous viral strains, both in humans and chimpanzees, strongly suggested a lack of protective immunity to HCV. Data supporting this conclusion also came from attempts to vaccinate chimpanzees with recombinant HCV envelope antigens expressed in eukaryotic cells.[129] Vaccinated chimpanzees were protected against intravenous infection with 10 chimpanzee infectious doses (CID) of the homologous virus but not against 64 CID of a closely related viral strain belonging to the same genotype and subtype (1a).[130] But the most striking evidence that the host is unable to clear the virus is the fact that HCV induces chronic infection in most infected individuals, in spite of a vigorous humoral and cellular immune response. Viruses that persist in their hosts must evolve successful strategies to survive by avoiding recognition by the immune system. Genetic variation constitutes an important strategy whereby HCV can evade specific cellular or humoral host immune responses.

To date, the major hindrance to the study of the protective immunity elicited by HCV has been the lack of

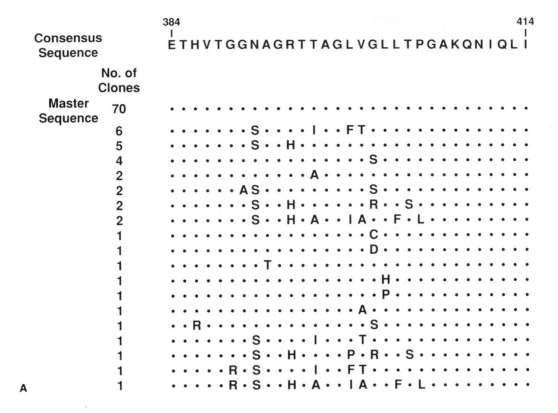

sensitive and reproducible in vitro systems for the growth of the virus in cell culture, although limited viral replication has been reported in some continuous cell lines.[131] In particular, this limitation has hampered the identification and characterization of neutralizing antibodies. Therefore, chimpanzees remain the most reliable and sensitive animal model for the study of HCV neutralization, although there are obvious limitations to their routine use, primarily because they are a costly and limited species. Direct evidence that neutralizing antibodies are produced in patients with chronic HCV infection was obtained with experiments conducted both in vivo in the chimpanzee model[125] and in vitro using a human T-lymphoid cell line.[132,133] However, the same studies also demonstrated that the effectiveness of the neutralizing antibodies is limited because they are isolate restricted and ineffective against other variant strains present in the complex HCV quasispecies. Other attempts to measure HCV-neutralizing antibodies include in vitro assays that measure the ability of antibodies to block the binding of virions or recombinant viral envelope to human cells. Zibert et al.[134] demonstrated that human sera obtained early after HCV infection contained antibodies specific for the HVR1 that could prevent binding of HCV to cells. A different in vitro system, based on the ability of the recombinant E2 envelope glycoprotein to bind to the surface of human lymphoid cells, recently resulted in the identification of the CD81 antigen as a specific E2-binding receptor expressed on the cell surface.[135] Using this system, low titers of antibodies that blocked binding of E2 to cells were detected in patients infected with different genotypes of HCV, and higher titers of such antibody correlated with protection of chimpanzees vaccinated with recombinant E1/E2 proteins from challenge with 10 CID of homologous virus.[136]

The experiments outlined above suggest that the limited spectrum of activity of the anti-HCV neutralizing antibodies is directly related to the quasispecies nature of this virus, with the continuous emergence of viral variants that can escape neutralization. Consistent with this concept, accumulating evidence suggests that the HVR1, the most variable region of the entire HCV genome, is a critical target of neutralizing antibodies. The first evidence that the HVR1 is subjected to the selective pressure of the immune system came from Weiner et al.,[137] who documented a temporal relationship between the appearance of isolate-restricted antibodies directed against linear HVR1 epitopes and sequential mutations within such epitopes; the mutated HVR1 was no longer recognized by antibodies present at previous time points. The fact that genetic variation within the HVR1 was sufficient to determine a lack of recognition by preexisting antibodies strongly suggested that this region contains epitopes recognized by putative neutralizing antibodies. Several subsequent studies confirmed that the HVR1[29,30,118,119,138–141] contains linear epitopes recognized by patient antibodies.[142–146] That an effective humoral immune pressure is required for driving HVR1 variability was demonstrated by the lack of genetic variation documented in pa-

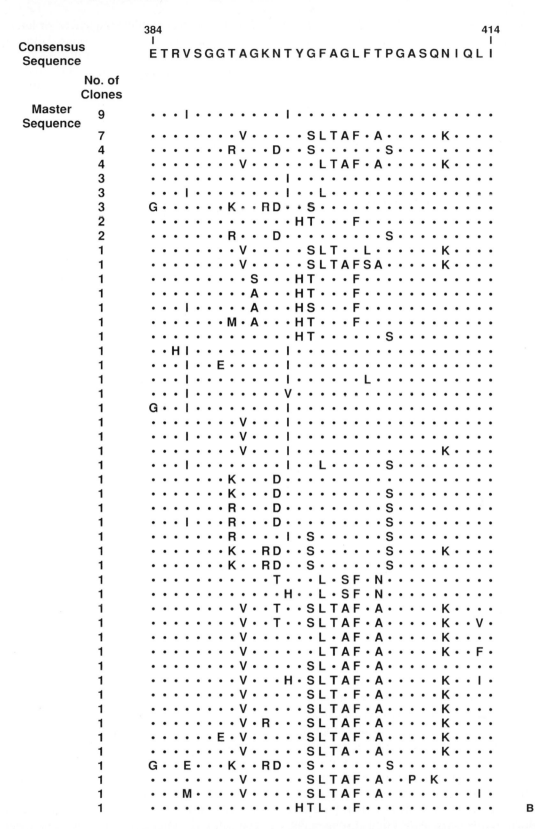

FIG. 4. Genetic diversity of two HCV strains derived from the NIH prospective study of posttransfusion non-A, non-B hepatitis[126] during the acute phase of hepatitis. Predicted amino acid sequence alignment based on 31 amino acids (in single-letter code) representing the HVR1 of the E2 gene, spanning map positions 384–414 of the HCV genome. The consensus sequence is shown at the top of the figure. **(A, preceeding page)** Strain H77 (104 molecular clones). The consensus sequence coincides with the master sequence.[125] **(B)** Strain M77 (81 molecular clones). The consensus sequence is not identical to the master sequence. Five additional different viral variants, each carrying a stop codon, are not shown in the alignment.

tients with agammaglobulinemia.[147] Additional evidence that the HVR1 could be implicated in HCV neutralization came from studies of the correlation between the antibody response to HVR1 and the outcome of HCV infection. In resolving hepatitis, clearance of HCV viremia was associated with the detection of early and high titers of antibodies to HVR1.[19,148–150] Interestingly, patients with acute self-limited hepatitis had antibodies directed against the N-terminus of the HVR1, whereas patients who progressed to chronicity had broadly reactive antibodies against the C-terminus of HVR1.[150] Similarly, Mondelli et al.[151] documented cross-reactive IgG1 antibodies directed to the C-terminus of HVR1 in both acute and chronic HCV infection.

Direct evidence that the HVR1 is a critical target of HCV-neutralizing antibodies was obtained in a study conducted in chimpanzees, which also provided the first in vivo model for the emergence of neutralization escape mutants.[125] A hyperimmune rabbit serum raised against a synthetic HVR1 peptide, corresponding to the sequence of the predominant strain contained within the H77 inoculum, was used for in vitro neutralization of HCV, followed by analysis of residual infectivity by intravenous inoculation of two HCV-seronegative chimpanzees. One animal did not show any signs of HCV infection, whereas the second developed a typical acute hepatitis C that progressed to chronicity. Analysis of the viruses recovered from the latter chimpanzee demonstrated that none of the molecular clones recovered from this animal was identical to the predominant H77 strain that was used to raise the hyperimmune rabbit anti-HVR1 serum. Instead, the viruses emerging in vivo were identical to two minor variants present within the H77 inoculum, which represented only 6% and 2%, respectively, of the original HCV quasispecies. Thus, the hyperimmune anti-HVR1 serum was able to neutralize the predominant clone but was ineffective against the two minor variants that emerged in vivo. These data support the concept that the genetic heterogeneity of the viral quasispecies is involved in immune escape.

Although several lines of evidence indicate that the quasispecies may be an important strategy whereby HCV establishes persistent infection by escaping the host immune recognition, alternative mechanisms have been suggested. McAllister et al.[152] recently studied the evolution of HVR1 in a cohort of Irish women, infected in 1977 from a batch of anti-D immunoglobulins contaminated with HCV, genotype 1b. Whereas the viral population in the infectious source was quite homogeneous, each anti-D recipient showed distinct HVR1 variants, none of which was detected in the original source. Phylogenetic analysis, using the extent of divergence at synonymous sites in the regions flanking the HVR1 to estimate the time of divergence of the HVR1 sequences, suggested that variant sequences had diverged many years before infection with the contaminated immuno-

globulin and that multiple sequences, or lineages, could persist and coexist for long periods during chronic infection. The authors concluded that the distinct HVR1 variants detected in individual patients were not the result of host immune pressure against HVR1.

The development of infectious molecular clones of HCV from the well-characterized strain H77[122,153] has recently provided a valuable tool for studying the effects of the host immune system on viral evolution and its relationship to HCV persistence. A recent study of experimental intrahepatic inoculation of two chimpanzees with the first infectious molecular clone of HCV, derived from strain H77,[154] provided evidence that persistent infection may develop despite the lack of a viral quasispecies in the inoculum and of mutations within the HVR1. Long-term follow-up demonstrated that the infection became chronic in both animals despite a very limited clonal variation. A single point mutation within the HVR1 first occurred at week 51 in one of the two chimpanzees, in the face of detectable anti-E1/E2 antibodies in both animals and anti-HVR1 in one animal. Thus, these data provide evidence that the development of chronic infection in chimpanzees is not necessarily associated with variations in the HVR1 and that the rate of mutations in this region does not differ from the rest of the viral genome. Also, in a separate study,[155] chronic infection developed in one of the two chimpanzees inoculated with a second infectious molecular clone of strain H77.[122] Antibodies to E2 became detectable and persisted in the animal in which the infection became chronic, whereas they did not appear in the animal in which the infection resolved. During the first year of follow-up, no amino acid changes occurred in the envelope proteins despite the appearance of anti-E1 and anti-E2 antibodies, whereas amino acid changes occurred in p7, NS3, NS5A, and NS5B. Similar results were obtained by Hong et al.[156] Overall, four of the five chimpanzees inoculated with monoclonal viruses derived from multiple cDNA clones developed persistent infection.

In contrast to the observations so far accumulated in humans, the results of these studies suggest that immune escape through HVR1 variation does not account for viral persistence in the chimpanzee model, although a role of mutations in other parts of the genome, where several changes occurred in the animals studied,[154–156] cannot be excluded. The reasons for this are not known, although it is important to underline that the experimental setting with an HCV molecular clone in an animal model is different from natural infection in humans. In general, the immune response of chimpanzees against HCV, particularly the antibody response against the E2 glycoprotein, is weaker in the chimpanzee model[129] than in humans. Moreover, whereas a molecular clone consists of a single viral species, the inoculum in natural infection is usually represented by a complex quasispecies. Regardless of these differences, however, the findings in the chimpanzee model may reflect the existence of alternative mechanisms of viral persistence.

The role of the HVR1 in HCV physiology was also recently investigated by intrahepatic inoculation of an infectious molecular clone containing a deletion of the entire HVR1 in to a naive chimpanzee.[157] Persistent viremia at very low titers was observed, and late antibody seroconversion (after 6 months) in the absence of liver inflammation was documented in this animal. The HVR1 deletion mutant virus was transmitted to a second chimpanzee, proving that it was fully viable (X. Forns, unpublished data, 2000). Thus, these data suggest that the HVR1 is not essential for viral replication, but without the HVR1 the virus seems to be attenuated in vivo. This observation is interesting, and additional studies of the host's immune response to the deletion mutant are warranted.

Cellular Immunity

The potential role o f the genetic heterogeniety of the HCV quasispecies in immune escape has also been investigated with regard to cell-mediated immunity. Unlike the humoral neutralizing immune response, cellular immune responses have been extensively investigated with in vitro systems based on the use of recombinant HCV proteins both for the stimulation of specific helper (CD4+) T cells and for performing CTL assays on CD8+ T cells derived either from peripheral blood or directly from the liver.[20,21] In contrast to patients with hepatitis B, who generally show vigorous CD4 T-cell responses only during the acute phase of hepatitis,[158] patients infected with HCV were found to exhibit strong and sustained CD4 T-cell responses directed against multiple HCV proteins both during the acute and the chronic phase of infection.[159] However, patients who cleared the virus after primary infection appeared to have more vigorous responses,[160,161] suggesting a role of effective CD4-mediated immunity in viral clearance. Similarly to the CD4 T-cell response, HCV-specific CTL activity has been documented both in acutely and in chronically infected humans,[20,21] and chimpanzees,[162] although studies during the acute phase of hepatitis in humans have been very limited. In a small number of acutely infected chimpanzees, an association between effective CTL responses and HCV clearance has recently been suggested.[163] However, in a more recent study performed in two chimpanzees during the incubation period and acute phase of hepatitis C, Thimme et al.[164] clearly demonstrated that HCV persisted despite a multispecific peripheral and intrahepatic T-cell response.

The role of the antigenic variation of HCV, particularly of the viral quasispecies, in providing a CTL-escape mechanism has been postulated. In a chronically infected chimpanzee, Weiner et al.[165] described the emergence of a single point mutation within a CTL epitope in the NS3 gene product, which was apparently sufficient to induce loss of recognition by specific CTLs extracted from the liver. Other authors have shown that CTLs directed against conserved epitopes may select for variants with enhanced ability to persist in the host.[166–168] In a recent study performed during the acute phase of HCV infection, an association between the in vivo emergence of HVR1 variants escaping CTL control and subsequent viral persistence[169] was documented. However, it has to be emphasized that the importance of CTL escape for HCV persistence remains controversial, because the HCV-specific CTL responses are multispecific and thus the loss of individual epitopes would be unlikely to confer a significant survival advantage to the emerging viral variants.

HCV Quasispecies and Outcome of Acute Hepatitis

A small proportion of patients infected with HCV experience an acute self-limited hepatitis with clearance of serum HCV RNA within 6 months of infection. The immunologic correlates of HCV clearance are still undefined. However, it is conceivable that the outcome of the disease is the result of the complex interactions between the virus and the host during the earliest phase of the infection. As stated above, several lines of evidence support the hypothesis that the antigenic variability, specifically the quasispecies nature of HCV, may allow the virus to circumvent the immune response, leading to chronic infection. However, studies of the evolution of the viral quasispecies during the acute phase of hepatitis are very limited, mainly because of difficulties in recruiting patients during the early phase of primary infection and the lack of long-term follow-up thereafter. The role of the HCV quasispecies in this setting has only recently been investigated.[170] The genetic complexity, the genetic diversity, and the evolution of the HCV quasispecies, in parallel with the levels of viral replication and the humoral immune response, were analyzed during the incubation period and acute phase of hepatitis C in serial serum samples from patients with different clinical outcomes. Three patients had fulminant hepatitis (FH), three had acute resolving hepatitis, and six had acute hepatitis that progressed to chronicity, associated with persistent viremia; among the latter six patients, the disease was mild and stable for over 20 years in three (slow progressors) and rapidly progressive leading to liver-related death within 5 years of the onset of infection in the remaining three (rapid progressors).

This study provided evidence that the evolutionary dynamics of the viral quasispecies during the acute phase of hepatitis C predicts whether the infection will resolve or become chronic; by contrast, analysis of the HCV quasispecies at a single time point within 2–3 weeks of transfusion did not differentiate between resolving and progressing hepatitis. Acute resolving hepatitis was associated with the emergence of a homogeneous viral population and relative evolutionary stasis before viral clearance, whereas progressing hepatitis correlated with genetic evolution within the first 4 months of infection. Consistent with selection by the immune system, the amino acid changes occurred almost exclusively within the HVR1 of the E2 gene and were temporally related to antibody seroconversion. The outcome of the disease was independent of the level of viremia and HCV genotype. A unique pattern was observed in patients with FH who, despite high levels of serum HCV RNA, showed the lowest degree of genetic diversity and a highly homogeneous viral population. These data are in agreement with a concept of negative pressure against amino acid changes, suggesting that in HCV-associated FH there is a trend to preserve the unique fitness of a particularly virulent viral strain.[171] The presence in FH of a dominant viral strain with great pathogenic potential has recently been confirmed by experimental transmission of HCV from a patient with FH to a chimpanzee.[172] The chimpanzee developed the most severe acute hepatitis hitherto documented in a large series of studies conducted in this animal model (R.H. Purcell, unpublished data); moreover, analysis of the HCV quasispecies recovered from the chimpanzee again exhibited a highly homogeneous viral population.

In another analysis of HVR1 and HCV,[173] three patients who developed chronic hepatitis C had oligoclonal viral populations of HVR1 quasispecies during the acute phase of hepatitis C that evolved toward viral diversification between 9 and 12 months after infection, with a different pattern of genetic evolution in each of the three patients studied.[173] Recently, Ray et al.[174] reported a higher degree of genetic complexity in intravenous drug users who developed chronic hepatitis compared with those who cleared viremia, but the analysis was limited to a single sample from each patient and the interval between time of sampling and time of seroconversion was highly heterogeneous (range, −14 to +41 months from the first seropositive sample). In addition to a higher quasispecies complexity, patients who progressed to chronicity showed a higher ratio of nonsynonymous (amino acid replacement) to synonymous (silent) nucleotide substitutions within the HVR1 compared with those who cleared the virus, whereas the ratio was lower within a segment of the E1. These data were interpreted as an indication of a possible role of the HVR1 as an immunologic decoy capable of stimulating a strong but ineffective immune response. However, the limited number of clones sequenced in this study for each patient (mean, 4.2) may not have been sufficient for providing an accurate representation of the HCV quasispecies. Also, the hypothesis of a decoy role for the HVR1 is difficult to reconcile with the results of other studies that demonstrated that clearance of HCV viremia was associated with an early and strong antibody response to HVR1.[19,148–150]

HCV Quasispecies and Natural History of Hepatitis C

The study of the HCV quasispecies and its relationship to the clinical course of HCV-associated disease has represented an area of intensive investigation over the past few years. Several groups have examined the relationship between the degree of viral quasispecies and the stage of HCV infection. Honda et al.[175] analyzed the HCV quasispecies in 28 patients with liver disease of varying severity, including patients with acute hepatitis, chronic persistent hepatitis, chronic active hepatitis, and cirrhosis, with or without HCC. The intrapatient genetic diversity, based on sequences of the core and E1 envelope regions of the HCV genome, increased significantly and progressively from patients with acute hepatitis to those with cirrhosis, suggesting that the degree of HCV quasispecies correlated with the progression of liver disease. In another subsequent study,[176] however, the genetic complexity and dive rsity of the HVR1 did not correlate with the stage of the disease, although this finding was not confirmed in other studies. Koizumi et al.[177] showed, by multivariate analysis, that viral diversity was independently related to the progression of liver disease and was not correlated with the duration of infection. By contrast, González-Peralta et al.[178] reported a correlation between an increase in genetic complexity and the estimated duration of HCV infection. Kao et al.[179] investigated the HCV quasispecies in sequential serum samples from two patients with different clinical courses of chronic hepatitis. In one patient, who developed an episode of acute exacerbation, the degree of viral diversity within the HVR1 was higher than that observed in the other patient, who did not manifest acute exacerbations during the course of the disease. In another study, Yuki et al.[180] found that the genetic complexity of the HCV quasispecies significantly correlated with the degree of aminotransferase elevation during the course of chronic hepatitis C. The effect of multiple exposures to HCV on the degree of viral quasispecies was investigated in 21 hemophiliacs with a history of multiple transfusions compared with 16 patients with posttransfusion hepatitis C resulting from a single HCV exposure. Although there was no significant difference in the number of viral strains within the HVR1, the average number of nucleotide substitutions per variant was significantly higher in hemophiliac patients.[181] Recently, the HCV quasispecies was also investigated in patients with compensated and decompensated alcoholic liver disease and in matched nonalcoholic controls. Overall, the number of variants was higher in alcoholic patients than in nonalcoholic controls, raising the question of whether the differences in quasispecies complexity may help to explain the poor IFN responsiveness in alcoholic patients.[182]

Most studies summarized above suggest that the heterogeneity of viral quasispecies correlates with the progression of HCV-related liver disease. However, the evidence is still preliminary. Only rarely were the genetic complexity and diversity of the HCV quasispecies both investigated in the same study. Another limitation of these studies is the fact that the duration of HCV infection was generally unknown. As the degree of quasispecies heterogeneity tends to increase over time, time is an important confounding factor that should be considered in the interpretation of the results reported to date.

HCV Quasispecies and Orthotopic Liver Transplantation

In patients undergoing orthotopic liver transplantation for HCV-related chronic liver disease, recurrence of HCV infection after surgery is almost universal. The study of these patients has provided a new model for understanding the role of the viral quasispecies in HCV transmission and pathogenicity. Martell et al.[183] analyzed the diversity of the viral sequences in samples obtained from two patients with end-stage liver cirrhosis before and after liver transplantation. In both cases, the complexity of the viral quasispecies diminished after transplantation, with conservation of the consensus sequences that were present before transplantation. Whether this decrease in complexity after liver transplantation was determined by the selective effect of the preexisting immune response of the graft recipient or, alternatively, by a lack of de novo selective pressure secondary to iatrogenic immunosuppression remains to be established.

Similar data were obtained by Gretch et al.,[184] who performed a longitudinal analysis of the viral quasispecies in five transplanted patients, all infected with HCV genotype 1. An average of 30 clones per sample was sequenced, with a follow-up ranging from 6 to 24 months. Before liver transplantation, the number of viral variants in the five subjects ranged from one to nine. After liver transplantation, a relatively homogeneous viral quasispecies emerged in all patients. Moreover, three patients who developed severe hepatitis with a rapidly progressive course after transplantation maintained the major viral variants that were present before transplantation, whereas the two patients with asymptomatic posttransplant HCV infection exhibited only variants that were present as minor components before the transplant. The role of the evolution of the HCV quasispecies in the severity of recurrent hepatitis after liver transplantation was recently investigated in 22 patients, all infected with HCV, genotype 1.[185] Although genetic diversification occurred in several regions of the viral genome after liver transplantation, the E1 and E2 genes showed the greatest changes. Interestingly, diversification was greater in patients with asymptomatic or moderate disease after liver transplantation than in those with severe disease.

HCV Quasispecies and Immune Suppression

Patients with immune suppression caused by drugs or viral infections represent a model for studying the role of the immune system in the evolution of HCV quasispecies. If the host immunity is deficient or suppressed, there is a trend toward a more homogeneous viral population, suggesting that viral diversity is driven by host immune pressure. The study of the HCV quasispecies in infants,[186] whose immune system is still immature, demonstrated the presence of a homogeneous viral population that progressively increased in viral diversity with age. A dramatic change in HCV quasispecies evolution was observed in the setting of bone marrow transplantation. Longitudinal analysis of three children showed a very high degree of diversity immediately before transplantation, which was interpreted as a dramatic increase secondary to the immunosuppressive regimen started 1 week earlier; however, no samples before immunosuppression were analyzed. After transplantation, a decrease in viral diversity was seen during the phase of immunosuppression, with the predominance of a single viral strain, followed by an increase over time, after the reconstitution of immune function.[187] In patients co-infected with HIV, discrepant results were reported. Sherman et al.[188] reported an increased diversity in the HVR1 in dually infected patients compared with those infected with HCV alone. The authors suggested a correlation between such increase in diversity and a poor response to IFN therapy. By contrast, Toyoda et al.[189] found no significant difference in genetic diversity and complexity among patients with or without HIV co-infection. However, when the patients were stratified according to circulating CD4+ cell counts, the diversity was significantly lower in patients with fewer than 50 cell/μL. These findings suggest that the decline in helper activity by CD4+ T cells results in a lowered immune pressure and, thereby, to the emergence of a more homogeneous HCV population. Similarly, a lower viral diversity in the HVR1 was reported in immunocompromised patients than in immunocompetent HCV-infected individuals.[190]

The evolution of the HCV quasispecies was also investigated in patients with humoral immunodeficiency. Little or no genetic heterogeneity in HVR1 was seen in agammaglobulinemic patients; similarly, the genetic variation in the HVR1 was significantly lower in patients with hypogammaglobulinemia due to common variable immunodeficiency.[191] Altogether, the data obtained from HCV-infected patients with either cellular or humoral immunodeficiency suggest that in the absence of immune selective pressures, the frequency of genetic variation is low.

Compartmentalization of the HCV Quasispecies

In recent years, it has been suggested that HCV may replicate not only within the liver but also at extrahepatic sites, although this issue remains controversial.[192] Two major lines of evidence have been provided for extrahepatic HCV replication: the diversification of the HCV quasispecies detected in different body compartments and the demonstration of negative-strand HCV RNA at extrahepatic sites. However, the latter evidence is the most questionable due to the inherent limitations of strand-specific assays. After the initial study by Sakamoto et al.,[193] who documented an identical HVR1 quasispecies in plasma and liver by SSCP analysis, most subsequent studies suggested that the HVR1 quasispecies in the liver differs from that circulating in serum or in peripheral blood mononuclear cells (PBMC).[194–200] By analyzing the 5'untranslated region in two patients co-infected with HIV, Laskus et al.[192] demonstrated HCV quasispecies divergence in different extrahepatic sites. Based on this evidence, together with the detection of negative-strand HCV RNA in the same tissues, the authors suggested the presence of bona fide extrahepatic HCV replication.

Conflicting data have been reported concerning the degree of genetic heterogeneity in the different compartments. Cabot et al.[195] found that in most patients with chronic hepatitis C, the complexity of the HCV quasispecies in the liver considerably exceeded that in serum. Similar results were subsequently reported in other studies.[201,202] By contrast, Navas et al.[198] found that both the genetic complexity and the genetic diversity of the HCV quasispecies in serum were higher than in liver tissue or in PBMC; phylogenetic analysis showed that the sequences from liver tissue and PBMC were more closely related to each other than to those from serum. The reasons for the discrepant results obtained in different studies are at present unknown, but they might be related to differences in the sensitivity of the techniques used in the different laboratories or in the selection of patients. The influence of the clinical characteristics of the patients on the results of HCV quasispecies analyses emerged from the results of a recent study by Sakai et al.[203] They evaluated the HCV quasispecies in the serum and in three different parts of the liver in eight patients with varying severity of chronic hepatitis C. The major findings of this study were that diversification of the HCV quasispecies correlated with the histopathologic stage. A significant difference in quasispecies composition between liver and serum was seen only in the two patients with cirrhosis, whereas common viral clones predominated in the six noncirrhotic patients. In the latter patients, the genetic diversity was higher in serum than in liver. Moreover, a significant difference in genetic diversity among the liver samples taken from the same patient was seen only in the four patients with fibrosis and advanced liver disease.

The HCV quasispecies has also been examined within the neoplastic tissue of patients with HCC. Kurosaki et al.[204] first reported a different HCV envelope quasispecies composition in paired noncancerous and cancerous lesions obtained from three of four patients studied. A larger number of HCV variants was documented in the cancerous lesions of seven patients with HCC.[205] De Mitri et al.[206] confirmed a different complexity of the HVR1 quasispecies between tumorous and nontumorous tissue, although in some of their patients the tissue of HCC harbored a less complex viral population. In these patients, the degree of HCV quasispecies was not influenced by the presence or absence of cirrhosis.

As discussed above, the results of the studies on HCV quasispecies compartimentalization are conflicting. Although most studies have provided evidence for the existence of a compartimentalization, a major unresolved question remains as to whether the different complexities of the viral quasispecies between liver and serum reflect HCV diversification within different niches within the liver, particularly in patients with a high degree of fibrosis, or active HCV replication in extrahepatic anatomic sites.

HCV Quasispecies and Viral Transmission

The existence of selective mechanisms in the transmission of the HCV quasispecies was suggested by a study of mother-to-child transmission.[207] Analysis of 10 clones obtained at the time of birth from both the mother and the newborn demonstrated the presence of nine different variants in the mother, whereas the viral population was totally homogeneous in the infant. Interestingly, the strain detected in the infant was not identical, albeit highly related, to any of the variants identified in the mother. Similar results were reported by Kudo et al.,[208] who found that the variants from the infants were not identical to those present in the mothers. Interestingly, antibody-bound HCV virions were found consistently in the mothers who did not transmit HCV to their offspring but less frequently in those who transmitted, suggesting that maternal antibodies may prevent viral transmission.

Evidence for a selective transmission of distinct variants contained within the quasispecies also came from studies of experimental transmission of HCV to chimpanzees. In a study of three animals that received a pedigreed serum from a chronically infected patient (H77), comparative sequence analysis showed a different representation of the HCV quasispecies after transmission.[125] The original master sequence was consistently transmitted, although in only one of three animals it remained dominant. The second most prevalent variant, representing 6% of the strains present in the inoculum, became dominant in the other two chimpanzees, whereas the third most prevalent variant (5%) was never recovered from any chimpanzee. Because all the animals received the same infectious dose (64 CID_{50}), these data suggested a selective transmission. Similarly, only one variant harbored by a patient with fulminant hepatitis C was successfully transmitted to a chimpanzee.[172]

A selective transmission was also reported by Sugitani et al.[209] in two chimpanzees inoculated with two different 10-fold dilutions of the same infected human serum, not previously titrated in vivo. At variance with the results reported above, however, only the dominant strain was transmitted in both animals, despite the presence of at least six different variants in the inoculum. In a report by Hijikata et al.,[210] a human plasma containing a complex HCV quasispecies was both inoculated into a chimpanzee and used to infect human lymphoid cell lines in vitro. Interestingly, only two of the seven clones present in the inoculum were recovered both in vivo and in vitro, suggesting a selective transmission of specific variants of the HCV quasispecies. Whether this selectivity is due to an inherently higher replicative capability or transmissibility remains to be established. Kojima et al.,[211] using the chimpanzee model, suggested that the presence of antibodies to HVR1 may exert an influence on the selective transmission of the HCV variants present in the inoculum.

HCV Quasispecies and Response to Antiviral Therapy

Although the HCV genotype has been associated with the response to IFN therapy,[100,212] the observation of different responses in patients with the same geno-type and the same titer of viremia suggests that other factors also may be responsible for the effectiveness of IFN therapy. Over the past few years, the HCV quasispecies has been intensively investigated to determine whether the degree of genetic complexity and diversity may influence the outcome of IFN therapy.

The first study that documented an association between the degree of the HCV quasispecies before starting therapy, particularly within the HVR1, and the response to interferon treatment was reported in 1992.[213] After this observation, several other studies confirmed that the genetic complexity of the HCV quasispecies before therapy correlates with the response to IFN.[144,177,214–220] In most of these studies, the target sequence used to assess the genetic heterogeneity of HCV was the HVR1 domain. In other reports,[221,222] however, no such association was found. For example, Hagiwara et al.[221] reported that the response to IFN therapy correlated with the levels of viremia before treatment and not to the genetic complexity of the quasispecies. Similarly, Shindo et al.[222] showed that the correlation between long-term response to IFN and low HVR1 heterogeneity could be demonstrated only when there were low levels of HCV viremia. Polyak et al.[223] reported that only the genetic diversity, but not the genetic complexity, was a predictor of response to IFN therapy.

The effects of IFN therapy on the evolution of the HCV quasispecies were analyzed in several studies. Consistent with the original observation by Okada et al.,[213] changes in the composition of the HCV quasispecies were demonstrated during IFN treatment,[224,225] suggesting the existence of selective mechanisms either directly related to the action of IFN or secondary to modulation of specific immune responses. Comparative analysis of the HCV quasispecies before and after therapy showed a significantly greater evolution, within the HVR1 in treated patients compared with untreated controls.[226] Similar results were reported by Pawlotsky et al.,[227] who observed profound changes in HVR1 quasispecies major variants in 70% of the patients during and after IFN therapy but no changes in untreated controls. Changes were less likely to occur in nonresponders. Consistent with positive selection, the average number of nonsynonymous substitutions within the HVR1 was significantly higher than that of synonymous substitutions.

In a recent study, the evolution of the HCV quasispecies, tracked by sequence analysis, was evaluated in serial serum samples obtained from 24 patients with chronic hepatitis C selected according to their different patterns of response to IFN therapy.[228] The results of this longitudinal study, based on more than 1,800 molecular clones, showed a significant decrease in genetic complexity and diversity of the HCV quasispecies within 2 weeks of starting therapy in long-term responders but not in nonresponders or in patients who had a breakthrough or a relapse after treatment, suggesting that the early evolution of the HCV quasispecies may predict a sustained complete response. Analysis of individual viral variants over time demonstrated that relapse was characterized by a loss of the dominant strain and by the emergence of new viral variants. By contrast, the viral population in nonresponders and in patients who experienced a breakthrough was characterized by the persistence of the original dominant strain, suggesting that some viral strains are inherently resistant to IFN therapy.

Recently, the HCV quasispecies has been investigated in nonresponder patients retreated with IFN for 2 months, followed by either IFN alone or IFN plus ribavirin.[229] The rate of HVR1 diversification was significantly higher during the early phase of retreatment in both groups of patients. Early quasispecies changes were also observed within the NS5A region, although the comparison between early and late retreatment phases did not show statistical difference. Consistent with a previous observation by Gonzáles-Peralta et al.,[230] the addition of ribavirin had no major effects on the quasispecies evolution. Similarly, data from another study provide evidence that ribavirin alone has no effect on HCV quasispecies[231]. In addition to the HVR1, other regions of the HCV genome have been selected for investigating the relationship between HCV quasispecies and response to IFN therapy. One such region was identified by Enomoto et al.[232] within the NS5A gene and designated IFN-sensitivity-determining region because it was associated with sensitivity of HCV genotype 1b to IFN treatment. Whereas patients with no amino acid substitutions within this region were resistant to IFN, patients with amino acid substitutions responded to the therapy.[233] In IFN-resistant patients, the sequence of the IFN-sensitivity-determining region was identical to that of prototype HCV genotype 1b.[234,235] A mechanism has been proposed whereby IFN sensitivity is regulated by the interaction of NS5A with the IFN-induced cellular protein kinase PKR.[236] Although these data may have important implications for predicting the response to IFN treatment in patients infected with genotype 1b, such correlation has not been confirmed in subsequent studies.[237–239] Another region of potential interest is the PKR-homologous site of E2, described above in the section on HCV genotypes, although the quasispecies in this region and its clinical relevance remains to be defined.

Despite the controversies, the evidence so far accumulated suggests that the degree of genetic diversity and complexity before therapy may predict the response to IFN. Although the composition and size of the HCV quasispecies changes during IFN treatment in non responders and in patients who experience a breakthrough, the dominant strain persists over time, suggesting that some strains are inherently resistant to IFN.

There have been some suggestions that specific regions of the viral genome determine the responsiveness of HCV to IFN. In conclusion, although some of the interesting observations discussed above require further confirmation, there is no doubt that the quasispecies represents a large reservoir of biologically different viral variants that may play a critical role in determining the response to antiviral therapy.

SUMMARY AND CONCLUSIONS

Over the last 10 years, the wide application of novel and sophisticated molecular techniques has dramatically advanced our knowledge of the biology of HCV and of the complex interactions between this virus and the host. The study of the genetic heterogeneity of HCV has represented a paradigm of the convergence between molecular biology and clinical medicine. Recent evidence indicates that the quasispecies nature of HCV constitutes a critical strategy for the virus to survive in the host. In fact, the quasispecies represents a rapidly moving target that the host immune system seems unable to fully control. Moreover, the large reservoir of genetic variants provided by the quasispecies poses a major challenge for the development of effective therapeutic and preventive measures. On the other hand, however, the fine molecular dissection of the HCV quasispecies has provided new hints for understanding why patients are unable to clear the virus and why some do not respond to antiviral therapy. These insights might eventually lead to novel strategies for the control of HCV infection.

In conclusion, more than a decade after its discovery, HCV still represents a complex public health problem. Despite the increasing understanding of the biologic and clinical aspects of HCV infection, this virus remains a major challenge to both virologists and physicians.

ABBREVIATIONS

CID	chimpanzee infectious doses
CTL	cytotoxic T lymphocytes
E1 and E2	envelope 1 and 2
eIF2α	initiation factor
FH	fulminant hepatitis
HCC	hepatocellular carcinoma
HCV	hepatitis C virus
HIV	human immunodeficiency virus
HVR1	hypervariable region 1
HVR2	hypervariable region 2
IFN	interferon
NC	noncoding
NS	nonstructural
ORF	open reading frame

PBMC   peripheral blood mononuclear cells
PKR   RNA-activated protein kinase
RT-PCR   reverse transcriptase-polymerase chain
           reaction
SSCP   single-stranded conformation
           polymorphism

REFERENCES

1. National Institutes of Health Consensus Development Conference Panel Statement: Management of hepatitis C. Hepatology 1997;26:2S–10S
2. Seeff LB. Natural history of viral hepatitis, type C. Semin Gastrointest Dis 1995;6:20–27
3. Di Bisceglie AM. Hepatitis C and hepatocellular carcinoma. Semin Liver Dis 1995;15:64–69
4. Detre KM, Belle SH, Lombardero M. Liver transplantation for chronic viral hepatitis. Viral Hepat Rev 1996;2:219–228
5. Alter MJ, Margolis HS, Krawczynski K, et al. The natural history of community-acquired hepatitis C in the United States. N Engl J Med 1992;327:1899–1902
6. Alter HJ. To C or not to C: These are the questions. Blood 1995;85:1681–1695
7. Di Bisceglie AM, Goodman ZD, Ishask KG, et al. Long-term clinical and histopathological follow-up of chronic posttransfusion hepatitis. Hepatology 1991;14:969–974
8. Farci P, Alter HJ, Wong D, et al. Long-term study of hepatitis C virus replication in non-A, non-B hepatitis. N Engl J Med 1991;325:98–104
9. Seeff LB. Natural history of hepatitis C. Hepatology 1997;26:21S–28S
10. Hoofnagle JH. Hepatitis C: The clinical spectrum of disease. Hepatology 1997;26:15S–20S
11. Seeff LB, Buskell-Bales Z, Wright EC, et al. Long-term mortality after transfusion-associated non-A, non-B hepatitis. N Engl J Med 1992;327:1906–1911
12. Tong MJ, el-Farra NS, Reikes AR, Co RL. Clinical outcomes after transfusion-associated hepatitis C. N Engl J Med 1995;332:1463–1466
13. Farci P, Alter HJ, Govindarajan S, et al. Lack of protective immunity against reinfection with hepatitis C virus. Science 1992;258:135–140
14. Prince AM, Brotman B, Huima T, et al. Immunity in hepatitis C infection. J Infect Dis 1992;165:438–443
15. Wyatt CA, Andrus L, Brotman B, et al. Immunity in chimpanzees chronically infected with hepatitis C virus: Role of minor quasispecies in reinfection. J Virol 1998;72:1725–1730
16. Lai ME, Mazzoleni AP, Argiolu F, et al. Hepatitis C virus in multiple episodes of acute hepatitis in polytransfused thalassemic children. Lancet 1994;343:388–390
17. Kao JH, Chen PJ, Lai MY, Chen DS. Superinfection of heterologous hepatitis C virus in a patient with chronic type C hepatitis. Gastroenterology 1992;105:583–587
18. Okamoto H, Mishiro S, Tokita H, et al. Superinfection of chimpanzees carrying hepatitis C virus of genotype II/1b with that of genotype III/2a or I/1a. Hepatology 1994;20:1131–1136
19. Kobayashi M, Tanaka E, Matsumoto A, et al. Antibody response to E2/NS1 hepatitis C virus protein in patients with acute hepatitis C. J Gastroenterol Hepatol 1997;12:73–76
20. Koziel MJ, Walker BD. Characteristics of the intrahepatic cytotoxic T lymphocyte response in chronic hepatitis C virus infection. Semin Immunopathol 1997;19:69–83
21. Chang K-M, Rehermann B, Chisari FV. Immunopathology of hepatitis C. Semin Immunopathol 1997;19:57–68
22. Shimizu YK, Feinstone SM, Kohara M, et al. Hepatitis C virus: Detection of intracellular virus particles by electron microscopy. Hepatology 1996;23:205–209
23. International Union of Microbiological Societies. Murphy FA, Fauquet CM, Bishop DHL, et al. eds. Virus Taxonomy, 7th ed. New York: Springer-Verlag, 1995, pp. 424–427
24. Houghton M. Hepatitis C virus. In: Fields BN, Knipe DM, Howley PM, Chanock RH, eds. Fields Virology, 3rd ed. Philadelphia: Lippincott-Raven, 1996, pp. 1035–1058
25. Tsukiyama-Kohara K, Kohara I, Nomoto A. Internal ribosome entry site within hepatitis C virus RNA. J Virol 1992;66:1476–1483
26. Tanaka T, Kato N, Cho M, Shimotohno K. A novel sequence found at the 3′terminus of hepatitis C virus genome. Biochem Biophys Res Commun 1995;215:744–749
27. Choo Q-L, Richman KH, Han JH, et al. Genetic organization and diversity of the hepatitis C virus. Proc Natl Acad Sci USA 1991;88:2451–2455
28. Holland J, Spindler K, Horodyski F, et al. Rapid evolution of RNA genomes. Science 1982;215:1577–1585
29. Ogata N, Alter HJ, Miller RH, Purcell RH. Nucleotide sequence and mutation rate of the H strain of hepatitis C virus. Proc Natl Acad Sci USA 1991;88:3392–3396
30. Okamoto H, Kojima M, Okada S-I, et al. Genetic drift of hepatitis C virus during an 8.2-year infection in a chimpanzee: Variability and stability. Virology 1992;190:894–899
31. Holland J, Domingo E, De La Torre JC, Steinhauer DA. Mutation frequencies at defined single codon sites in vesicular stomatitis virus can be increased only slightly by chemical mutagenesis. J Virol 1990;64:3960–3962
32. Martell M, Esteban JL, Quer J, et al. Hepatitis C virus (HCV) circulates as a population of different but closely related genomes: Quasispecies nature of HCV genome distribution. J Virol 1992;66:3225–3229
33. Nowak MA. Variability of HIV infections. J Theor Biol 1992;155:1–20
34. Weiner AJ, Brauer MJ, Rosemblatt J, et al. Variable and hypervariable domains are found in the regions of HCV corresponding to the flavivirus envelope and NS1 proteins and the pestivirus envelope glycoproteins. Virology 1991;180:842–848
35. Hijikata M, Kato N, Ootsuyama Y, et al. Hypervariable regions in the putative glycoprotein of hepatitis C virus. Biochem Biophys Res Commun 1991;175:220–228
36. Okamoto H, Mishiro S. Genetic heterogeneity of hepatitis C virus. Intervirology 1994;43:68–76
37. Bukh J, Miller RH, Purcell RH. Genetic heterogeneity of hepatitis C virus: Quasispecies and genotypes. Semin Liver Dis 1995;15:41–63
38. Simmonds P. Variability of hepatitis C virus. Hepatology 1995;21:570–583
39. Chan S-W, McOmish F, Holmes EC, et al. Analysis of a new hepatitis C virus type and its phylogenetic relationship to existing variants. J Gen Virol 1992;73:1131–1141
40. Simmonds P, Holmes E C, Cha T-A, et al. Classification of hepatitis C virus into six major genotypes and a series of subtypes by phylogenetic analysis of the NS-5 region. Gen Virol 1993;74:2391–2399
41. Maertens G, Stuyver L. Genotypes and genetic variation of hepatitis C virus. In: Harrison TJ, Zuckerman A, eds. The Molecular Medicine of Viral Hepatitis. Chichester, England: Medical Science Series, John Wiley & Sons Ltd; 1997, pp. 183–233
42. Forns X, Bukh J. Methods for determining the hepatitis C virus genotype. Viral Hepat Rev 1998;4:1–19
43. Tokita H, Okamoto H, Tsuda F, et al. Hepatitis C virus variants from Vietnam are classifiable into the seventh, eighth and ninth major genetic groups. Proc Natl Acad Sci USA 1994;91:11022–11026

44. Tokita H, Okamoto H, Luengrojanakul P, et al. Hepatitis C virus variants from Thailand classifiable into five novel genotypes in the sixth (6b), seventh (7c, 7d) and ninth (9b, 9c) major genetic groups. J Gen Virol 1995;76 :2329–2335

45. Mizokami M, Gojobori T, Ohba K-I, et al. Hepatitis C virus types 7, 8 and 9 should be classified as type 6 subtypes. J Hepatol 1996;24:622–624

46. Simmonds P, Mellor J, Sakuldamrongpanich T, et al. Evolutionary analysis of variants of hepatitis C virus found in South-East Asia: Comparison with classifications based upon sequence similarity. J Gen Virol 1996;77:3 013–3024

47. Bukh J, Purcell RH, Miller RH. At least 12 genotypes of hepatitis C virus predicted by sequence analysis of the putative E1 gene of isolates collected worldwide. Proc Natl Acad Sci USA 1993;90:8234–8238

48. Simmonds P, Holmes EC, Cha T-A, et al. Classification of hepatitis C virus into six major genotypes and a series of subtypes by phylogenetic analysis of the NS-5 region. J Gen Virol 1993;74: 2391–2399

49. Purcell RH. The hepatitis C virus: Overview. Hepatology 1997; 26:11S–14S

50. Mondelli MU. Clinical Implications of Viral Genotypes. International Consensus Conference on Hepatitis C. European Association for the Study of the Liver, Paris, 1999

51. Okamoto H, Sugiyama Y, Okada S, et al. Typing hepatitis C virus by polymerase chain reaction with type-specific primers: Application to clinical surveys and tracing infectious sources. J Gen Virol 1992;73:673–679

52. Ichimura H, Tamura I, Kurimura O, et al. Hepatitis C virus genotypes, reactivity to recombinant immunoblot assay 2 antigens and liver disease. J Med Virol 1994;43:212–215

53. Hadiwandowo S, Tsuda F, Okamoto H, et al. Hepatitis B virus subtypes and hepatitis C virus genotypes in patients with chronic liver disease or on maintenance hemodialysis in Indonesia. J Med Virol 1994;43:182–186

54. Bréchot C. Hepatitis C virus genetic variability: clinical implications. Am J Gastroenterol 1994;89:41S–47S

55. Silini EM, Bono F, Cividini A, et al. Differential distribution of hepatitis C virus genotypes in patients with and without liver function abnormalities. Hepatology 1995;21:285–290

56. Puoti C, Magrini A, Stati T, et al. Clinical, histological, and virological features of hepatitis C virus carriers with persistently normal or abnormal alanine transaminase levels. Hepatology 1997;26:1393–1398

57. Guadagnino V, Stroffolini T, Rapicetta M, et al. Prevalence, risk factors, and genotype distribution of hepatitis C virus infection in the general population: A community-based survey in southern Italy. Hepatology 1997;26:1006–1011

58. Silini EM, Mondelli MU. Significance of hepatitis C virus genotypes. Viral Hepat Rev 1995;1:111–120

59. Jarvis LM, Ludlam CA, Ellender JA, et al. Investigation of the relative infectivity and pathogenicity of different hepatitis C virus genotypes in hemophiliacs. Blood 1996;87:3007–3011

60. Smith DB, Davidson F, Yap P-L, et al. Levels of hepatitis C virus in blood donors infected with different virus genotypes. J Infect Dis 1996;173:727–730

61. Lau JYN, Davis GL, Prescott LE, et al. Distribution of hepatitis C virus genotypes determined by line probe assay in patients with chronic hepatitis C seen at tertiary referral centers in the United States. Ann Intern Med 1996;24:868–876

62. Gane EJ, Naoumov NV, Quian K-P, et al. A longitudinal analysis of hepatitis C virus replication following liver transplantation. Gastroenterology 1996;110:167–177

63. Pozzato G, Moretti M, Franzin F, et al. Severity of liver disease with different hepatitis C viral clones. Lancet 1991;338: 509

64. Pozzato G, Kaneko S, Moretti M, et al. Different genotypes of hepatitis C virus are associated with different severity of chronic liver disease. J Med Virol 1994;43:291–296

65. Qu D , Li J-S, Vitvitski L, et al. Hepatitis C virus genotypes in France: Comparison of clinical features of patients infected with HCV type I and type II. J Hepatol 1994;21:70–75

66. Pistello M, Maggi F, Vatteroni L, et al. Prevalence of hepatitis C virus genotypes in Italy. J Clin Microbiol 1994;32:232–234

67. Zein NN, Poterucha JJ, Gross JB Jr, et al. Increased risk of hepatocellular carcinoma in patients infected with hepatitis C genotype 1b. Am J Gastroenterol 1996;91:2560–2562

68. Cathomas G, McGandy CE, Terracciano LM, et al. Detection and typing of hepatitis C RNA in liver biopsies and its relation to histopathology. Virchows Arch 1996;429:353–358

69. Booth JC, Doster GR, Levine T, et al. The relationship of histology to genotype in chronic HCV infection. Liver 1997;17: 144–151

70. Kobayashi M, Tanaka E, Sodeyama T, et al. The natural course of chronic hepatitis C: A comparison between patients with genotypes 1 and 2 hepatitis C viruses. Hepatology 1996;23:695–699

71. Mita E, Hayashi N, Kanazawa Y, et al. Hepatitis C virus genotype and RNA titer in the progression of type C chronic liver disease. J Hepatol 1994;21:468–473

72. Kobayashi M, Kumada H, Chayama K, et al. Prevalence of HCV genotype among patients with chronic liver diseases in the Tokyo metropolitan area. J Gastroenterol 1994;29–583–587

73. Yamada M, Kakumu S, Yoshioka K, et al. Hepatitis C virus genotypes are not responsible for development of serious liver disease. Dig Dis Sci 1994;39:234–239

74. Naoumov NV, Chokshi S, Metivier E, et al. Hepatitis C virus infection in the development of hepatocelluler carcinoma in cirrhosis. J Hepatol 1997;27:331–336

75. Guido M, Rugge M, Thung SN, et al. Hepatitis C virus serotypes and liver pathology. Liver 1996;16:353–357

76. Ravaggi A, Rossini A, Mazza C, et al. Hepatitis C virus genotypes in northern Italy: Clinical and virological features. J Clin Microbiol 1996;34:2822–2825

77. Lee DS, Sung YC, Whang YS. Distribution of HCV genotypes among blood donors, patients with chronic liver disease, hepatocellular carcinoma, and patients on maintenance hemodialysis in Korea. J Med Virol 1996;49:55–60

78. Mangia A, Cascavilla I, Lezzi G, et al. HCV genotypes in patients with liver disease of different stages and severity. J Hepatol 1997;26:1173–1178

79. Kleter B, Brouwer JT, Nevens F, et al. Hepatitis C virus genotypes: Epidemiological and clinical associations. Benelux Study Group on Treatment of Chronic Hepatitis C. Liver 1998;18: 32–38

80. Nousbaum J-B, Pol S, Nalpas B, et al. Hepatitis C virus type 1b (II) infection in France and Italy. Ann Intern Med 1995;122: 161–168

81. Lopez-Labrador FX, Ampurdanes S, Forns X, et al. Hepatitis C virus (HCV) genotypes in Spanish patients with HCV infection: Relationship between HCV genotype 1b, cirrhosis and hepatocellular carcinoma. J Hepatol 1997;27:959–965

82. Bruno S, Silini E, Crosignani A, et al. Hepatitis C virus genotypes and risk of hepatocellular carcinoma in cirrhosis: A prospective study. Hepatology 1997;25:754–758

83. Benvegnù L, Pontisso P, Cavalletto D, et al. Lack of correlation between hepatitis C virus genotypes and clinical course of hepatitis C virus-related cirrhosis. Hepatology 1997;25:211–215

84. Serfaty L, Aumaitre H, Chazouilleres O, et al. Determinants of outcome of compensated hepatitis C virus-related cirrhosis. Hepatology 1998;27:1435–1440

85. Silini E, Bottelli R, Asti M, et al. Hepatitis C virus genotypes and risk of hepatocellular carcinoma in cirrhosis: A case control study. Gastroenterology 1996;111:199–205

86. Hatzakis A, Katsoulidou A, Kaklamani E, et al. Hepatitis C virus 1b is the dominant genotype in HCV-related carcinogenesis: A case-control study. Int J Cancer 1996;68:51–53

87. Donato F, Tagger A, Chiesa R, et al. Hepatitis B and C virus infection, alcohol drinking and hepatocellular carcinoma; A case-control study in Italy. Hepatology 1997;26:579–584

88. Féray C, Gigou M, Samuel D, et al. Influence of the genotypes of hepatitis C virus on the severity of recurrent liver disease after liver transplatation. Gastroenterology 1995;108:1088–1096

89. Gane EJ, Portmann BC, Naoumov NV, et al. Long-term outcome of hepatitis C infection after liver transplantation. N Engl J Med 1996;334:815–820

90. Caccamo L, Gridelli B, Sampietro M, et al. Hepatitis C virus genotypes and reinfection of the graft during long-term follow-up in 35 liver transplant recipients. Transplant Int 1996;9:204S-209S

91. Belli LS, Silini E, Alberti A, et al. Hepatitis C virus genotypes, hepatitis, and hepatitis C virus recurrence after liver transplantation. Liver Transplant Surg 1996;2:200–205

92. Gordon FD, Poterucha JJ, Germer J, et al. Relationship between hepatitis C genotype and severity of recurrent hepatitis C after liver transplantation. Trasplantation 1997;63:1419–1423

93. Zhou S, Terrault NA, Ferrell L, et al. Severity of liver disease in liver transplantation recipients with hepatitis C virus infection: Relationship to genotype and level of viremia. Hepatology 1996; 24:1041–1046

94. Vargas HE, Laskus T, Wang LF, et al. The influence of hepatitis C virus genotypes on the outcome of liver transplantation. Liver Transplant Surg 1998;4:22–27

95. Laskus T, Wanf LF, Rakela J, et al. Dynamic behavior of hepatitis C virus in chronically infected patients receiving liver graft from infected donors. Virology 1996;220:171–176

96. Poynard T, Bedossa P, Opolon P, et al. Natural history of liver fibrosis progression in patients with chronic hepatitis C. Lancet 1997;349:825–832

97. Cacciola I, Pollicino T, Squadrito G, et al. Occult hepatitis B virus infection in patients with chronic hepatitis C liver disease. N Engl J Med 1999;341:22–26

98. McHutchinson JG, Gordon ST, Schiff ER, et al. Interferon alfa-2b alone or in combination with ribavirin as initial treatment for chronic hepatitis C. N Engl J Med 1998;339:1485–1492

99. Davis GL, Mur RE, Rustgi V, et al. Interferon alfa-2b alone or in combination with ribavirin for the treatment of relapse of chronic hepatitis C. N Engl J Med 1998;339:1493–1499

100. Davis GL, Lau JYN. Factors predictive of a beneficial response to therapy of hepatitis C. Hepatology 1997;26:122S–127S

101. Taylor DR, Shi ST, Romano PR, et al. Inhibition of the interferon-inducible protein kinase PKR by HCV E2 protein. Science 1999;285:107–110

102. Eigen M. Self organization of matter and the evolution of biological macromolecules. Naturwissenschaften 1972;58:465:523

103. Eigen M, Schuster P. The Hypercycle. A Principle of Natural Self-Organization. Berlin: Springer, 1979

104. Eigen M, Biebricher CK. Sequence space and quasispecies distribution. In: Domingo E, Holland JJ, Ahlquist P, eds. RNA Genetics. Boca Raton, FL: CRC Press, 1988, pp. 211–245

105. Domingo E, Holland JJ. High error rates, population equilibrium and evolution of RNA replication systems. In: Domingo E, Holland JJ, Ahlquist P, eds. RNA Genetics, Vol 3. Boca Raton, FL: CRC, 1988, pp 3–36

106. Holland JJ, De La Torre JC, Steinhauer DA. RNA virus populations as quasispecies. Curr Top Microbiol Immunol 1992; 176:1–20

107. Domingo E. Biological significance of viral quasispecies. J Viral Hepat 1996;2:2 47–261

108. Steinhauer DA, Holland JJ. Rapid evolution of RNA viruses. Annu Rev Microbiol 1987;41:409–433

109. Domingo E, Sabo D, Taniguchi T, Weissmann C. Nucleotide sequence heterogeneity of an RNA phage population. Cell 1978; 13:735–744

110. Branch AD, Benenfeld BJ, Paul CP, et al. Analysis of ultraviolet-induced RNA-RNA cross-links: A means for probing RNA structure-function relationships. Methods Enzymol 1989;180:418–442

111. Gretch DR, Polyak SJ. The Quasispecies Nature of Hepatitis C Virus: Research Methods and Biological Implications. Hepatitis C Virus: Genetic Heterogeneity and Viral Load. GEMHEP. Paris: John Libbey Eurotext, 1997, pp. 57–69

112. Gómez J, Martell M, Quer B, et al. Hepatitis C viral quasispecies. J Viral Hepat 1999;6:3–16

113. Orita M, Iwahana H, Kanazawa H, et al. Detection of polymorphisms of human DNA by gel electrophoresis as single-strand conformation polymorphisms. Proc Natl Acad Sci USA 1989; 86:2766–2770

114. Moribe T, Hayashi N, Kanazawa Y, et al. Hepatitis C viral complexity detected by single-strand conformation polymorphisms and response to interferon therapy. Gastroenterology 1995;108:789–795

115. Lu M, Funsch B, Wiese M, Roggendorf M. Analysis of hepatitis C virus quasispecies populations by temperature gradient gel electrophoresis. J Gen Virol 1995;76:881–887

116. Wilson JJ, Polyak SJ, Day TD, Gretch DR. Characterization of simple and complex hepatitis C virus quasispecies by heteroduplex gel shift analysis: Correlation with nucleotide sequencing. J Gen Virol 1995;76:1763–1771

117. Forns X, Purcell RH, Bukh J. Quasispecies in viral persistence and pathogenesis of hepatitis C virus. Trends Microbiol 1999;7: 402–410

118. Higashi Y, Kakumu S, Yoshioka K, et al. Dynamics of genome change in the E2/NS1 region of hepatitis C virus in vivo. Virology 1993;197:659–668

119. Kato N, Ootsuyama Y, Tanaka T, et al. Marked sequence diversity in the putative envelope proteins of hepatitis C viruses. Virus Res 1992;22:107–123

120. Murakawa K, Esumi M, Kato T, et al. Heterogeneity within the nonstructural protein 5-encoding region of hepatitis C viruses from a single patient. Gene 1992;117:229–232

121. Tanaka T, Kato N, Nakagawa M, et al. Molecular cloning of hepatitis C virus genome from a single Japanese carrier: Sequence variation within the same individual and among infected individuals. Virus Res 1992;23:39–53

122. Yanagy M, Purcell RH, Emerson SU, Bukh J. Transcripts from a single full-length cDNA clone of hepatitis C virus are infectious when directly transfected into the liver of a chimpanzee. Proc Natl Acad Sci USA 1997;94:8738–8743

123. Farci P, Alter HJ, Wong DC, et al. Prevention of hepatitis C virus infection in chimpanzees after antibody-mediated in vitro neutralization. Proc Natl Acad Sci USA 1994;91:7792–7796

124. Yanagi M, St. Claire M, Shapiro M, et al. Transcripts of a chimeric cDNA clone of hepatitis C virus genotype 1b are infectious in vivo. Virology 1998;244:161–172

125. Farci P, Shimoda A, Wong D, et al. Prevention of hepatitis C virus infection in chimpanzees by hyperimmune serum against the hypervariable region 1 of the envelope 2 protein. Proc Natl Acad Sci USA 1996;93:15394–15399

126. Koziol DE, Holland PV, Alling DW, et al. Antibody to hepatitis B core antigen as a paradoxical marker for non-A, non-B hepatitis agents in donated blood. Ann Intern Med 1986;104:488–495

127. Domingo E. RNA virus evolution and the control of viral disease. Progr Drug Res 1989;33:93–133

128. Domingo E, Martinez-Salas E, Sobrino F, et al. The quasispecies (extremely heterogeneous) nature of viral RNA genome populations: biological relevance—a review. Gene 1985;40:1–8

129. Choo QL, Kuo G, Ralston R, et al. Vaccination of chimpanzees against infection by the hepatitis C virus. Proc Natl Acad Sci USA 1994;91:1294–1298

130. Houghton M, Choo Q-L, Chien D, et al. Development of an HCV vaccine. In Rizzetto M, Purcell RH, Gerin JL, Verme G, eds. Viral Hepatitis and Liver Disease. Turin: Minerva Meolia 1997; pp. 656–659

131. Shimizu YK, Iwamoto A, Hijikata M, et al. Evidence for in vitro replication of hepatitis C virus genome in a human T-cell line. Proc Natl Acad Sci USA 1992;89:5477–5481

132. Shimizu YK, Igarashi H, Kiyohara T, et al. A Hyperimmune serum against a synthetic peptide corresponding to the hypervariable region 1 of hepatitis C virus can prevent viral infection in cell cultures. Virology 1996;223:409–412

133. Shimizu YK, Hijikata M, Iwamoto A, et al. Neutralizing antibodies against hepatitis C virus and the emergence of neutralization escape mutants. J Virol 1994;68:1494–1500

134. Zibert A, Schreier E, Roggendorf M. Antibodies in human sera specific to hypervariable region 1 of hepatitis C virus can block viral attachment. Virology 1994;208:653–661

135. Pileri P, Uematsu Y, Campagnoli S, et al. Binding of hepatitis C virus to CD81. Science 1998;282:938–941

136. Rosa D, Campagnoli S, Moretto C, et al. A quantitative test to estimate neutralizing antibodies to hepatitis C virus: Cytofluorometric assessment of envelope glycoprotein E2 binding to target cells. Proc Natl Acad Sci USA 1996;93:1759–1763

137. Weiner AJ, Geysen HM, Christopherson C, et al. Evidence for immune selection of hepatitis C virus (HCV) putative envelope glycoprotein variants: Potential role in chronic HCV infection. Proc Natl Acad Sci USA 1992;89:3468–3472

138. Kato N, Ootsuyama Y, Sekiya H, et al. Genetic drift in hypervariable region 1 of the viral genome in persistent hepatitis C virus infection. J Virol 1994;68:4776–4784

139. Kumar U, Brown J, Monjardino J, Thomas HC. Sequence variation in the large envelope glycoprotein (E2/NS1) of hepatitis C virus during chronic infection. J Infect Dis 1993;167:726–730

140. Kurosaki M, Enomoto N, Marumo F, Sato C. Rapid sequence variation of the hypervariable region of hepatitis C virus during the course of chronic infection. Hepatology 1993;18:1293–1299

141. Sakamoto N, Enomoto N, Kurosaki M, et al. Sequential change of the hypervariable region of the hepatitis C virus genome in acute infection. J Med Virol 1994;42:103–108

142. Kato N, Sekiya H, Ootsuyama Y, et al. Humoral immune response to hypervariable region 1 of the putative envelope glycoprotein (gp70) of hepatitis C virus. J Virol 1993;67:3923–3930

143. Lesniewski RR, Boardway KM, Casey JM, et al. Hypervariable 5′-terminus of hepatitis C virus E2/NS1 encodes antigenically distinct variants. J Med Virol 1993;40:150–156

144. Scarselli E, Cerino A, Esposito G, et al. Occurrence of antibodies reactive with more than one variant of the putative envelope glycoprotein (E2; gp70) hypervariable region 1 in hepatitis C viremic patients. J Virol 1995;69:4407–4412

145. Taniguchi S, Okamoto H, Sakamoto M, et al. A structurally flexible and antigenically variable N-terminal domain of the hepatitis C virus (E2/NS1) protein: Implication for an escape from antibody. Virology 1993;195:297–301

146. van Doorn LJ, Capriles I, Maertens G, et al. Sequence evolution of the hypervariable region in the putative envelope region E2/NS1 of hepatitis C virus is correlated with specific humoral immune response. J Virol 1995;69:773–778

147. Kumar U, Monjardino J, Thomas HC. Hypervariable region of hepatitis C virus envelope glycoprotein (E2/NS1) in an agammaglobulinemic patient. Gastroenterology 1994;106:1072–1075

148. Zibert A, Meisel H, Kraas W, et al. Early antibody response against hypervariable region 1 is associated with acute self-limiting infectioms of hepatitis C virus. Hepatology 1997;25:1245–1249

149. Allander T, Beyene A, Jacobson SH, et al. Patients infected with the same hepatitis C virus strain display different kinetics of the isolate-specific antibody response. J Infect Dis 1997;175:26–31

150. Zibert A, Kraas W, Meisel H, et al. Epitope mapping of antibodies directed against hypervariable region 1 in acute self-limiting and chronic infections due to hepatitis C virus. J Virol 1997;71:4123–4127

151. Mondelli MU, Cerino A, Lisa A, et al. Antibody responses to hepatitis C virus hypervariable region 1: Evidence for cross-reactivity and immune-mediated sequence variation. Hepatology 1999;30:537–545

152. McAllister J, Casino C, Davidson F, et al. Long-term evolution of the hypervariable region of hepatitis C virus in a common-source-infected cohort. J Virol 1998;72:4893–4905

153. Kolykhalov AA, Agapov EV, Blight K, et al. Transmission of hepatitis C by intrahepatic inoculation with transcribed RNA. Science 1997;277:570–574

154. Major ME, Mihalik K, Fernandez J, et al. Long-term follow-up of chimpanzees inoculated with the first infectious clone for hepatitis C virus. J Virol 1999;73:3317–3325

155. Bukh J, Yanagi M, Emerson SU, Purcell RH. Course of infection and evolution of monoclonal hepatitis C virus (HCV) strain H77 in chimpanzees transfected with RNA transcripts from an infectious cDNA clone. Hepatology 1998;28:319A

156. Hong Z, Beaudet-Miller M, Lanford RE, et al. Generation of transmissible hepatitis C virions from a molecular clone in chimpanzees. Virology 1999;256:36–44

157. Forns X, Emerson SU, Purcell RH, Bukh J. Deletion mutant of hepatitis C virus (HCV) molecular infectious clone lacking the hypervariable region 1 (HVR1) is viable but attenuated in vivo. Hepatology 1999;30:422A

158. Chisari FV. Im munobiology and pathogenesis of viral hepatitis. In: Rizzetto M, Purcell RH, Gerin Jl, Verme G, eds. Viral Hepatitis and Liver Disease. Turin: Minerva Medica, 1997, pp. 405–415

159. Botarelli P, Brunetto MR, Minutello MA, et al. T-lymphocyte response to hepatitis C virus in different clinical courses of infection. Gastroenterology 1993;104:580–587

160. Missale G, Bertoni R, Lamonaca V, et al. Different clinical behaviors of acute hepatitis C virus infection are associated with different vigor of the anti-viral cell-mediated immune response. J Clin Invest 1996;98:706–714

161. Diepolder HM, Zachoval R, Hoffmann RM, et al. Possible mechanism involving T-lymphocyte response to non-structural protein 3 in viral clearance in acute hepatitis C virus infection. Lancet 1995;346:1006–1007

162. Erickson AL, Houghton M, Choo QL, et al. Hepatitis C virus-specific CTL responses in the liver of chimpanzees with acute and chronic hepatitis C. J Immunol 1993;151:4189–4199

163. Cooper S, Erickson AL, Adams EJ, et al. Analysis of a successful immune response against hepatitis C virus. Immunity 1999;10:439–449

164. Thimme R, La Jolla CA, Bukh J, et al. HCV persists despite a multispecific peripheral and intrahepatic T cell response in acutely infected chimpanzees. Hepatology 1999;30:422A

165. Weiner A, Erickson AL, Kansopon J, et al. Persistent hepatitis C virus infection in a chimpanzee is associated with emergence of a cytotoxic T lymphocyte escape variant. Proc Natl Acad Sci USA 1995;92:2755–2759

166. Chang K-M, Rehermann B, McHutchison JG, et al. Immunological significance of cytotoxic T lymphocyte epitope variants in patients chronically infected by the hepatitis C virus. J Clin Invest 1997;100:2376–2385

167. Kaneko T, Moriyama T, Udaka K, et al. Impaired induction of cytotoxic T lymphocytes by antagonism of a weak agonist borne by a variant hepatitis C virus epitope. Eur J Immunol 1997;27:1782–1787

168. Wang H, Eckels DD. Mutations in immunodominant T cell epitopes derived from the nonstructural 3 protein of hepatitis C virus have the potential for generating escape variants that may have important consequences for T cell recognition. J Immunol 1999;162:4177–4183

169. Tsai S-L, Chen Y-M, Chen M-H, et al. Hepatitis C virus variants circumventing cytotoxic T-lymphocyte activity as a mechanism of chronicity. Gastroenterology 1998;115:954–966

170. Farci P, Shirmoda A, Colana A, et al. The outcome of acute hepatitis C predicted by the evolution of the viral quasispecies. Science 2000;288:339–344

171. Farci P, Alter HJ, Shimoda A, et al. Hepatitis C virus-associated fulminant hepatic failure. N Engl J Med 1996;335:631–634

172. Farci P, Munoz SJ, Shimoda A, et al. Experimental transmission of hepatitis C virus-associated fulminant hepatitis to a chimpanzee. J Infect Dis 1999;179:1007–1011

173. Manzin A, Solforosi L, Petrelli E, et al. Evolution of hypervariable region 1 of hepatitis C virus in primary infection. J Virol 1998;72:6271–6276

174. Ray SC, Wang Y-M, Laeyendecker O, et al. Acute hepatitis C virus structural gene sequences as predictors of persistent viremia: Hypervariable region 1 as a decoy. J Virol 1999;73:2938–2946

175. Honda M, Kaneko S, Sakai A, et al. Degree of diversity of hepatitis C virus quasispecies and progression of liver disease. Hepatology 1994;20:1144–1151

176. Naito M, Hayashi N, Moribe T, et al. Hepatitis C viral quasispecies in hepatitis C virus carriers with normal liver enzymes and patients with type C chronic liver disease. Hepatology 1995; 22:407–412

177. Koizumik, Enomoto N, Kurosaki M, et al. Diversity of quasispecies in various disease stages of chronic hepatitis C virus infection and its significance in interferon treatment. Hepatology 1995;22:30–35

178. González-Peralta RP, Quian K, She JY, et al. Clinical implications of viral quasispecies heterogeneity in chronic hepatitis C. J Med Virol 1996;49:242–247

179. Kao JH, Chen PJ, Lai MY, et al. Quasispecies of hepatitis C virus and genetic drift of the hypervariable region in chronic type C hepatitis. J Infect Dis 1995;172:261–264

180. Yuki N, Hayashi N, Moribe T, et al. Relation of disease activity during chronic hepatitis C infection to complexity of hypervariable region 1 quasispecies. Hepatology 1997;25:439–444

181. Toyoda H, Fukuda Y, Koyama Y, et al. Nucleotide sequence diversity of hypervariable region 1 of hepatitis C virus in Japanese hemophiliacs with chronic hepatitis C and patients with chronic posttransfusion hepatitis C. Blood 1996;88:1488–1493

182. Sherman KE, Rouster SD, Mendenhall C, Thee D. Hepatitis cRNA quasispecies complexity in patients with alcoholic liver disease. Hepatology 1999;30:265–270

183. Martell M, Esteban JI, Quer J, et al. Dynamic behavior of hepatitis C virus quasispecies in patients undergoing orthotopic liver transplantation. J Virol 1994;68:3425–3436

184. Gretch DR, Polyak SJ, Wilson JJ, et al. Tracking hepatitis C virus quasispecies major and minor variants in symptomatic and asymptomatic liver transplant recipients. J Virol 1996;70:7622–7631

185. Sullivan DG, Wilson JJ, Carithers RL Jr, et al. Multigene tracking of hepatitis C virus quasispecies after liver transplantation: correlation of genetic diversification in the envelope region with asymptomatic or mild disease patterns. J Virol 1998;72:10036–10043

186. Lawal Z, Petrik J, Wong VS, et al. Hepatitis C virus genomic variability in untreated and immunosuppressed patients. Virology 1997;228:107–111

187. Ni Y-H, Chang M-H, Chen P-J, et al. Decreased diversity of hepatitis C virus quasispecies during bone marrow transplantation. J Med Virol 1999;58:132–138

188. Sherman KE, Andreatta C, O'Brien J, et al. Hepatitis C in human immunodeficiency virus-coinfected patients: Increased variability in the hypervariable envelope coding domain. Hepatology 1996;23:688–694

189. Toyoda H, Fukuda Y, Koyama Y, et al. Effect of immunosuppression on composition of quasispecies population of hepatitis C virus in patients with chronic hepatitis C coinfected with human immunodeficiency virus. J Hepatol 1997;26:975–982

190. Odeberg J, Yun Z, Sönnerborg A, et al. Variation of hepatitis C virus hypervariable region 1 in immunocompromised patients. J Infect Dis 1997;175:938–943

191. Booth JCL, Kumar U, Webster D, et al. Comparison of the rate of sequence variation in the hypervariable region of E2/NS1 region of hepatitis C virus in normal and hypogammaglobulinemic patients. Hepatology 1998;27:223–227

192. Laskus T, Radkowski M, Wang L-F, et al. Hepatitis C virus quasispecies in patients infected with HIV-1: Correlation with extrahepatic viral replication. Virology 1998;248:164–171

193. Sakamoto N, Enomoto N, Kurosaki M, et al. Comparison of the hypervariable region of hepatitis C virus genomes in plasma and liver. J Med Virol 1995;46:7–11

194. Fuji K, Hino K, Okazaki M, et al. Differences in hypervariable region 1 quasispecies of hepatitis C virus between human serum and peripheral blood mononuclear cells. Biochem Biophys Res Commun 1996;225:771–776

195. Cabot B, Esteban JI, Martell M, et al. Structure of replicating hepatitis C virus (HCV) quasispecies in the liver may not be reflected by analysis of circulating HCV virions. Virol 1997;71:1732–1734

196. Shimizu YK, Igarashi H, Kanematu T, et al. Sequence analysis of the hepatitis C virus genome recovered from serum, liver, and peripheral blood mononuclear cells of infected chimpanzees. J Virol 1997;71:5769–5773

197. Maggi F, Fornai C, Vatteroni ML, et al. Differences in hepatitis C virus quasispecies composition between liver, peripheral blood mononuclear cells and plasma. J Gen Virol 1997;78:1521–1525

198. Navas S, Martin J, Quiroga JA, et al. Genetic diversity and tissue compartmentalization of the hepatitis C virus genome in blood mononuclear cells, liver, and serum from chronic hepatitis C patients. J Virol 1998;72:1640–1646

199. Maggi F, Fornai C, Morrica A, et al. Divergent evolution of hepatitis C virus in liver and peripheral blood mononuclear cells of infected patients. J Med Virol 1999;57:57–63

200. Okuda M, Hino K, Korenaga M, et al. Differences in hypervariable region 1 quasispecies of hepatitis C virus in human serum, peripheral blood mononuclear cells, and liver. Hepatology 1999;29:217–222

201. Fan X, Solomon H, Poulos JE, et al. Comparison of genetic heterogeneity of hepatitis C viral RNA in liver tissue and serum. Am J Gastroenterol 1999;94:1347–1354

202. Jang SJ, Wang L-F, Radkowski M, et al. Differences between hepatitis C virus 5′untranslated region quasispecies in serum and liver. J Gen Virol 1999;80:711–716

203. Sakai A, Kaneko S, Masao H, et al. Quasispecies of hepatitis C virus in serum and in three different parts of the liver of patients with chronic hepatitis. Hepatology 1999;30:556–561

204. Kurosaki M, Enomoto N , Sakamoto N, et al. Detection and analysis of replication hepatitis C virus RNA in hepatocellular carcinoma tissues. J Hepatol 1995;22:527–535

205. Horie C, Iwahana H, Horie T, et al. Detection of different quasispecies of hepatitis C virus core region in cancerous and noncancerous lesions. Biochem Biophys Res Commun 1996;26:674–681

206. De Mitri MS, Mele L, Chen CH, et al. Comparison of serum and liver hepatitis C virus quasispecies in HCV-related hepatocellular carcinoma. J Hepatol 1998;29:887–892

207. Weiner AJ, Thaler MM, Crawford K, et al. A unique, predominant hepatitis C virus variant found in an infant born to a mother with multiple variants. J Virol 1993;67:4365–4368

208. Kudo T, Yanase Y, Ohshiro M, et al. Analysis of mother-to-infant transmission of hepatitis C virus: Quasispecies nature and buoyant densities of maternal virus populations. J Med Virol 1997;51:225–230

209. SugitaniM, Shikata T. Comparison of amino acid sequences in hypervariable region-1 of hepatitis C virus clones between human inocula and the infected chimpanzee sera. Virus Res 1998; 56:177–182.

210. Hijikata M, Mizuno K, Rikihisa T, et al. Selective transmission of hepatitis C virus in vivo and in vitro. Arch Virol 1995; 140:1623–1628

211. Kojima M, Osuga T, Tsuda F, et al. Influence of antibodies to the hypervariable region of E2/NS1 glycoprotein on the selective replication of hepatitis C virus in chimpanzees. Virology 1994,204:665–672

212. Fried MW, Hoofnagle JH. Therapy of hepatitis C. Semin Liver Dis 1995;15:82–91

213. Okada S, Akahane Y, Suzuki H, et al. The degree of variability in the amino terminal region of the E2/NS1 protein of hepatitis C virus correlates with responsiveness to interferon therapy in viremic patients. Hepatology 1992;16:619–624

214. Kanazawa Y, Hayashi N, Mita E, et al. Influence of viral quasispecies on effectiveness of interferon therapy in chronic hepatitis C patients. Hepatology 1994;20:1121–1130

215. Mizokami M, Lau JYN, Suzuki K, et al. Differential sensitivity of hepatitis C virus quasispecies to interferon-therapy. J Hepatol 1994;21:884–886

216. Yeh BI, Han KH, Oh SH, et al. Nucleotide sequence variation in the hypervariable region of the hepatitis C virus in the sera of chronic hepatitis C patients undergoing controlled interferon-therapy. J Med Virol 1996;49:95–102

217. González-Peralta RP, Qian K, She JY, et al. Clinical implications of viral quasispecies heterogeneity in chronic hepatitis C. J Med Virol 1996;49:242–247

218. Toyoda H, Kumada T, Nakano S, et al. Quasispecies nature of hepatitis C virus and response to alpha interferon: Significance as a predictor of direct response to interferon. J Hepatol 1997; 26:6–13

219. Le Guen B, Squadrito G, Nalpas B, et al. Hepatitis C virus genome complexity correlates with response to interferon therapy: A study in French patients with chronic hepatitis C. Hepatology 1997;25:1250–1254

220. Pawlotsky JM, Pellerin M, Bouvier M, et al. Genetic complexity of the hypervariable region 1 (HVR1) of hepatitis C virus (HCV): Influence on the characteristics of the infection and responses to interferon alfa therapy in patients with chronic hepatitis C. J Med Virol 1998;54:256–264

221. Hagiwara H, Hayashi N, Kasahara A, et al. Treatment with recombinant interferon-alpha 2a for patients with chronic hepatitis C: Predictive factors for biochemical and virologic response. Osaka Liver disease Study Group. Scand J Gastroenterol 1996; 31:1021–1026

222. Shindo M, Hamada K, Koya S, et al. The clinical significance of changes in genetic heterogeneity of the hypervariable region 1 in chronic hepatitis C with interferon therapy. Hepatology 1996; 24:1018–1023

223. Polyak SJ, Faulkner G, Carithers RL Jr, et al. Assessment of hepatitis C virus quasispecies heterogeneity by gel shift analysis:

224. Yun ZB, Odeberg J, Lundeberg J, et al. Restriction of hepatitis C virus heterogeneity during prolonged interferon-alpha therapy in relation to changes in virus load. J Infect Dis 1996;173:992–996

225. Sakuma I, Enomoto N, Kurosaki M, et al. Selection of hepatitis C virus quasispecies during interferon treatment. Arch Virol 1996;141:1921–1932

226. Polyak SJ, McArdle S, Liu S-L, et al. Evolution of hepatitis C virus quasispecies in hypervariable region 1 and the putative interferon sensitivity-determining region during interferon therapy and natural infection. J Virol 1998;72:4288–4296

227. Pawlotsky JM, Germanidis G, Frainais PO, et al. Evolution of the hepatitis C virus second envelope protein hypervariable region in chronically infected patients receiving alpha interferon therapy. J Virol 1999;73:6490–6499

228. Farci P, Strazzera R, De Gioannis D, et al. Evolution of HCV quasispecies in the different patterns of response to interferon therapy in chronic hepatitis C. Proceedings of the 6th International Symposium on Hepatitis C and Related Viruses, Bethesda, MD, 6–9 June 1999, p. 80

229. Gerotto M, Sullivan DG, Polyak SJ, et al. Effect of retreatment with interferon alone or interferon plus ribavirin on hepatitis C virus quasispecies diversification in nonresponder patients with chronic hepatitis C. J Virol 1999;73:7241–7247

230. González-Peralta RP, Liu WZ, Davis GL, et al. Modulation of hepatitis C virus quasispecies heterogeneity by interferon-alpha and ribavirin therapy. J Viral Hepat 1997;4:99–106

231. Lee J-H, von Wagner M, Roth WK, et al. Effect of ribavirin on virus load and quasispecies distribution in patients infected with hepatitis C virus. J Hepatol 1998;29:29–35

232. Enomoto N, Sakuma I, Asahina Y, et al. Comparison of full-length sequences of interferon-sensitive and resistant hepatitis C virus 1b. J Clin Invest 1995;96:224–230

233. Enomoto N, Sakuma I, Asahina Y, et al. Mutations in the nonstructural protein 5A gene and response to interferon in patients with chronic hepatitis C virus 1b infection. N Engl J Med 1996;334:77–81

234. Tao Q, Wei L, Chang J, et al. Relationship between interferon therapy and variability in nonstructural gene 5b of hepatitis C virus. J Gastroenterol 1998;33:684–693

235. Saiz JC, Lopez-Labrador FX, Ampurdanes S, et al. The prognostic relevance of the nonstructural A gene interferon sensitivity determining region is different in infections with genotype 1b and 3a isolates of hepatitis C virus. J Infect Dis 1998;177: 839–847

236. Gale MJ, Jr., Korth MJ, Tang NM, et al. Evidence that hepatitis C virus resistance to interferon is mediated through repression of the PKR protein kinase by the nonstructural A protein. Virology 1997;230:217–227

237. Squadrito G, Leone F, Sartori M, et al. Mutations in the nonstructural A region of hepatitis C virus and response of chronic hepatitis C to interferon alfa. Gastroenterololy 1997;113: 67–72

238. Odeberg J, Yun Z, Sonnerborg A, et al. Variation in the hepatitis C virus NS5a region in relation to hypervariable region 1 heterogeneity during interferon treatment. J Med Virol 1998;6: 33–38

239. Pawlotsky JM, Germanidis G, Neumann AU, et al. Interferon resistance of hepatitis C virus genotype 1b: Relationship to nonstructural 5A gene quasispecies mutations. J Virol 1998;72: 279–280

correlation with response to interferon therapy. J Infect Dis 1997;175:1101–1107

Interaction between the Hepatitis C Virus and the Immune System

BARBARA REHERMANN, M.D.

ABSTRACT: The hepatitis C virus (HCV) causes a wide spectrum of liver diseases ranging from symptomatic or asymptomatic acute infection with self-limited disease to persistent infection with chronic active hepatitis and an increased risk of liver cirrhosis and hepatocellular carcinoma. The outcome of HCV infection (i.e., viral clearance or persistence) and the manifestation and degree of liver disease is the result of complicated interactions between the virus and the immune response of the host. Remarkably, most de novo HCV infections are clinically inapparent and characterized by a high incidence (70%) of chronically evolving hepatitis, which suggests that HCV may have evolved strategies to not induce, overcome, or evade efficient immune responses of the host. This may be a multifactorial process, influenced by viral tissue tropism, replication, sequence variation and by functional alteration of infected cells. The interaction between HCV and the specific humoral and cellular immune response of the host, the role of the liver as the primary site of viral replication, the target of the host's immune response, and potential mechanisms of viral escape are discussed.

KEY WORDS: liver, hepatitis C, T cell, cytotoxic, immune response

HEPATITIS C VIRUS INFECTION AND CELL AND TISSUE TROPISM

Infection with the hepatitis C virus (HCV) is generally thought to occur via parenteral or percutaneous routes and HCV virions spread via the bloodstream to the liver, the primary site of HCV replication. As early as 2 days after infection of chimpanzees, HCV RNA is detectable in the liver,[1] and during chronic infection, the liver has been shown to contain high levels of HCV RNA. However, as discussed in E. Gowan's article in this two-issue series in *Seminars in Liver Diseases*, the

---

Objectives
Upon completion of this article, the reader should be able to 1) summarize components and functions of the innate and adaptive, cellular and humoral immune response in antiviral defense; 2) characterize the HCV-specific cellular immune response in acute, self-limited and chronic hepatitis C; 3) discuss potential mechanisms of HCV persistence.

Accreditation
The Indiana University School of Medicine is accredited by the Accreditation Council for Continuing Medical Education to provide continuing medical education for physicians.

Credit
The Indiana University School of Medicine designates this educational activity for a maximum of 1.0 hours credit toward the AMA Physicians Recognition Award in category one. Each physician should claim only those hours of credit that he/she actually spent in the educational activity.

Disclosure
Statements have been obtained regarding the author's relationships with financial supporters of this activity. There is no apparent conflict of interest related to the context of participation of the author of this article.

Liver Diseases Section, NIDDK, National Institutes of Health, Bethesda, Maryland.

Reprint requests: Barbara Rehermann, M.D., Liver Diseases Section, NIDDK, National Institutes of Health, Bldg. 10, Room 9B16, 10 Center Drive, Bethesda, MD 20892. E-mail: Rehermann@nih.gov

Published by Thieme Medical Publishers, Inc., 333 Seventh Avenue, New York, NY 10001, USA. Tel.: +1(212) 584-4662. 0272-8087,p;2000,20,02,127,142,ftx,en;sld00052x

number of virions produced on a per cell basis is estimated to be low[2] and most infected hepatocytes display little or no hepatocellular damage,[3] which provides evidence for a noncytopathic nature of HCV. Using reverse transcriptase polymerase chain reaction techniques with a high specificity for the negative-strand HCV RNA, HCV is also commonly detected in lymph nodes and pancreas and less frequently in adrenal glands, bone marrow, thyroid tissue, and spleen.[4] Whether HCV also replicates in peripheral blood mononuclear cells is still controversial.[5–7]

It has recently been suggested that HCV is selectively associated with low-density lipoproteins (LDL) in type II mixed cryoglobulins[8] and that this complex facilitates viral entry into cells by selective binding to the LDL receptor and endocytosis.[9] A second HCV binding protein and candidate receptor is human CD81, a tetraspanin with four transmembrane segments that is expressed on most human cells except for red blood cells and platelets.[10] It has been shown to bind to the HCV E2 protein coated on beads[11] and to HCV RNA containing particles in chimpanzee infectious plasma. Binding is species specific and can be inhibited by anti-E2 antibodies and by serum from protected chimpanzee vaccinees. Importantly, it is still to be demonstrated whether either of these receptors provides a route of entry that causes productive infection of hepatocytes. Even in the absence of viral replication, however, uptake and processing of viral antigens may lead to display of viral peptides on major histocompatibility complex (MHC) molecules, recognition of these hepatocytes by virus-specific T cells, and may thus contribute to pathogenesis of liver disease.

HUMORAL IMMUNE RESPONSE

The humoral immune response against HCV is targeted against epitopes within all viral proteins.[12–15] As in other viral infections, antibody binding could potentially interfere with viral entry into host cells and replication. Antibody binding could also opsonize virions for elimination by macrophages and transport to secondary lymphatic organs to induce efficient cellular immune responses. In other viral infections, it has recently been shown that not only specific but also natural antibodies (i.e., the innate immune response) may contribute to these effects.[16] The relevance of unspecific and specific antibodies for the outcome of HCV infection, however, is difficult to assess because of the lack of an in vitro cell culture system or a small animal model of infection that would allow analysis of virus neutralization and infection.

Although individuals vary in both antibody specificity and timing of anti-HCV seroconversion, HCV-specific antibodies are generally detectable in the serum between 7 and 31 weeks after infection.[17] This response appears to be rather late when compared with humoral responses against other viruses[18–21] and to the cellular immune response to HCV.[22] Evidence for a protective role of HCV-specific antibodies stems from limited studies in which chimpanzee-infectious HCV was neutralized in vitro by incubation with antibody. Thus far, the hypervariable region 1 (HVR1) of the HCV E2 protein has been identified as target for neutralizing antibodies.[23–25] This region exhibits high-sequence variability,[26–31] and it has been suggested that viral escape mutants are selected by the humoral immune response. For example, a hyperimmune rabbit serum directed against the HVR1 sequence that was predominant in a plasma sample of a chronically infected patient blocked replication of HCV obtained from this same sample but not from a plasma sample obtained from the same patient 13 years later. Notably, the later sample contained a different predominant HVR1 sequence.[25] Similarly, Farci et al.[24] showed that hyperimmune rabbit serum raised against the predominant HVR1 sequence of the earlier sample could neutralize homologous HCV. However, neutralization was not complete, and escape mutants emerged that had already constituted minor variants in the initial inoculum.

In addition to the HVR1 sequence, neutralizing antibodies also appear to be targeted to other sequences within the envelope glycoproteins. Vaccination with recombinant envelope proteins expressed in mammalian cells elicited high titers of glycoprotein-specific antibodies that protected chimpanzees from low-dose homologous HCV.[32] In this experiment, the strongest correlate of protection was the level of specific antibodies capable of inhibiting binding of the HCV E2 ectodomain to the candidate HCV receptor CD81 expressed by the cell line Molt-4.[11,33] This neutralization of binding (NOB) assay was also used to detect high titers of antibodies that interfered with binding to the HCV E2 protein in sera of patients who resolved chronic hepatitis C.[34] Thus, data suggest that the epitope responsible for priming of NOB antibody responses is conserved between different viral genotypes.

Despite these observations, however, the role of antibodies in the outcome of HCV infection remains unclear. On the one hand, several studies suggest that an early antibody response to the NH_2 terminus of HVR1 is associated with a self-limited course of infection[35–37] and that more complex initial quasispecies distribution and viral complexity of the HVR1 is associated with HCV persistence.[38] On the other hand, however, a recent study on HCV-infected chimpanzees reports that HCV clearance occurred in the absence of any antibody response to the envelope proteins.[39] Moreover, two independent studies demonstrated that HCV persistence in 12 chimpanzees was not associated with sequence changes in the envelope proteins and specifically the HVR-1 region.[39,40] Similarly, an analysis of HCV variations in acutely infected and prospectively followed patients demonstrates that a correlation between HCV clearance and nonsynonymous changes in E1 was complemented by a similar correlation between HCV persistence and nonsynonymous changes in HVR1/E2, suggesting that HVR1 may act as an immunologic decoy and that additional mechanisms are involved in establishing and maintaining viral persistence.[38]

CELLULAR IMMUNE RESPONSE

Immunology of the Liver

The liver as the primary site of HCV replication represents a unique microenvironment with distinct immunologic characteristics. Its location between gastrointestinal tract and peripheral lymphoid organs and its fenestrated endothelium allows contact with many antigenic substances. These consist of dietary antigens derived from the gut that reach the liver via the portal vein, new substances generated during intrahepatic metabolism, and antigens from pathogenic organisms such as HCV that invade the liver. This may explain the observations that the liver has the capacity to induce immunologic tolerance,[41,42] and immune responses against pathogens.

Most importantly, even the uninfected average liver of 1,200–1,500 g contains approximately 10^9–10^{10} lymphocytes, and a high percentage is considered to represent truly resident lymphocytes. Because liver and gut are derived from the endoderm, both organs can support tissue-specific lymphocyte differentiation as evidenced by expression of genes such as recombinase activation genes 1 and 2 that are otherwise only expressed by immature thymocytes undergoing gene rearrangement.[43-46] Similarly, CD45, CD34, and CD7 expression indicate the presence of hematopoietic stem cells and early lymphoid progenitors in the liver,[47] and indeed, hematopoesis can take place in the fetal liver and in liver grafts.[48]

The lymphocyte population of the liver, however, differs considerably from that found in the blood. Specifically, the CD4:CD8 ratio is reversed, and the CD8+ T-cell population is extremely heterogeneous and contains a large percentage of unconventional lymphocytes that are not frequently found in the peripheral blood.[47] These include CD4−CD8− double-negative T cells,[49-51] CD4+CD8+ double-positive T cells,[47] T cells that display the γδ T-cell receptor instead of the αβ T-cell receptor that characterizes peripheral blood T cells,[52] and cells that express both the natural killer (NK) cell marker CD56 and the T-cell marker CD3.[53]

The latter have been termed NKT cells and have distinct functional characteristics, such as the ability to recognize nonpeptide antigens presented by nonclassical MHC molecules.[54]

Innate Immune Response

The innate immune response does not only constitute the earliest phase of immune defense but also regulates the adaptive immune response.[55] Although it is known that the liver, the primary site of HCV replication, is significantly enriched for cells of the innate immune response, the relevance of this antigen-nonspecific immune response has not been sufficiently studied during HCV infection yet. An important question is, for example, whether HCV may have developed strategies to avoid stimulation of the innate immune response, which could explain the asymptomatic onset of *de novo* infection and the generally weak adaptive immune response during persistent infection.

In general, innate immune responses occur early, within the first days, after viral infections and can directly activate intracellular mechanisms that inhibit viral replication, gene expression, or protein synthesis. Many viruses produce double stranded RNA in infected cells, a potent inducer of interferon (IFN)α/β.[56] IFNα/β interferes with the replication of viruses such as vesicular stomatitis virus, influenza virus, vaccinia virus, herpes simplex virus, picornavirus, and reovirus[57] by induction of 2′5′-oligoadenylate synthetase and double-stranded RNA-dependent protein kinase (PKR), enzymes that both inhibit protein synthesis in infected cells.[57] Interestingly, defined sequences within two proteins of HCV, namely E2 and NS5A, have been shown to bind to protein kinase and to alter its function (see below).

Other cytokines that are part of the innate immune response and can be produced by macrophages, NK cells, and polymorphonuclear leukocytes include interleukin (IL)-12, tumor necrosis factor (TNF)α, IL-1α, IL-1β, IL-6, IL-10, transforming growth factor (TGF)-β, IL-12, IL-15, and IL-18. Many of these proteins modify distribution and migration of immune cells[56,58] and activate the main cells of the innate response (i.e., macrophages and NK cells).[59]

It is important to note that the liver is the organ with the highest proportion of CD56+ NK-like cells in the body (22–40%).[47] Depending on coexpression of the T-cell marker CD3, these cells are termed NK cells (CD56+CD3−) or NKT cells (CD56+CD3+). NK cells are activated by INFα/β and lyse target cells via perforin. They can also be stimulated through their cell surface receptors for immunoglobulins to mediate antibody-dependent cellular cytotoxicity and to produce the cytokines IFNγ, TNF, granulocyte-macrophage colony-stimulating factor (GM-CSF), and the beta chemokines macrophage inflammatory protein (MIP)-1α, MIP-1β, and RANTES (regulated upon activation, normal T cell expressed and secreted). MIP-1α[60] and TNF[61,62] are also potent inducers of NK cell chemotaxis and thus promote accumulation of even more NK cells within the liver. Because NK cell responses of cytotoxicity and IFNγ production occur within the first several hours to days after primary infections, these cells could efficiently lyse virus-infected cells before assembly and release of virions. However, NK cell function is inhibited by MHC class I molecules that stimulate inhibitory (killing inhibitory receptor) receptors on NK cell surfaces and deliver negative signals.[63] Interestingly, MHC class I expression on hepatocytes is upregulated during HCV infection.[64,65] If this effect occurs early during acute HCV infection (which has not been demonstrated yet), it may represent a viral strategy to avoid recognition by NK cells and to escape from an innate immune responses.

Adaptive Cellular Immune Response in Acute Self-limited Hepatitis C

It is generally assumed that the HCV-specific adaptive immune response is primed in lymph nodes and possibly in the bone marrow, which was recently reported as an alternative pathway for priming of MHC class I restricted CD8+ antiviral T cells.[66,67] This assumption is based on the observation that virus infected nonhematopoietic cells, although recognized by virus-specific T cells, are not capable of directly stimulating primary T-cell-mediated immunity due to a lack or low level expression of adhesion and costimulatory molecules and the absence of MHC class II expression.[67] Thus, professional antigen-presenting cells such as dendritic cells in lymph nodes and/or bone marrow are required to initiate antiviral T-cell responses. Although most cells present peptides that are derived from intracellularly synthesized viral proteins, a process that requires productive infection, these professional antigen-presenting cells do have an additional alternative processing pathway and can present peptides from extracellular antigens on MHC class I molecules. Thus, these cells may acquire viral antigen by phagocytosis of apoptotic virus-infected cells.[67] Although the relevance of this pathway for the induction immune responses against hepatitis viruses remains to be demonstrated, the noncytopathic nature of HCV may correlate well with the weak induction of immune responses.

Naive T cells express L-selectin, an adhesion molecule that directs them to the high endothelial venules in lymph nodes. Upon recognition of antigens via their specific T-cell receptor, antigen-specific T cells then become activated, down-regulate L-selectin, and leave the lymph node via efferent lymph vessels. An HCV-specific response of CD4+ and CD8+ T cells is generally detectable in the blood of HCV-infected chimpanzees within the first weeks after infection (T. Arichi et al., unpublished observation, 1999).

The adaptive cellular immune response is thought to play a particularly important role in the host's defense against noncytopathic viruses such as HCV because of its ability to recognize viral antigens in HCV-infected cells throughout the body due to the ubiquitous distribution of MHC class I expression and because of its ability to induce and to maintain immunologic memory. These functions are attributed to antigen-specific helper (T_H) and CD8+ cytotoxic T cells (CTL). CD4+ T_H cells recognize viral peptides presented by other cells in the context of MHC class II molecules and CD8+ T cells respond to peptides presented on MHC class I molecules. Whereas peptides presented by MHC class II molecules are derived from phagocytosed and proteolytically cleaved viral proteins, peptides presented on MHC class I molecules stem from viral proteins that are endogenously synthesized in HCV infected cells (Fig. 1).

Upon activation via their specific T-cell receptors, HCV-specific T_H cells fulfill a variety of immunoregulatory functions, most of them mediated by T_H1 and T_H2 cytokines.[68,69] Specifically, they provide help for activation and differentiation of B cells or for induction[70] and stimulation of virus-specific cytotoxic T cells. Together with CTL, T_H cells may also secrete IFNγ and TNF-α that inhibit replication and gene expression of several viruses such as hepatitis B,[71] cytomegalovirus,[72] and rotavirus.[73] Finally, T_H cells and CTL, the main effector cells, can induce apoptosis and lysis of virus-infected cells.[74]

Recent studies suggest that the human leukocyte antigen (HLA) class II restricted T_H cell response is particularly important for the outcome of acute HCV infection.[75–80] Specifically, patients with acute self-limited hepatitis C have been demonstrated to mount an early, vigorous, and multispecific T-helper response that is readily detectable in the peripheral blood. If, in contrast, this immune response is weak, less efficient, or not maintained for a sufficient length of time, patients proceed to persistent infection and chronic hepatitis.[80] Thus, the intensity, epitope specificity, and cytokine profile of the T-cell response during the early stages of HCV infection seem to be predictive for the outcome of HCV infection.

The most frequently recognized HCV T_H epitopes are located within the HCV core 21–40 NS3 1253–1272, NS4 1767–1786, and NS4 1909–1929 amino acid sequences.[79] Remarkably, all these immunodominant epitopes are highly conserved among HCV genotypes and bind promiscuously and with high affinity to a large panel of different HLA class II molecules. Thus, they

Presentation by MHC I molecules

Presentation by MHC II molecules

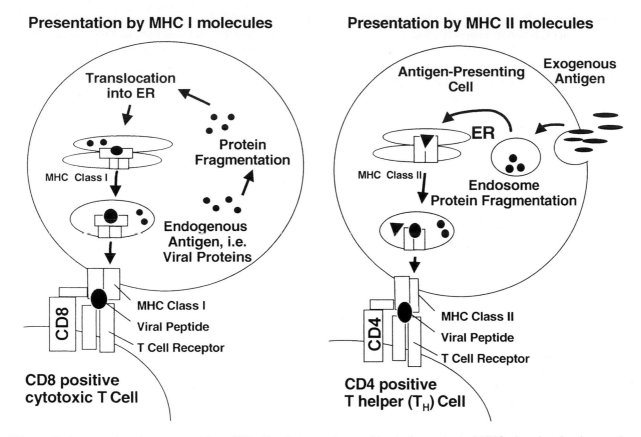

FIG. 1. Pathways of antigen processing. CD8+ T cells recognize peptides in the context of MHC class I molecules on virus-infected cells. Peptides are derived from intracellulary synthesized and processed viral proteins. CD4+ T cells recognize peptides in the MHC class II binding grove of antigen-presenting cells. These peptides are derived from viral proteins that are internalized by the antigen-presenting cell.

are ideal candidates for preventive or therapeutic T-cell-based vaccines.

Because T_H cells that mediate this HCV-specific immune response frequently display a T_H1 or T_H0 cytokine profile and IFNγ as the predominant T_H1 cytokine and IL-2 as the predominant T_H0 cytokine support differentiation and proliferation of CD8+ T cells, it is not surprising that early, vigorous, and multispecific CTL responses have also been associated with a self-limited outcome of HCV infection.[81] In chimpanzees, termination of acute infection correlated precisely with the onset of an early and multispecific intrahepatic CTL response, whereas chronically evolving hepatitis C was associated with a delayed and weaker T-cell response targeted against fewer epitopes.[82] As recently described in HIV infection,[83] it is therefore possible that qualitative differences in the initial immune response to a given pathogen, reflected by the diversity of the primary cytotoxic T-cell response, determine the outcome of HCV infection. Because of different HLA haplotypes and the shaping of the T-cell repertoire during thymus ontogeny,[84] it is conceivable that both epitope specificity and the size of HCV-specific T-cell

populations vary between individuals and that these differences may be further aggrevated by different antigenic composition and quantity of the virus and by its route of infection.

Similar to T_H epitopes, CTL epitopes have been identified in all viral proteins.[85–91] Because many epitopes can be recognized in the context of several HLA haplotypes, HLA class I supertype families have been defined. Importantly, the A2-like,[92] B7-like,[93] B44-like,[94] and A3-like supertypes[95] cover the HLA haplotypes of more than 80% of the world population—an important consideration for the applicability of potential T-cell-based vaccines.

Interestingly, a recent study by Scognamiglio et al.[96] demonstrated HCV-specific T cells in the blood of 7 of 29 (24%) healthy family members of HCV-infected patients. These cells were capable of mounting an immediate IFNγ response upon antigen-specific T-cell receptor ligation and did not require *in vitro* proliferation, restimulation, or the addition of specific cytokines. Thus, they represent potent effector cells that may be sustained by and confer protection upon frequent reexposure to HCV.

Adaptive Cellular Immune Response in Chronic Hepatitis C

As described above, lack or loss of a multispecific and vigorous T_H cell response in the early phase of infection is associated with chronic evolution of infection. Similarly, the CTL response is weaker in chronically evolving than in self-limited hepatitis C, and repetitive *in vitro* stimulation with HCV-derived peptides is required to expand CTL from the peripheral blood.[87,97] Thus, the frequency of progenitor CTL in the circulation is rather low. For example, T cells specific for two HCV NS3 epitopes constitute between 0.01 and 1.2 % of all peripheral blood CD8+ T cells.[98] For comparison, between 7 and 44% of peripheral blood CD8-positive T cells have been demonstrated to be Epstein-Barr virus specific in acute EBV infection and 50–70% of activated CD8+ T cells were lymphocytic choriomeningitis virus specific during the acute phase of LCMV infection.[99] Although the reasons for the weak cellular immune response of patients with chronic hepatitis C have not been determined, the strength of the CTL response against influenza virus[97] and Epstein Barr virus[100] was comparable with that of healthy non-HCV-infected patients and renders the hypothesis of generalized immune suppression unlikely.

At the site of inflammation, the infected liver, the frequency of CD8+ T cells was found to be at least 30-fold higher than in the blood.[98] Importantly, all the intrahepatic HCV NS3-specific CD8+ T cells were CD69+,[98] suggesting that they were activated and presumably exert a certain control over viral load but do at the same time also contribute to immunopathogenesis of liver disease. Along this line it has been shown that a stronger polyclonal CTL response in the peripheral blood[101] and the liver[102] is associated with lower levels of HCV viremia, but it is also known that long-standing immune-mediated liver injury may eventually result in liver cirrhosis and hepatocellular carcinoma.[103]

Recruitment of T Cells to the Liver

How are activated HCV-specific T cells recruited to the liver? Chemokines are important molecules for the selective attraction of specific subsets of leukocytes and expression of the chemokine receptors CXCR3 and CCR5 has been found to be higher on lymphocytes isolated from the liver than from the peripheral blood.[104] Chemokine receptor expression and tissue-specific migration is related to the activation status of T cells. Whereas naive T cells only express CXCR4, most memory/activated T cells express CXCR3. Moreover, T_H1 and T_H2 cells express distinct patterns of chemokine receptors that can further be modulated by inflammatory cytokines such as IFNα and TGF-β.[105] The chemokine receptor CXCR3, for example, is expressed at high levels on T_H0 and T_H1 cells and at low levels on T_H2 cells, whereas CCR3, CCR4 and CCR8 constitute T_H2 cell specific markers.[106]

What are the ligands for chemokine receptors expressed on different T cell subsets? CXCR3 and CCR5[105] bind to two molecules with chemoattractant and proinflammatory functions,[107] namely IFN-inducible protein-10 (IP-10) and monokine-induced by IFNγ (MIG). These chemokines of the CXC family are preferentially expressed by hepatic sinusoidal endothelial cells and macrophages. Thus, expression of the CXCR3 ligands IP-10 and MIG would lead to a preferential T_H1 cell recruitment, whereas expression of CCR3 or CCR4 ligands such as eotaxin would lead to preferential T_H2 cell recruitment. Indeed, expression of IP-10 and MIG are upregulated by the T_H1 cytokine IFNγ together with IL-1 and TNFα liver,[104,108,109] resulting in a potent amplification cascade in the inflamed liver.

CCR5 is also the receptor for three other chemokines of the CC chemokine family (i.e., MIP-1α), MIP-1β, and RANTES). MIP-1α and MIP-1β are predominantly expressed by vascular endothelium within portal tracts in both normal and hepatitis C liver. Interestingly, cytotoxic CD8+ T cells also release MIP-1α, MIP-1β, and RANTES, which are stored with granzyme A in their cytotoxic granules.[110,111] Thus, in addition to mediating cytotoxic function, CD8+ T cells may be able to attract additional T_H cells and CD8+ T cells via MIP-1α–CCR5 interaction. These findings may be of therapeutic value. For example, treatment with anti-CCR5 and anti-MIP-1α antibodies reduced the infiltration of CCR5-positive CD8-positive T lymphocytes into the liver and consequently protected against liver damage in graft versus host disease.[112] Thus, chemokine-induced migration of CCR5 expressing CD8+ T cells into the portal areas of the liver plays a significant role in the pathogenesis of liver injury.[112]

Because certain adhesion molecules are constitutively expressed even in the noninflamed liver, this mechanism traps activated peripheral blood T cells in the liver regardless of the antigen specificity.[113] Binding of circulating T cells to specific chemokines and adhesion molecules expressed on sinusoidal endothelial cells and Kupffer cells[113] is facilitated by the low blood flow and branched structure of the intrahepatic vascular bed and by the mobility of the Kupffer cells.[114] Accordingly, a large percentage of influenza-specific T cells has been detected in the liver and in the lung of influenza virus-infected mice.[115] Once activated T cells are trapped the liver, they undergo activation induced cell death, presumably induced by T-cell activation in the absence of sufficient costimulation. Under such conditions, apoptosis occurs within 18 hours.[113] Thus, activated cells are continuously recruited from the peripheral blood,[116] and the normal liver can be regarded as a sink for activated T cells and may contribute to homeostasis of the T-cell repertoire after pathogen-induced expansion of antigen-specific T-cell clones.

Mechanisms of Immune-mediated Liver Injury

Within the HCV-infected liver, a certain local and functional compartmentalization of antigen-specific cells has been observed. Although CD4+ T_H cells are found in the portal areas,[117] CD8+ T cells infiltrate the hepatic lobules.[118] B cells, on the other hand, are predominantly seen in germinal centers of lymphoid follicles located in the portal tracts.[119,120] These lymphoid follicles belong to the triade of characteristic histologic features that allow differentiation between hepatitis C and other kinds of liver disease (bile duct damage and steatosis are the other components of this triade). Studies on the effector function of intrahepatic T cells revealed that the intrahepatic T_H cell response is focused on the HCV NS4 protein and mediated by T cells that express a selective T-cell receptor not found in the peripheral blood compartment.[121] The predominant use of Vβ5.1 by intrahepatic T cells[122] also indicates oligoclonal expansion and a restricted specificity for a common immunodominant HCV antigen.

Immune-mediated liver disease is thought to be initiated by these HCV-specific liver-infiltrating T cells but amplified by antigen-nonspecific cells. Presentation of HCV antigens on infected hepatocytes, recognition by CTL, and induction of liver injury seems to be enhanced by HCV-induced expression of HLA-A, B and C and intercellular adhesion molecule (ICAM-1) molecules.[64] In more aggressive forms of HCV infection, even CD68+ macrophages and monocytes are found. These activated cells are thought to mediate and enhance antigen presentation and the inflammatory process as a whole.[123,124] Indeed, in regions of active inflammation,[125] CD8+ T cells can be found surrounding Fas antigen-expressing hepatocytes,[64] and the generation of acidophil Councilman bodies is interpreted as CTL-induced hepatocyte apoptosis.[120]

Destruction of infected hepatocytes may occur in several ways: HCV-infected hepatocytes can be killed by HCV-specific CTL clones via Fas ligand, TNFα, and/or perforin-based mechanisms. Fas ligand-induced apoptosis of hepatocytes is especially feasible because expression of Fas, a mediator of apoptosis,[125] is upregulated on HCV-infected hepatocytes and on uninfected bystander cells in response to inflammatory cytokines[126] and because Fas-ligand is expressed on activated liver-infiltrating T cells.[127] TNFα is predominantly produced by macrophages[128] but also released

by[88] and expressed on the surface of CTL.[129] Finally, perforin-mediated mechanisms may contribute to lysis of antigen-presenting, Fas-, and TNFα-resistant cells.[130]

After exerting their effector functions, the majority of these liver-infiltrating HCV-specific T cells undergo programmed cell death. Especially, T_H1 cells, which are preferentially attracted into HCV-infected livers, are sensitive to Fas - FasL-induced apoptosis, whereas T_H2 effectors express high levels of FAP-1, a Fas-associated phophatase that presumably inhibits Fas signaling.[131] The loss of lymphocytes by intrahepatic sequestration and apoptosis has been estimated to be as high as 2×10^8 cells (i.e., 0.1% of the total body lymphocytes per day).[132]

ANIMAL MODELS

Chimpanzee

The chimpanzee (*Pan troglodyte*) is the only proven animal model for HCV infection and disease. It is genetically more than 98.5% identical to humans, an important fact for immune response studies because many HCV epitopes are presented and recognized by both chimpanzee and human MHC molecules and T-cell receptors, respectively. Chimpanzee studies provided the first evidence for HCV transmission and allowed amplification of the virus for cloning and molecular characterization of the genome[133] and insights into the physical nature of the virus.[134] Currently, the chimpanzee is also an important model for studies on viral sequence and quasispecies evolution,[40] the kinetics of virus–host interaction, and the mechanisms of recovery from infection, especially because infectious RNA transcripts from a functional molecular clone allowed infection/pathogenesis studies with a single well-defined viral polyprotein sequence.[135-138] Finally, the chimpanzee is also the only model to test prophylactic and therapeutic vaccines.

Many aspects of HCV infection are similar in humans and chimpanzees, including the level of viremia, the timing of serum alanine aminotransferase (ALT) elevations that peak approximately 10–14 weeks after infection, and humoral and cellular immune responses.[135] There are, however, some differences. For example, the onset of hepatitis C in chimpanzees is typically milder than in humans. This is reflected in the degree of hepatic injury measured by ALT levels or histopathology[139,140] both in acute and in chronic HCV infection. Although about 25% of patients with transfusion-associated hepatitis C become jaundiced, there are no reports of jaundice in HCV-infected chimpanzees. Similarly, chimpanzees rarely develop significant chronic liver disease,[141] although both chronic hepatitis and hepatocellular carcinoma have been reported.[142] This observation may be biased, however, by the young age at which many animals were infected, the short observation period, and also by the fact that asymptomatic self-limited HCV infections of humans are generally not diagnosed. Indeed, the incidence of viral clearance with complete recovery from disease and the incidence of a mild course of chronic HCV infection was significantly higher than expected, when long-term follow-up studies after documented exposure were performed.[143–145] Thus, it is possible that the full clinical spectrum of HCV infection in humans has not been observed in studies on select individuals based on virologic or disease status.

Mice

Although HCV does not infect mice, several mouse models have proven valuable in hepatitis C research. Mice that are transgenic for HLA-A2, the most frequent MHC class I molecule, for example, have efficiently been used to identify HLA-A2-restricted HCV epitopes.[146–148] These epitopes were endogenously processed and also recognized by patients with hepatitis C. Despite species differences, the T-cell repertoire of mice is obviously plastic enough to allow a similar response when human or murine/human chimeric MHC class I molecules are presenting a given peptide. Thus, mice transgenic for human MHC molecules represent a good model system to develop immunotherapeutic vaccines. For example, a multiepitope vaccine has been shown to induce simultaneous CTL responses to a pool of five different epitopes in mice transgenic for human HLA alleles,[148] and a prophylactic DNA vaccine was demonstrated to induce HCV core-specific CTL that protected from HCV-recombinant vaccinia infection.[149]

Transgenic mice that express individual or several HCV proteins have been used to analyze the biosynthesis of HCV proteins and their pathogenic role. Liver-specific expression of HCV core and E2 proteins under the control of either the mouse major urinary protein promoter or the albumin promoter resulted in the predominantly cytoplasmic presence of HCV core protein with occasional nuclear staining and both cytoplasmic and membrane expression of the E2 protein. Importantly, the livers of two independent mouse lineages remained histologically normal for the entire observation period (i.e., until 6 and 18 months of age, respectively).[150,151] Although these studies suggest that HCV structural proteins are not directly cytopathic, transgenic mice expressing HCV core under the control of a regulatory region from the hepatitis B virus did develop progressive hepatic steatosis.[152] As early as 2 months after birth, Sudan III positive vacuolating lesions appeared in the cytoplasm of hepatocytes. At the age of 16 months, adenomas with fat droplets in the cytoplasm were present, and ultimately one fourth of the male transgenic mice developed hepatocellular carcinoma.[153] This effect was specific for the expression of HCV core as a transgene, because transgenic mice that carried HCV E1 and E2 under the same transcription control region did not display any neoplastic lesions in the liver.[154]

Finally, immunodeficient mice have been used to adoptively transfer HCV-infected human cells. Specifically, severe combined immunodeficiency (SCID) mice have been inoculated intraperitoneally with hematopoietic cells from HCV-infected subjects[155] and HCV-infected human liver fragments have been transplanted under the kidney capsule of beige, nude, x-linked immunodeficient mice[156] that had been preconditioned by lethal total body irradiation and reconstituted with SCID mouse bone marrow cells. In the latter mice, circulating HCV RNA was detectable in the blood 8 days after transplantation, and the level peaked between days 18 and 25. However, because infection of murine host cells has not been detected and the immune response of the animals is severely impaired, this model cannot be used for the analysis of complex virus–host interactions.

POTENTIAL MECHANISMS OF HCV PERSISTENCE

As described above, the current literature suggests that once chronic infection is established, the HCV-specific immune response exerts some control over viral load but in most cases is unable to terminate persistent infection and/or to resolve chronic hepatitis. Thus, the analysis and discussion of immunologic and virologic correlates that may facilitate HCV persistence seems to

---

TABLE 1.   Potential Mechanisms of Viral Persistence

1. Quantitative or qualitative insufficiency of the virus specific immune response
   a. Inadequate innate immune response
   b. Insufficient induction of the adaptive response due to
      • Low level of viral antigen expression
      • Type of antigen-presenting cell
      • Virus infection of antigen-presenting cells
      • Cytokine profile of T_H cells
      • Lack or low frequency of neutralizing antibodies
   c. Inability to maintain the adaptive response
      • Incomplete activation and expansion of virus-specific CTL
      • Insufficient T-cell help
2. Viral evasion of otherwise efficient immune responses
   a. Replication in immunoprivileged sites
   b. Viral interference with antigen processing
   c. Viral suppression of host immune responses
   d. Viral sequence variation, selection of quasispecies
      • Escape from humoral immune response
      • Escape from cellular immune response
   e. Viral insusceptibility to cytokine mediated inhibition of replication and gene expression

be a necessary step toward the development of efficient vaccines and therapies (Table 1).

One frequently discussed hypothesis is that HCV avoids the induction of a strong innate or adaptive immune response during the early infection. This may explain the virus' remarkable ability to establish clinically inapparent de novo infections that present without any symptoms of acute hepatitis but ultimately evolve into persistent infection in most cases. Generally, the intensity of the immune response depends on cytopathic effects of the virus, antigenic load, costimulatory signals, the type of the antigen-presenting cell, and on the differentiation and cytokine profile of T-helper cells. Each of these factors may not be optimal in acute HCV infection, because for example, display of HCV antigens is relatively low. It has also been shown that dendritic cells from HCV-infected individuals exhibited an impaired allostimulatory capacity[157] with lower expression of CD86 and IL-12 than dendritic cells of normal uninfected controls. With small doses of antigen or insufficient costimulation, however, T-cell activation and proliferation may be suboptimal,[158] which may be reflected by the relatively low number of HCV-specific cytotoxic T cells in the peripheral blood of chronically infected patients.

Second, HCV may have evolved strategies to actively suppress an efficient immune response of the host. For example, tightly regulated tetracycline-inducible expression of all HCV proteins in a continuous human cell line interfered specifically with IFNα-induced signal transduction through the Jak-STAT pathway.[159] In an *in vivo* model, expression of HCV core by recombinant vaccinia viruses suppressed the generation of vaccinia virus-specific cytotoxic T cells in mice.[160] Although the mechanisms of this inhibitory HCV core-specific effect have not been identified, numerous regulatory roles of HCV core that affect signal transduction by interaction with the lymphotoxin-β receptor,[161,162] expression of viral and cellular genes,[163,164] replication of hepatitis B virus[165] cell growth, proliferation, and sensitivity to apoptosis have been described.[166]

In addition, two separate proteins of HCV have been shown to interfere with the antiviral actions of interferon, a dominant cytokine of both the innate and adaptive immune responses. Liver-infiltrating HCV-specific T cells are T_H1 dominant and have been shown to produce IFNγ and TNF-α, cytokines that are known to suppress replication and gene expression of other viruses such as hepatitis B virus,[167] cytomegalovirus,[168] HIV,[169] or rotavirus.[73] In hepatitis B virus infection, these cytokines are known to clear hepatocytes from the infecting virus without causing liver disease.[167,170,171] Thus, it is possible that HCV is less susceptible to these cytokines. IFN induces antiviral genes such as PKR at the transcriptional level and PKR inhibits protein synthesis by phosphorylation of the translation initiation factor eIF2α. Strikingly, an E2 sequence of the IFN-resistant HCV genotypes 1a and 1b but not the IFN-sensitive genotypes HCV 2a, 2b, and 3a exhibits homology with the phosphorylation sites of the IFN-inducible protein kinase PKR and the translation initiation factor eIF2α.[172] This HCV sequence has been shown to bind to and inhibit the kinase activity of PKR. Similarly, a particular sequence within the HCV nonstructural protein NS5A (amino acids 2209–2248) has also been shown to block PKR activation and phosphorylation of eIF-2α.[173–178] Although it is striking that two different HCV proteins are capable to interact specifically with an IFN-inducible protein, it remains controversial whether these observations may contribute to viral persistence in vivo. For example, an association between the HCV NS5A sequence, termed the interferon sensitivity-determining region, and IFN resistance or sensitivity in infected patients was not confirmed in all study populations.[179–181] Similarly, it is controversial whether HCV proteins that are expressed at a low level in infected cells may be able to inhibit PKR, which constitutes a highly abundant cellular protein completely (see also A. Branch's article in this two-issue series in *Seminars in Liver Disease*). A small animal model or tissue culture system that allows HCV infection and expression of HCV proteins at physiologic levels would be helpful to provide a definite answer.

Finally, the high genetic variability of HCV may be an important factor that contributes to viral persistence. Genetic diversity of HCV manifests in the presence of six different genotypes[14] that have evolved in different regions of the world and a multitude of different viral quasispecies that can be isolated from any chronically infected patient at any given time point.[13] The high propensity of the virus to mutate is due to its high replication rate, with an estimated half-life of circulating HCV of only 3 hours, at least in patients with high levels of viral load.[15] The lack of proofreading activity of the viral RNA polymerase further contributes to the continuous generation of viral variants at an estimated rate of 0.4 to 1.2×10^{-3} base substitutions per site per year.[182–184] Because a small quasispecies repertoire size before IFN therapy is necessary to achieve sustained HCV RNA clearance,[180,185,186] viral variation may be important for the establishment and maintenance of persistent infection to adapt quickly to selection humoral or cellular immune selection pressure. For example, more complex initial quasispecies with sequence changes in E1 and HVR1 of E2 have been reported in patients who develop persistent infection than in patients who clear HCV.[38] Sequence variations in T-cell epitopes have also been found (e.g., the emergence of an HCV mutant that was able to escape an HCV-specific CTL response was reported in a chimpanzee with chronic evolution of HCV infection).[187] Similarly, viral variations in T-cell epitopes of patients with acute and chronic hepatitis

C[188–190] have been described. Despite many efforts, however, it is still unknown whether the emergence of viral variants is the cause or consequence of persistent infection. Thus, prospective analysis of viral sequence evolution and the kinetics of virus–host interaction in both clinically symptomatic and asymptomatic patients with de novo HCV infection is required to definitely answer this question.

ABBREVIATIONS

ALT	alanine aminotransferase
CTL	cytotoxic T lymphocyte
HCV	hepatitis C virus
HVR1	hypervariable region 1
IFN	interferon
IP-10	interferon-inducible protein-10
IL	interleukin
LDL	low-density lipoprotein
MIP-1α	macrophage inflammatory protein 1a
MIP-1β	macrophage inflammatory protein 1b
NK	natural killer cell
NOB	neutralization of binding
PKR	double-stranded RNA-dependent protein kinase
RANTES	factor regulated on activation, normal T cell expressed and secreted
SCID	severe combined immunodeficiency
TGF	transforming growth factor
TNF	tumor necrosis factor
T_H	T helper cell

REFERENCES

1. Negro F, Pacchioni D, Shimizu Y, et al. Detection of intrahepatic replication of hepatitis C virus RNA by in situ hybridization and comparison with histopathology. Proc Natl Acad Sci USA 1992;89:2247–2251
2. Honda M, Brown EA, Lemon SM. Stability of a stem-loop involving the initiator AUG controls the efficiency of internal initiation of translation on hepatitis C virus RNA. RNA 1996;2:955–968
3. Ballardini G, Groff P, Pontisso P, et al. Hepatitis C virus (HCV) genotype, tissue HCV antigens, hepatocellular expression of HLA-A,B,C, and intercellular adhesion-1 molecules. Clues to pathogenesis of hepatocellular damage and response to interferon treatment in patients with chronic hepatitis C. J Clin Invest 1995;95:2067–2075
4. Laskus T, Radkowski M, Wang LF, Vargas H, Rakela J. Search for hepatitis C virus extrahepatic replication sites in patients with acquired immunodeficiency syndrome: Specific detection of negative-strand viral RNA in various tissues. Hepatology 1998;28:1398–1401
5. Negro F, Levrero M. Does the hepatitis C virus replicate in cells of the hematopoietic lineage? Hepatology 1998;28:261–264
6. Lanford RE, Chavez D, Chisari FV, Sureau C. Lack of detection of negative-strand hepatitis C virus RNA in peripheral blood mononuclear cells and other extrahepatic tissues by the highly strand-specific rTth reverse transcriptase PCR. J Virol 1995;69:8079–8083
7. Okuda M, Hino K, Korenaga M, Yamaguchi Y, Katoh Y, Okita K. Differences in hypervariable region 1 quasispecies of hepatitis C virus in human serum, peripheral blood mononuclear cells, and liver. Hepatology 1999;29:217–222
8. Agnello V. The etiology and pathophysiology of mixed cryoglobulinemia secondary to hepatitis C virus infection. Springer Semin Immunopathol 1997;19:111–129
9. Agnello V, Abel G, Elfahal M, Knight GB, Zhang QX. Hepatitis C virus and other flaviviridae viruses enter cells via low density lipoprotein receptor. Proc Natl Acad Sci USA 1999;96:12766–12771
10. Levy S, Todd SC, Maecker HT. CD81 (TAPA-1): A molecule involved in signal transduction and cell adhesion in the immune system. Annu Rev Immunol 1998;16:89–109
11. Pileri P, Uematsu Y, Campagnoli, S, et al. Binding of hepatitis C virus to CD81. Science 1998;282:938–941
12. Lemon S, Honda M. Internal ribosome entry sites within the RNA genomes of hepatitis C virus and other flaviviruses. Semin Virol 1997;8:274–288
13. Bukh J, Miller RH, Purcell RH. Genetic heterogeneity of hepatitis C virus: Quasispecies and genotypes. Semin Liver Dis 1995;15:41–63
14. Simmonds P. Variability of hepatitis C virus. Hepatology 1995;21:570–583
15. Neumann AU, Lam NP, Dahari H, et al. Hepatitis C viral dynamics in vivo and the antiviral efficacy of interferon-alpha therapy. Science 1998;282:103–107
16. Ochsenbein AF, Fehr T, Lutz C, et al. Control of early viral and bacterial distribution and disease by natural antibodies. Science 1999;286:2156–2159
17. Chien DY, Choo QL, Tabrizi A, et al. Diagnosis of hepatitis C virus (HCV) infection using an immunodominant chimeric polyprotein to capture antibodies: Reevaluation of the role of HCV in liver disease. Proc Natl Acad Sci USA 1992;89:10011–10015
18. Alberti A, Cavalletto D, Pontisso P, Chemello L, Tagariello G, Belussi F. Antibody response to pre-S2 and hepatitis B virus induced liver damage. Lancet 1988;1:1421–1424
19. Battegay M, Moskophidis D, Waldner H, et al. Impairment and delay of neutralizing antiviral antibody responses by virus-specific cytotoxic T cells. J Immunol 1993;151:5408–5415
20. Koup RA, Ho DD. Shutting down HIV. Nature 1994;370:416
21. Modlin J. Poliovirus. In: Mandell GL, Dolin R, eds. Principles and Practice of Infectious Diseases. Vol. 2. Philadelphia: Churchill Livingstone, 2000, pp 1895–1903
22. Arichi T, Major M, Wedemeyer H, et al. A vigorous HCV-helicase specific T helper response dominates in the liver of a chimpanzee during acute, self-limited hepatitis C. Hepatology 1999;30:453A
23. Simmonds P, Rose KA, Graham S, et al. Mapping of serotype-specific, immunodominant epitopes in the NS-4 region of hepatitis C virus (HCV): Use of type-specific peptides to serologically differentiate infections with HCV types 1, 2, and 3. J Clin Microbiol 1993;31:1493–1503
24. Farci P, Shimoda A, Wong D, et al. Prevention of hepatitis C virus infection in chimpanzees by hyperimmune serum against the hypervariable region 1 of the envelope 2 protein. Proc Natl Acad Sci USA 1996;93:15394–15399
25. Shimizu YK, Igarashi H, Kiyohara T, et al. A hyperimmune serum against a synthetic peptide corresponding to the hypervariable region 1 of hepatitis C virus can prevent viral infection in cell cultures. Virology 1996;223:409–412
26. Kato N, Ootsuyama Y, Ohkohsi S, et al. Characterization of hypervariable regions in the putative envelope protein of hepatitis C virus. Biochem Biophys Res Commun 1992;189:119–127

27. Hijikata M, Kato N, Ootsuyama Y, Nakagawa M, Ohkoshi S, Shimotohno K. Hypervariable regions in the putative glycoprotein of hepatitis C virus. Biochem Biophys Res Commun 1991; 175:220–228

28. Sekiya H, Kato N, Ootsuyama Y, Nakazawa T, Yamauchi K, Shimotohno K. Genetic alterations of the putative envelope proteins encoding region of the hepatitis C virus in the progression to relapsed phase from acute hepatitis: Humoral immune response to hypervariable region 1. Int J Cancer 1994;57:664–670

29. Weiner AJ, Brauer MJ, Rosenblatt J, et al. Variable and hypervariable domains are found in the regions of HCV corresponding to the flavivirus envelope and NS1 proteins and the pestivirus envelope glycoproteins. Virology 1991;180:842–848

30. Weiner AJ, Geysen HM, Christopherson C, et al. Evidence for immune selection of hepatitis C virus (HCV) putative envelope glycoprotein variants: Potential role in chronic HCV infections. Proc Natl Acad Sci USA 1992;89:3468–3472

31. Akatsuka T, Donets M, Scaglione L, et al. B cell epitopes on the hepatitis C virus nucleocapsid protein determined by human monospecific antibodies. Hepatology 1993;18:503–510

32. Choo QL, Kuo G, Ralston R, et al. Vaccination of chimpanzees against infection by the hepatitis C virus. Proc Natl Acad Sci USA 1994;91:1294–1298

33. Rosa D, Campagnoli S, Moretto C, et al. A quantitative test to estimate neutralizing antibodies to the hepatitis C virus: Cytofluorimetric assessment of envelope glycoprotein 2 binding to target cells. Proc Natl Acad Sci USA 1996;93:1759–1763

34. Ishii K, Rosa D, Watanabe Y, et al. High titers of antibodies inhibiting the binding of envelope to human cells correlate with natural resolution of chronic hepatitis C. Hepatology 1998;28: 1117–1120

35. Allander T, Beyene A, Jacobson SH, Grillner L, Persson MA. Patients infected with the same hepatitis C virus strain display different kinetics of the isolate-specific antibody response. J Infect Dis 1997;175:26–31

36. Zibert A, Kraas W, Meisel H, Jung G, Roggendorf M. Epitope mapping of antibodies directed against hypervariable region 1 in acute self-limiting and chronic infections due to hepatitis C virus. J Virol 1997;71:4123–4127

37. Zibert A, Meisel H, Kraas W, Schulz A, Jung G, Roggendorf M. Early antibody response against hypervariable region 1 is associated with acute self-limiting infections of hepatitis C virus. Hepatology 1997;25:1245–1249

38. Ray SC, Wang YM, Laeyendecker O, Ticehurst JR, Villano SA, Thomas DL. Acute hepatitis C virus structural gene sequences as predictors of persistent viremia: Hypervariable region 1 as a decoy. J Virol 1999;73:2938–2946

39. Bassett SE, Thomas DL, Brasky KM, Lanford RE. Viral persistence, antibody to E1 and E2, and hypervariable region 1 sequence stability in hepatitis C virus-inoculated chimpanzees. J Virol 1999;73:1118–1126

40. Major ME, Mihalik K, Fernandez J, et al. Long-term follow-up of chimpanzees inoculated with the first infectious clone for hepatitis C virus. J Virol 1999;73:3317–3325

41. Cantor HM, Dumont AE. Hepatic suppression of sensitization to antigen absorbed into the portal system. Nature 1967;215: 744–745

42. Wang C, Sun J, Wang L, Li L, Horvat M, Sheil R. Combined liver and pancreas transplantation induces pancreas allograft tolerance. Transplant Proc 1997;29:1145–1146

43. Collins C, Norris S, McEntee G, et al. RAG1, RAG2 and pre-T cell receptor alpha chain expression by adult human hepatic T cells: Evidence for extrathymic T cell maturation. Eur J Immunol 1996;26:3114–3118

44. Lynch S, Kelleher D, McManus R, O'Farrelly C. RAG1 and RAG2 expression in human intestinal epithelium: Evidence of

extrathymic T cell differentiation. Eur J Immunol 1995;25: 1143–1147

45. Guy-Grand D, Vanden Broecke C, Briottet C, Malassis-Seris M, Selz F, Vassalli P. Different expression of the recombination activity gene RAG-1 in various populations of thymocytes, peripheral T cells and gut thymus-independent intraepithelial lymphocytes suggests two pathways of T cell receptor rearrangement. Eur J Immunol 1992;22:505–510

46. Lundqvist C, Baranov V, Hammarstrom S, Athlin L, Hammarstrom ML. Intra-epithelial lymphocytes. Evidence for regional specialization and extrathymic T cell maturation in the human gut epithelium. Int Immunol 1995;7:1473–1487

47. O'Farrelly C, Crispe IN. Prometheus through the looking glass: Reflections on the hepatic immune system. Immunol Today 1999;20:394–398

48. Schlitt HJ, Schafers S, Deiwick A, et al. Extramedullary erythropoiesis in human liver grafts. Hepatology 1995;21:689–696

49. Huang L, Sye K, Crispe IN. Proliferation and apoptosis of B220+CD4-CD8-TCR alpha beta intermediate T cells in the liver of normal adult mice: Implication for lpr pathogenesis. Int Immunol 1994;6:533–540

50. Huang L, Soldevila G, Leeker M, Flavell R, Crispe IN: The liver eliminates T cells undergoing antigen-triggered apoptosis in vivo. Immunity 1994;1;741–749

51. Masuda T, Ohteki T, Abo T, et al. Expansion of the population of double negative CD4-8- T alpha beta- cells in the liver is a common feature of autoimmune mice. J Immunol 1991;147: 2907–2912

52. Bandeira A, Itohara S, Bonneville M, et al. Extrathymic origin of intestinal intraepithelial lymphocytes bearing T-cell antigen receptor gamma delta. Proc Natl Acad Sci USA 1991;88:43–47

53. MacDonald HR. NK1.1+ T cell receptor-alpha/beta+ cells: New clues to their origin, specificity, and function. J Exp Med 1995; 182:633–638

54. Bendelac A, Lantz O, Quimby ME, Yewdell JW, Bennink JR, Brutkiewicz RR. CD1 recognition by mouse NK1+ T lymphocytes. Science 1995;268:863–865

55. Biron CA. Role of early cytokines, including alpha and beta interferons (IFN- alpha/beta), in innate and adaptive immune responses to viral infections. Semin Immunol 1998;10:383–390

56. Ishikawa R, Biron CA. IFN induction and associated changes in splenic leukocyte distribution. J Immunol 1993;150:3713–3727

57. Vilcek JSG. Interferons and other cytokines. In: Fields BN, Howley PM, eds. Fundamental Virology. Vol. 11. Philadelphia: Lippincott-Raven, 1996, pp 341–365

58. Salazar-Mather TP, Ishikawa R, Biron CA. NK cell trafficking and cytokine expression in splenic compartments after IFN induction and viral infection. J Immunol 1996;157:3054–3064

59. MacMicking J, Xie QW, Nathan C. Nitric oxide and macrophage function. Annu Rev Immunol 1997;15:323–350

60. Salazar-Mather TP, Orange JS, Biron CA. Early murine cytomegalovirus (MCMV) infection induces liver natural killer (NK) cell inflammation and protection through macrophage inflammatory protein 1alpha (MIP-1alpha)-dependent pathways. J Exp Med 1998;187:1–14

61. Pilaro AM, Taub DD, McCormick KL, et al. TNF-alpha is a principal cytokine involved in the recruitment of NK cells to liver parenchyma. J Immunol 1994;153:333–342

62. Orange JS, Salazar-Mather TP, Opal SM, Biron CA. Mechanisms for virus-induced liver disease: Tumor necrosis factor-mediated pathology independent of natural killer and T cells during murine cytomegalovirus infection. J Virol 1997;71:9248–9258

63. Lanier LL. NK cell receptors. Annu Rev Immunol 1998;16: 359–393

64. Ballardini G, Groff P, Pontisso P, et al. Hepatitis C virus (HCV) genotype, tissue HCV antigens, hepatocellular expression of

HLA-A, B, C, and intercellular adhesion-1 molecules. J Clin Invest 1995;95:2967–2975

65. Barbatis C, Morton JA, Fleming KA, McMichael A, McGee JO. Immunohistochemical analysis of HLA (A,B,C) antigens in liver disease using a monoclonal antibody. Gut 1981;22:985–991

66. Albert ML, Sauter B, Bhardwaj N. Dendritic cells acquire antigen from apoptotic cells and induce class I- restricted CTLs. Nature 1998;392:86–89

67. Sigal LJ, Crotty S, Andino R, Rock KL. Cytotoxic T-cell immunity to virus-infected non-haematopoietic cells requires presentation of exogenous antigen. Nature 1999;398:77–80

68. Kim J, Woods A, Becker-Dunn E, Bottomly K. Distinct functional phenotypes of cloned Ia-restricted helper T cells. J Exp Med 1985;162:188–201

69. Mosmann TR, Cherwinski H, Bond MW, Giedlin MA, Coffman RL. Two types of murine helper T cell clone. I. Definition according to profiles of lymphokine activities and secreted proteins. J Immunol 1986;136:2348–2357

70. Ridge JP, Di Rosa F, Matzinger P. A conditioned dendritic cell can be a temporal bridge between a cD4+ T-helper and a T-killer cell. Nature 1998;393:474–478

71. Guidotti LG, Rochford R, Chung J, Shapiro M, Purcell R, Chisari FV. Viral clearance without destruction of infected cells during acute HBV infection. Science 1999;284:825–829

72. Pavic I, Polic B, Crnkovic I, Lucin P, Jonjic S, Koszinowski UH. Participation of endogenous tumour necrosis factor alpha in host resistance to cytomegalovirus infection. J Gen Virol 1993;74:2215–2223

73. Franco MA, Tin C, Rott LS, Van Cotte JL, McGhee JR, Greenberg HB. Evidence for CD8+ T-cell immunity to murine rotavirus in the absence of perforin, fas and gamma interferon. J Virol 1997;71:479–486

74. Franco A, Guidotti LG, Hobbs MV, Pasquetto V, Chisari FV. Pathogenetic effector function of CD4-positive T helper 1 cells in hepatitis B virus transgenic mice. J Immunol 1997;159:2001–2008

75. Ferrari C, Valli A, Galati L, et al. T-cell response to structural and nonstructural hepatitis C virus antigens in persistent and self-limited hepatitis C virus infections. Hepatology 1994;19:286–295

76. Diepolder HM, Zachoval R, Hoffmann RM, et al. Possible mechanism involving T lymphocyte response to non-structural protein 3 in viral clearance in acute hepatitis C virus infection. Lancet 1995;346:1006–1007

77. Diepolder HM, Gerlach J-T, Zachoval R, et al. Immunodominant CD4+ T-cell epitope within nonstructural protein 3 in acute hepatitis C virus infection. J Virol 1997;71:6011–6019

78. Missale G, Bertoni R, Lamonaca V, et al. Different clinical behaviors of acute hepatitis C virus infection are associated with different vigor of the anti-viral cell-mediated immune response. J Clin Invest 1996;98:706–714

79. Lamonaca V, Missale G, Urbani S, et al. Conserved hepatitis C virus sequences are highly immunogenic for CD4(+) T cells: Implications for vaccine development. Hepatology 1999;30:1088–1098

80. Gerlach JT, Diepolder HM, Jung MC, et al. Recurrence of hepatitis C virus after loss of virus-specific CD4(+) T-cell response in acute hepatitis C. Gastroenterology 1999;117:933–941

81. Chang KM, Gruener NH, Southwood S, et al. Identification of HLA-A3 and -B7-restricted CTL response to hepatitis C virus in patients with acute and chronic hepatitis C. J Immunol 1999;162:1156–1164

82. Cooper S, Erickson AL, Adams EJ, et al. Analysis of a successful immune response against hepatitis C virus. Immunity 1999;10:439–449

83. Pantaleo G, Demarest JF, Schacker T, et al. The qualitative nature of the primary immune response to HIV infection is a prognosticator of disease progression independent of the initial level of plasma viremia. Proc Natl Acad Sci USA 1997;94:254–258

84. von Boehmer H. The developmental biology of T lymphocytes. Annu Rev Immunol 1988;6:309–326

85. Rehermann B, Chisari FV. Cell mediated immune response to the hepatitis C virus. Curr Top Microbiol Immunol 2000;242:299–325

86. Battegay M, Fikes J, Di Bisceglie AM, et al. Patients with chronic hepatitis C have circulating cytotoxic T cells which recognize hepatitis C virus-encoded peptides binding to HLA-A2.1 molecules. J Virol 1995;69:2462–2470

87. Cerny A, McHutchison JG, Pasquinelli C, et al. Cytotoxic T lymphocyte response to hepatitis C virus-derived peptides containing the HLA A2.1 binding motif. J Clin Invest 1995;95:521–530

88. Koziel MJ, Dudley D, Afdhal N, et al. HLA class I-restricted cytotoxic T lymphocytes specific for hepatitis C virus. Identification of multiple epitopes and characterization of patterns of cytokine release. J Clin Invest 1995;96:2311–1221

89. Koziel MJ, Dudley D, Wong JT, et al. Intrahepatic cytotoxic T lymphocytes specific for hepatitis C virus in persons with chronic hepatitis. J Immunol 1992;149:3339–3344

90. Koziel JM, Dudley D, Afdhal N, et al. Hepatitis C virus (HCV)-specific cytotoxic T lymphocytes recognize epitopes in the core and envelope proteins of HCV. J Virol 1993;67:7522–7532

91. Erickson AL, Houghton M, Choo Q-L, et al. Hepatitis C virus-specific CTL responses in the liver of chimpanzees with acute and chronic hepatitis C. J Immunol 1993;151:4189–4199

92. Del Guercio MF, Sidney J, Hermanson G, et al. Binding of a peptide antigen to multiple HLA alleles allows definition of an A2-like supertype. J Immunol 1995;154:685–693

93. Sidney J, Del Guercio MF, Southwood S, et al. Several HLA alleles share overlapping peptide specificities. J Immunol 1995;154:247–259

94. Sidney J, Grey HM, Kubo RT, Sette A. Practical, biochemical and evolutionary implications of the discovery of HLA class I supermotifs. Immunol Today 1996;17:261–266

95. Sidney J, Grey HM, Southwood S, et al. Definition of an HLA-A3-like supermotif demonstrates the overlapping peptide-binding repertoires of common HLA molecules. Hum Immunol 1996;45:79–93

96. Scognamiglio P, Accapezzato D, Casciani A, et al. Presence of effector CD8+ T cells in hepatitis C virus-exposed healthy seronegative donors. J Immunol 1999;162:6681–6689

97. Rehermann B, Chang KM, McHutchison JG, Kokka R, Houghton M, Chisari FV. Quantitative analysis of the peripheral blood cytotoxic T lymphocyte response, disease activity and viral load in patients with chronic hepatitis C virus infection. J Clin Invest 1996;98:1432–1440

98. He XS, Rehermann B, Lopez-Labrador FX, et al. Quantitative analysis of hepatitis C virus-specific CD8(+) T cells in peripheral blood and liver using peptide-MHC tetramers. Proc Natl Acad Sci USA 1999;96:5692–5697

99. Murali-Krishna K, Altman JD, Suresh M, et al. Counting antigen-specific CD8 T cells: A reevaluation of bystander activation during viral infection. Immunity 1998;8:177–187

100. Hiroishi K, Kita H, Kojima M, et al. Cytotoxic T lymphocyte response and viral load in hepatitis C virus infection. Hepatology 1997;25:705–712

101. Rehermann B, Chang KM, McHutchison J, et al. Differential cytotoxic T lymphocyte responsiveness to the hepatitis B and C viruses in chronically infected patients. J Virol 1996;70:7092–7102

102. Nelson DR, Marousis CG, Davis GL, et al. The role of hepatitis C virus-specific cytotoxic T lymphocytes in chronic hepatitis C. J Immunol 1997;158:1473–1481

103. Nakamoto Y, Guidotti LG, Kuhlen CV, Fowler P, Chisari FV. Immune pathogenesis of hepatocellular carcinoma. J Exp Med 1998;188:341–350

104. Shields PL, Morland CM, Salmon M, Qin S, Hubscher SG, Adams DH. Chemokine and chemokine receptor interactions provide a mechanism for selective T cell recruitment to specific liver compartments within hepatitis C-infected liver. J Immunol 1999;163:6236–6243

105. Sallusto F, Lenig D, Mackay CR, Lanzavecchia A. Flexible programs of chemokine receptor expression on human polarized T helper 1 and 2 lymphocytes. J Exp Med 1998;187:875–883

106. Bonecchi R, Bianchi G, Bordignon PP, et al. Differential expression of chemokine receptors and chemotactic responsiveness of type 1 T helper cells (Th1s) and Th2s. J Exp Med 1998;187:129–134

107. Mukaida N, Hishinuma A, Zachariae CO, Oppenheim JJ, Matsushima K. Regulation of human interleukin 8 gene expression and binding of several other members of the intercrine family to receptors for interleukin-8. Adv Exp Med Biol 1991;305:31–38

108. Goebeler M, Yoshimura T, Toksoy A, Ritter U, Brocker EB, Gillitzer R. The chemokine repertoire of human dermal microvascular endothelial cells and its regulation by inflammatory cytokines. J Invest Dermatol 1997;108:445–451

109. Luster AD, Unkeless JC, Ravetch JV. Gamma-interferon transcriptionally regulates an early-response gene containing homology to platelet proteins. Nature 1985;315:672–676

110. Cocchi F, DeVico AL, Garzino-Demo A, Arya SK, Gallo RC, Lusso P. Identification of RANTES, MIP-1 alpha, and MIP-1 beta as the major HIV-suppressive factors produced by CD8+ T cells. Science 1995;270:1811–1815

111. Wagner L, Yang OO, Garcia-Zepeda EA, et al. Beta-chemokines are released from HIV-1-specific cytolytic T-cell granules complexed to proteoglycans. Nature 1998;391:908–911

112. Murai M, Yoneyama H, Harada A, et al. Active participation of CCR5(+)CD8(+) T lymphocytes in the pathogenesis of liver injury in graft-versus-host disease. J Clin Invest 1999;104:49–57

113. Mehal WZ, Juedes AE, Crispe IN. Selective retention of activated CD8+ T cells by the normal liver. J Immunol 1999;163:3202–3210

114. MacPhee PJ, Schmidt EE, Groom AC. Intermittence of blood flow in liver sinusoids, studied by high-resolution in vivo microscopy. Am J Physiol 1995;269:G692–G698

115. Flynn KJ, Belz GT, Altman JD, Ahmed R, Woodland DL, Doherty PC. Virus-specific CD8+ T cells in primary and secondary influenza pneumonia. Immunity 1998;8:683–691

116. Nuti S, Rosa D, Valiante NM, Saletti G. Caratozzolo M. Dellabona P. Barnaba V, Abrignani S. Dynamics of intrahepatic lymphocytes in chronic hepatitis C: enrichment for Valpha24+ T cells and rapid elimination of effector cells by apoptosis. Eur J Immunol 1998;28:3448–3455

117. Wejstal R, Norkrans R, Weiland O, et al. Lymphocyte subsets and B2 microglobulin expression in chronic hepatitis C/nonA-nonB: Effect of interferon-alpha treatment. Clin Exp Immunol 1992;87:340–345

118. Yuk K, Shimizu M, Aoyama S, et al. Analysis of lymphocyte subsets in liver biopsy specimens with lymphoid follicle like structures. Acta Hepatol Jpn 1986;27:720–725

119. Gonzalez-Peralta RP, Fang JWS, Davis GL, et al. Immunopathobiology of chronic hepatitis C virus infection. Hepatology 1994;20:232A

120. Onji M, Kikuchi T, Kumon I, et al. Intrahepatic lymphocyte subpopulations and HLA class I antigen expression by hepatocytes in chronic hepatitis C. Hepatogastroenterology 1992;39:340–343

121. Minutello MA, Pileri P, Unutmaz D, et al. Compartmentalization of T-lymphocyte to the site of disease: Intrahepatic CD4+ T-cells specific for the protein NS4 of hepatitis C virus in patients with chronic hepatitis. J Exp Med 1993;178:17–26

122. Kashii Y, Shimizu Y, Nambu S, et al. Analysis of T-cell receptor V beta repertoire in liver-infiltrating lymphocytes in chronic hepatitis C. J Hepatol 1997;26:462–470

123. Marrogi AJ, Cheles MK, Gerber MA. Chronic hepatitis C. Analysis of host immune response by immunohistochemistry. Arch Pathol Lab Med 1995;119:232–237

124. Mosnier JF, Scoaze JY, Marcellin P, Degott C, Benahmou JP, Feldmann G. Expression of cytokine-dependent immune adhesion molecules by hepatocytes. Gastroenterology 1994;107:1457–1468

125. Hiramatsu N, Hayashi N, Katayama K, et al. Immunohistochemical detection of Fas antigen in liver tissue of patients with chronic hepatitis C. Hepatology 1994;19:1354–1359

126. Mita E, Hayashi N, Iio S, et al. Role of Fas ligand in apoptosis induced by hepatitis C virus infection. Biochem Biophys Res Commun 1994;204:468–474

127. Lohman BL, Razvi ES, Welsh RM. T-lymphocyte downregulation after acute viral infection is not dependent on CD95 (Fas) receptor-ligand interactions. J Virol 1996;70:8199–8203

128. Vassalli P. The pathophysiology of tumor necrosis factors. Annu Rev Immunol 1992;10:411–452

129. Kinkhabwala M, Sehajpal P, Skolnik E, et al. A novel addition to the T cell repertory: Cell surface expression of tumor necrosis factor/cachectin by activated normal human T cells. J Exp Med 1990;171:941–946

130. Ando K, Hiroishi K, Kaneko T, et al. Perforin, fas/fas ligand, and TNF-alpha pathways as specific and bystander killing mechanisms of hepatitis C virus-specific human CTL. J Immunol 1997;158:5283–5291

131. Zhang Z, Brunner T, Carter L, et al. Unequal death in T helper cell (Th)1 and Th2 effectors: Th1, but not Th2, effectors undergo rapid Fas/FasL-mediated apoptosis. J Exp Med 1997;185:1837–1849

132. Nuti S, Rosa D, Valiante NM, et al. Dynamics of intra-hepatic lymphocytes in chronic hepatitis C: Enrichment for V alpha24+ T cells and rapid elimination of effector cells by apoptosis. Eur J Immunol 1998;28:3448–3455

133. Hollinger FB, Gitnick GL, Aach RD, et al. Non-A, and non-B hepatitis transmission in chimpanzees: A project of the transfusion-transmitted viruses study group. Intervirology 1978;10:60–68

134. He LF, Alling D, Popkin T, Shapiro M, Alter HJ, Purcell RH. Determining the size of non-A, non-B hepatitis virus by filtration. J Infect Dis 1987;156:636–640

135. Kolykhalov A, Agapov E, Blight K, Mihalik K, Feinstone S, Rice C. Transmission of hepatitis C by intrahepatic inocculation with transcribed RNA. Science 1997;277:570–574

136. Yanagi M, Purcell RH, Emerson SU, Bukh J. Hepatitis C virus: An infectious molecular clone of a second major genotype (2a) and lack of viability of intertypic 1a and 2a chimeras. Virology 1999;262:250–263

137. Yanagi M, Purcell RH, Emerson SU, Bukh J. Transcripts from a single full-length cDNA clone of hepatitis C virus are infectious when directly transfected into the liver of a chimpanzee. Proc Natl Acad Sci USA 1997;94:8738–8743

138. Beard MR, Abell G, Honda M, et al. An infectious molecular clone of a Japanese genotype 1b hepatitis C virus. Hepatology 1999;30:316–324

139. Alter HJ, Purcell RH, Holland PV, Popper H. Transmissible agent in non-A, non-B hepatitis. Lancet 1978;1:459–463

140. Popper H, Dienstag JL, Feinstone SM, Alter HJ, Purcell R. The pathology of viral hepatitis lin chimpanzees. Arch A Pathol Anat Histol 1980;387:91–106

141. Bassett SE, Brasky KM, Lanford RE. Analysis of hepatitis C virus-inoculated chimpanzees reveals unexpected clinical profiles. J Virol 1998;72:2589–2599

142. Walker CM. Comparative features of hepatitis C virus infection in humans and chimpanzees. Springer Semin Immunopathol 1997;19:85–98

143. Kenney-Walsh E. Clinical outcomes after hepatitis C infection from contaminated anti-D immune globulin. Irish Hepatology Research Group. N Engl J Med 1999;340:1228–1233

144. Takaki A, Wiese M, Maertens G, Depla E, Seifert U, Liebetrau A, Miller J, Manns MP, Rehermann B. Cellular immune responses persist and humoral responses decrease two decades after recovery from a single-source outbreak of hepatitis C. Nature Medicine 2000;6:578–582

145. Wiese M. Thema: Virushepatitis. Der Kassenarzt 1996;5:36–38

146. Shirai M, Arichi T, Nishioka M, et al. CTL responses of HLA-A2.1-transgenic mice specific for hepatitis C viral peptides predict epitopes for CTL of humans carrying HLA-A2.1. J Immunol 1995;154:2733–2742

147. Wentworth PA, Sette A, Celis E, et al. Identification of A2-restricted hepatitis C virus-specific cytotoxic T lymphocyte epitopes from conserved regions of the viral genome. Int Immunol 1996;8:651–659

148. Oseroff C, Sette A, Wentworth P, et al. Pools of lipidated HTL-CTL constructs prime for multiple HBV and HCV CTL epitope responses. Vaccine 1998;16:823–833

149. Arichi T, Saito T, Major ME, et al. Prophylactic DNA vaccine for hepatitis C virus (HCV) infection: HCV-specific cytotoxic T lymphocyte induction and protection from HCV-recombinant vaccinia infection in an HLA-A2.1 transgenic mouse model. Proc Natl Acad Sci USA 2000;97:297–302

150. Kawamura T, Furusaka A, Koziel MJ, et al. Transgenic expression of hepatitis C virus structural proteins in the mouse. Hepatology 1997;25:1014–1021

151. Pasquinelli C, Shoenberger JM, Chung J, et al. Hepatitis C virus core and E2 protein expression in transgenic mice. Hepatology 1997;25:719–727

152. Moriya K, Yotsuyanagi H, Shintani Y, et al. Hepatitis C virus core protein induces hepatic steatosis in transgenic mice. J Gen Virol 1997;78:1527–1531

153. Moriya K, Fujie H, Shintani Y, et al. The core protein of hepatitis C virus induces hepatocellular carcinoma in transgenic mice. Nat Med 1998;4:1065–1067

154. Koike K, Moriya K, Ishibashi K, et al. Expression of hepatitis C virus envelope proteins in transgenic mice. J Gen Viol 1995;76:3031–3038

155. Bronowicki JP, Loriot MA, Thiers V, Grignon Y, Zignego AL, Brechot C. Hepatitis C virus persistence in human hematopoietic cells injected into SCID mice. Hepatology 1998;28:211–218

156. Galun E, Burakova T, Ketzinel M, et al. Hepatitis C virus viremia in SCID → BNX mouse chimera. J Infect Dis 1995;172:25–30

157. Kanto T, Hayashi N, Takehara T, et al. Impaired allostimulatory capacity of peripheral blood dendritic cells recovered from hepatitis C virus-infected individuals. J Immunol 1999;162:5584–5591

158. Cai Z, Sprent J. Influence of antigen dose and costimulation on the primary response of CD8+ T cells in vitro. J Exp Med 1996;183:2247–2257

159. Heim MH, Moradpour D, Blum HE. Expression of hepatitis C virus proteins inhibits signal transduction through the Jak-STAT pathway. J Virol 1999;73:8469–8475

160. Large MK, Kittlesen DJ, Hahn YS. Suppression of host immune response by the core protein of hepatitis C virus: Possible implications for hepatic C virus persistence. J Immunol 1999;162:931–938

161. Matsumoto M, Hsieh TY, Zhu N, et al. Hepatitis C virus core protein interacts with the cytoplasmic tail of lymphotoxin-beta receptor. J Virol 1997;71:1301–1309

162. Chen CM, You LR, Hwang LH, Lee YH. Direct interaction of hepatitis C virus core protein with the cellular lymphocotoxin-beta receptor modulates the signal pathway of the lymphotoxin-beta receptor. J Virol 1997;71:9417–9426

163. Ray RB, Meyer K, Steele R, Shrivastava A, Aggarwal BB, Ray R. Inhibition of tumor necrosis factor (TNF-alpha)-mediated apoptosis by hepatitis C virus core protein. J Biol Chem 1998;273:2256–2259

164. Ray RB, Lagging LM, Meyer K, Steele R, Ray R. Transcriptional regulation of cellular and viral promoters by the hepatitis C virus core protein. Virus Res 1995;37:209–220

165. Shih CM, Lo SJ, Miyamura T, Chen SY, Lee YH. Suppression of hepatitis B virus expression and replication by hepatitis C virus core protein in HuH-7 cells. J Virol 1993;67:5823–5832

166. Ray RB, Lagging LM, Meyer K, Ray R. Hepatitis C virus core protein cooperates with ras and transforms primary rat embryo fibroblasts to tumorigenic phenotype. J Virol 1996;70:4438–4444

167. Guidotti LG, Ishikawa T, Hobbs MV, Matzke B, Schreiber R, Chisari FV. Intracellular inactivation of the hepatitis B virus by cytotoxic T lymphocytes. Immunity 1996;4:35–36

168. Pavic I, Polic B, Crnkovic I, Lucin P, Jonjic S, Koszinowski UH. Participation of endogenous tumor necrosis factor alpha in host resistance to cytomegalovirus infection. J Gen Virol 1993;74:2215–2223

169. Cocchi F, deVico AL, Garzino-Demo A, Arya SK, Gallo RC, Lusso P. Identification of Rantes, MIP-1alpha and MIP-1beta as the major HIV-suppressive factors produced by CD8+ T cells. Science 1995;270:1811–1815

170. Heise T, Guidotti LG, Chisari FV. La autoantigen specifically recognizes a predicted stem-loop in hepatitis B virus RNA. J Virol 1999;73:5767–5776

171. Heise T, Guidotti LG, Cavanaugh VJ, Chisari FV. Hepatitis B virus RNA-binding proteins associated with cytokine-induced clearance of viral RNA from the liver of transgenic mice. J Virol 1999;73:474–481

172. Taylor DR, Shi ST, Romano PR, Barber GN, Lai MM. Inhibition of the interferon-inducible protein kinase PKR by HCV E2 protein. Science 1999;285:107–110

173. Gale M Jr, Kwieciszewski B, Dossett M, Nakao H, Katze MG. Antiapoptotic and oncogenic potentials of hepatitis C virus are linked to interferon resistance by viral repression of the PKR protein kinase. J Virol 1999;73:6506–6516

174. Tan SL, Nakao H, He Y, et al. NS5A, a nonstructural protein of hepatitis C virus, binds growth factor receptor-bound protein 2 adaptor protein in a Src homology 3 domain/ligand-dependent manner and perturbs mitogenic signaling. Proc Natl Acad Sci USA 1999;96:5533–5538

175. Gale MJ Jr, Korth MJ, Katze MG. Repression of the PKR protein kinase by the hepatitis C virus NS5A protein: A potential mechanism of interferon resistance. Clin Diagn Virol 1998;10:157–162

176. Gale M Jr Blakely CM, Kwieciszewski B, et al. Control of PKR protein kinase by hepatitis C virus nonstructural 5A protein: Molecular mechanisms of kinase regulation. Mol Cell Biol 1998;18:5208–5218

177. Gale M Jr, Katze MG. Molecular mechanisms of interferon resistance mediated by viral-directed inhibition of PKR, the interferon-induced protein kinase. Pharmacol Ther 1998;78:29–46

178. Gale MJ Jr, Korth MJ, Tang NM, et al. Evidence that hepatitis C virus resistance to interferon is mediated through repression of the PKR protein kinase by the nonstructural 5A protein. Virology 1997;230:217–227

179. Chung RT, Monto A, Dienstag JL, Kaplan LM. Mutations in the NS5A region do not predict interferon-responsiveness in american patients infected with genotype 1b hepatitis C virus. J Med Virol 1999;58:353–358

180. Pawlotsky JM, Germanidis G, Neumann AU, Pellerin M, Frainais PO, Dhumeaux D. Interferon resistance of hepatitis C virus genotype 1b: Relationship to nonstructural 5A gene quasi-species mutations. J Virol 1998;72:2795–2805

181. Paterson M, Laxton CD, Thomas HC, Ackrill AM, Foster GR. Hepatitis C virus NS5A protein inhibits interferon antiviral activity, but the effects do not correlate with clinical response. Gastroenterology 1999;117:1187–1197

182. Ogata N, Alter HJ, Miller RH, Purcell RH. Nucleotide sequence and mutation rate of the H strain of hepatitis C virus. Proc Natl Acad Sci USA 1991;88:3392–3396

183. Okamoto H, Kojima M, Okada S, et al. Genetic drift of hepatitis C virus during an 8.2-year infection in a chimpanzee: Variability and stability. Virology 1992;190:894–899

184. Smith DB, Pathirana S, Davidson F, et al. The origin of hepatitis C virus genotypes. J Gen Virol 1997;78:321–328

185. Pawlotsky JM, Pellerin M, Bouvier M, et al. Genetic complexity of the hypervariable region 1 (HVR1) of hepatitis C virus (HCV): Influence on the characteristics of the infection and responses to interferon alfa therapy in patients with chronic hepatitis C. J Med Virol 1998;54:256–264

186. Toyoda H, Kumada T, Nakano S, et al. Quasispecies nature of hepatitis C virus and response to alpha interferon: Significance as a predictor of direct response to interferon. J Hepatol 1997;26:6–13

187. Weiner A, Erickson AL, Kansopon J, et al. Persistent hepatitis C virus infection in a chimpanzee is associated with emergence of a cytotoxic T lymphocyte escape variant. Proc Natl Acad Sci USA 1995;92:2755–2759

188. Chang KM, Rehermann B, McHutchison JG, et al. Immunological significance of cytotoxic T lymphocyte epitope variants in patients chronically infected by the hepatitis C virus. J Clin Invest 1997;100:2376–2385

189. Tsai SL, Chen YM, Chen MH, et al. Hepatitis C virus variants circumventing cytotoxic T lymphocyte activity as a mechanism of chronicity. Gastroenterology 1998;115:954–965

190. Kaneko T, Moriyama T, Udaka K, et al. Impaired induction of cytotoxic T lymphocytes by antagonism of a weak agonist borne by a variant hepatitis C virus epitope. Eur J Immunol 1997;27:1782–1787

The Lymphoid System in Hepatitis C Virus Infection: Autoimmunity, Mixed Cryoglobulinemia, and Overt B-Cell Malignancy

FRANCO DAMMACCO, M.D.,[1] DOMENICO SANSONNO, M.D.,[2]
CLAUDIA PICCOLI, B.Sc.,[1] VITO RACANELLI, M.D.,[1]
FRANCESCA PAOLA D'AMORE, B.Sc.,[1]
and GIANFRANCO LAULETTA, M.D.[1]

ABSTRACT: Like other hepatotropic viruses, hepatitis C virus (HCV) shares the property of inducing hepatocellular damage, possibly through induction of immune mechanisms that lead to hepatocellular necrosis. After infection of hepatocytes, and possibly other cells, humoral and cellular responses occur aimed at prevention of virus dissemination and elimination of infected cells. The early activated mechanisms include production of nonspecific and specific antibodies that represent the first-line of defense against invading foreign pathogens. As a consequence, circulating immune complexes are promptly formed, and antigen uptake and processing by specialized cells are enhanced. A major fraction of circulating immunoglobulins (Igs) are part of the spectrum of the so-called natural antibodies, which include anti-idiotypic antibodies and molecules with rheumatoid factor (RF) activity. They mainly belong to the IgM class, are polyclonal, and have no intrinsic pathogenetic potential. In 20–30% of HCV-infected patients, RFs share characteristics of high affinity molecules, are monoclonal in nature, and result in the production of cold-precipitating immune complexes and mixed cryoglobulinemia. It has been shown that anti-idiotypic antibodies and polyclonal and monoclonal RF molecules have the same cross-reactive idiotype, called WA, suggesting that their production is highly restricted. This strongly indicates that they arise from stimulation with the same antigen, likely HCV. It has also been speculated that B-1 (CD5$^+$) and B-2 (CD5$^-$) B-cell subsets, which use a limited number of V_H germline genes, underlie the production of low-affinity polyclonal and high-affinity monoclonal antibodies, respectively. The persistent production of monoclonal RF molecules implies the existence of a further mechanism capable

Objectives
Upon completion of this article, the reader should be able to 1) summarize the spectrum of autoantibodies that appear during HCV infection, 2) define intrahepatic B-cell clonal expansion as the underlying mechanism(s) sustaining an indolent stage of chronic B-cell lymphoproliferation (i.e., mixed cryoglobulinemia), and 3) emphasize the possible link between HCV infection and frank B-cell malignancy (i.e., non-Hodgkin's lymphoma).

Accreditation
The Indiana University School of Medicine is accredited by the Accreditation Council for Continuing Medical Education to provide continuing medical education for physicians.

Credit
The Indiana University School of Medicine designates this educational activity for a maximum of 1.0 hours credit toward the AMA Physicians Recognition Award in category one. Each physician should claim only those hours of credit that he/she actually spent in the educational activity.

Disclosure
Statements have been obtained regarding the authors' relationships with financial supporters of this activity. There is no apparent conflict of interest related to the context of participation of the author of this article.

[1]Department of Biomedical Sciences and Human Oncology, Section of Internal Medicine and Clinical Oncology, University of Bari Medical School, Bari, Italy; and [2]Chair of Internal Medicine, University of Foggia Medical School, Foggia, Italy.
Reprint requests: Franco Dammacco, M.D., Department of Biomedical Sciences and Human Oncology, Section of Internal Medicine and Clinical Oncology, University of Bari Medical School, Policlinico, Piazza G. Cesare 11, 70124 Bari, Italy. E-mail: dimoclin@cimedoc.uniba.it

of restricting the reactivity and reflects a distinct selection of a cell population that can be maintained throughout life because they are continuously exposed to antigen pressure. Either polyclonal or monoclonal profiles of B-cell expansion are demonstrable in the liver of most HCV-infected patients. The occurrence of B-cell clonal expansion is strictly related to intrahepatic production of RF molecules, and this suggests that liver is a microenvironment, other than lymphoid tissue, in which a germinal centerlike reaction is induced. The frequent detection of oligoclonal B-cell expansion may, indeed, represent a key pathobiologic feature that sustains nonmalignant B-cell lymphoproliferation. The preferential expansion of one clone would in turn lead to a monoclonal pattern that could favor stochastic oncogenic events. It can be postulated that HCV is the stimulus not only for the apparent benign lymphoproliferative process underlying a wide spectrum of clinical features, but also for the progression to frank lymphoid malignancy in a subgroup of patients. Current data indicate a higher prevalence of overt B-cell non-Hodgkin's lymphoma in HCV-infected patients, especially in some geographic areas.

KEY WORDS: autoimmunity, hepatitis C virus, lymphoproliferation

The discovery of hepatitis C virus (HCV) has led to a new classification of chronic hepatitis and to a better understanding of acute and chronic inflammatory liver disease. A growing number of clinical and biologic observations have strongly emphasized the possible role of HCV in causing a variety of extrahepatic disorders. Indeed, HCV has been associated with dermatologic, hematologic, endocrinologic, rheumatic, and autoimmune disorders.[1]

A strong association betweeen HCV and mixed cryoglobulinemia has been established.[2] Mixed cryoglobulinemia is a systemic vasculitis secondary to deposition in the small and medium-sized blood vessels of cryoglobulins (cold-precipitable immune complexes) and complement. It is considered an indolent B-cell lymphoproliferative disorder with a potential switching over to frank malignancy. Indeed, an association between HCV infection and non-Hodgkin's lymphoma (NHL) has been recently reported,[3] and this has led to hypothesize that a relationship possibly exists between HCV infection and malignant lymphoproliferation. In this context, clinical and experimental evidence are discussed on the following questions: Is there any association between autoantibodies and HCV infection? Is liver a site of autoantibody production? Is there a different role for B-cell subsets? Can HCV trigger B-cell expansion? Is mixed cryoglobulinemia related to intrahepatic B-cell expansion? Is there a role for HCV in B-cell NHL?

AUTOIMMUNITY IN HCV INFECTION

In a number of disease conditions, liver damage is assumed to be initiated by an immune-mediated reaction against several antigens expressed on the surface of hepatocytes. These reactions are directed against self-proteins displayed on liver cell membranes, and acute and chronic liver damage may be produced as a consequence of host response against autoantigens likely to be exposed after an exogenous trigger. Production of autoantibodies is thought to be the result of impaired immunologic functions. Indeed, B- and T-cell loss of normal immunosuppressive effect in the liver microenvironment, release of antigens normally sequestered in liver cells, loss of Kupffer cell functions, and cross-reacting antigens released after hepatocyte damage are the main mechanisms postulated in the initiation of an autoimmune reaction.[4]

Identification of infections and other triggering events has led to the belief that in many instances autoimmunity may be explained by an extrinsic process(es). In particular, the possible role of HCV in the initiation of autoimmune disorders has been emphasized in the light of the temporal relationship between HCV infection and development of autoimmune phenomena.[5]

Prevalence of *rheumatoid factor* (RF) autoantibodies ranges from 24 to 76% in chronically HCV-infected patients, and their frequency seems to increase with the severity of liver disease.[6] RFs are a consistent marker of immunologic disturbance in HCV infection in that they play a major pathogenetic role in extrahepatic-associated diseases. They are directed against the C-terminal part of the constant region of immunoglobulin (Ig)G heavy chain and react with native IgG but more strongly with aggregated or denatured IgG in immune complexes. They are mainly of IgM isotype and contribute to the disease process by activating the complement pathway. The occurrence of RF activity with titers higher than 100 IU/mL closely correlates with HCV RNA in the serum and is a good indication of the probability of isolating a cryoglobulin.[7,8] In virtually all HCV-positive patients, cryogenic immune complexes include in their structure RF molecules that bind the Fc portion of IgG *(a crystallizable fragment obtained by its papain digestion that consists of the C-terminal half of two heavy chains linked by disulfide bonds)* specifically directed against HCV proteins.[9]

Anti-idiotypic antibodies have been found in almost 80% of chronically HCV-infected patients and in all patients with acute hepatitis C.[10] Anti-idiotypic IgM molecules directed against IgG with anti-HCV reactivity are polyclonal in nature and have no cryogenic property. Apparently, they do not influence the clinical course of the disease and do not correlate with clinical variables. However, their identification implies a remarkable derangement of immune regulation. The persistent production of autoantibodies and the induction of IgM molecules with IgG anti-idiotypic activity suggest a failure in the down-regulation of the anti-idiotypic network. Thus, the production of autoantibodies, instead of attenuating and eventually turning off the immune reaction, perpetuates it through the production of immune complexes with intrinsic potentially pathogenetic features.

During the immune response against a xenogenic antigen, B cells bearing antigen-specific receptors are stimulated to proliferate and differentiate into antibody-secreting plasma cells within germinal centers.[11] A few B cells bearing the appropriate antigen receptor are usually stimulated to undergo clonal proliferation, and somatic hypermutation of the rearranged Ig variable *(V; N-terminal region of the light or heavy chain of an Ig molecule that differs greatly in amino acid sequence among different Ig chains)* genes and Ig class switching are initiated.

To persist, mature B cells require maintained expression of B-cell receptor *(BCR; a membrane–bound Ig as a part of a complex of molecules including Igα and Igβ, a disulfide-linked dimer. Igα and Igβ are noncovalently associated with membrane-bound Ig. The two functions of BCR are internalization of bound antigen for subsequent presentation and cellular activation)*. In vivo ablation of surface Ig using the technique of inducible gene targeting to delete the rearranged heavy-chain V gene in mature B cells leads not only to diminished BCR expression, but also to decreased major histocompatibility complex (MHC) antigen expression, upregulation of Fas, and rapid cell death by apoptosis.[12] This means that peripheral B cells need continual signaling to avoid apoptosis while they recirculate awaiting the encounter with foreign antigens.[13]

In contrast to conventional antigens, whose binding is relatively infrequent, superantigens *(a group of antigens that stimulate large numbers of T cells)* can bind to B cells bearing Ig receptors of a given heavy chain variable (V_H)-gene family, thereby resulting in higher binding frequencies. Such interactions may involve sequences from V_H framework regions 1 and 3 *(FR1 and FR3; region segments exhibiting a lesser degree of variability that separate complementarity-determining regions)* and complementarity-determining region 2 *(CDR2; a portion of an Ig molecule that determines the binding of one specific antigen)*.[14]

In the three-dimensional structure of V_H, FR1 and FR3 binding motifs are created that are separate from the classical binding site.[15] Recent data show that the CD5 molecule on B cells is an endogenous ligand selective for B-cell surface Ig FR sequences.[16] F(ab′)$_2$ fragments *(the antigen-binding fragments produced by papain digestion of an Ig molecule)* bind B cells irrespective of antibody specificity, and the binding can be inhibited by anti-CD5 antibodies.[17] Interaction of V_H FR structures with CD5 may sustain maintenance and selective expansions of B cells and may generate distinct activation signals at different stages of B-cell development.[18] A role for CD5 molecule as a candidate selective ligand is further suggested by its physical and functional coupling to the BCR.[16] Thus, CD5 accessory molecules in the BCR complex may have a unique potential to modulate BCR signals after interactions with antigens and/or superantigens.[19] CD5+ (B-1) B cells provide a consistent source of autoantibody-producing cells, and CD5-F(ab′)$_2$ region interaction provides effective autostimulatory growth and mediates selection of autoreactive repertoires. They express a restricted set of IgV genes that have no substantial diversification from the germline DNA. Indeed, the use of germline V genes seems to be a property of cells derived from CD5+ B-cell lineage.[20]

B cells can be divided into three subsets called B-1a, B-1b, and B-2 cells. B-1a and B-1b are believed to be separate self-replenishing lineages identical in functional and many phenotypic properties but differing in expression of the CD5 antigen, which is found only on the B-1a cells. B-2 cells, which are CD5−, constitute most mature B cells.[21] A major difference between the CD5+ and CD5− B cells is the frequency with which heavy chain variable-determining-joining (V_HDJ_H) rearrangements accumulate mutations. It seems that CD5+/IgM+ B cells are mutated significantly less often than CD5−/IgM+ B cells, supporting the finding that CD5+ cells home less efficiently to the germinal center, where it is thought that hypermutation primarily occurs. Characteristic of these cells are autoantibodies of IgM isotype that include a very restricted pattern of V genes[19] and are thought to be primarily involved in the immune response to T-independent antigens.[22]

In contrast, it appears that circulating RF-producing cells are mainly CD5 negative and display a high rate of somatic mutations that cluster in CDR regions.[23] The latter characteristics favor the view that RFs result from an antigen-driven process that usually takes place in germinal centers as a T-dependent mechanism. Somatic mutations in the V genes encoding self-reactive antibodies enhance the affinity of the expressed IgM molecules, thus contributing to augmented cell stimulation, B-cell maturation, and acquisition of high pathogenetic potential.[24]

Many other organ and nonorgan-specific autoantibodies have been described in anti-HCV-positive patients. *Anti-GOR antibody,* directed to a host-derived epitope named GOR, occurs in anti-HCV-positive patients with a frequency ranging from 20 to 70%.[25] There is a close correlation between immune response to GOR and HCV core peptides, which suggests that the GOR antibody is probably caused by cross-recognition related to partial sequence homology between GOR and the aminoterminal portion of the core protein. The GOR autoreactivity, however, may not be due to molecular mimicry with the core protein in that anti-GOR antibodies are found in patients negative for anti-core antibody, and this indicates that humoral responses to GOR and core are independently regulated.[26] The clinical significance of anti-GOR antibody is poorly defined, though a positive correlation has been recorded between anti-GOR reactivity and the necroinflammatory activity of liver disease.[27]

Smooth muscle autoantibodies (SMA) are a heterogeneous collection of antibodies of different specificity that react with cytoskeleton antigens of smooth muscle cells. They are mainly directed against actin, a globular 46-kDa protein, which displays a monomeric (G-actin) or polymeric (F-actin) structure. SMA are also directed against tubulin, which is a constituent of 25-nm microtubules, and against desmin and vimentin, which are proteins of 10-nm intermediate filaments.[28]

In chronic hepatitis C, the frequency of SMA is 15–20%, the bulk of which is formed by antibodies with non-anti-actin smooth muscle reactivity, whereas the occurrence of F-actin autoantibodies is the standard diagnostic marker of type 1 autoimmune hepatitis (AIH) in that its diagnostic significance reaches up to 80% sensitivity and virtually 100% specificity at titers higher than 1:40.[29]

The prevalence of serum *antinuclear autoantibody* (ANA) ranges between 6 and 13%, which is significantly higher compared with normal individuals or patients with hepatitis B virus infection (1–4%).[30] Though subspecificities of ANA reactivities have not been assessed, ANA in HCV-positive patients have distinct features, including low titer (1:40–1:80) and speckled immunofluorescent pattern (mainly anti-centromere and less frequently anti-nucleolar or anti-mitotic spindle apparatus pattern).[31] ANA with homogeneous pattern is a distinctive feature of AIH, and its potential diagnostic usefulness has been emphasized.[32]

Liver/kidney microsomal (LKM) autoantibodies have been characterized using indirect immunofluorescence by their reaction with the cytoplasm of hepatocytes and proximal renal tubules.[33] LKM-1 autoantibodies are a serologic marker of type 2 AIH[34] and must be distinguished from LKM-2 antibodies, which occur in drug-induced hepatitis caused by thienylic acid,[35] and LKM-3 antibodies found in patients with chronic hepatitis D.[36] LKM-1 antibodies are detected in up to 10% of patients with chronic hepatitis C.[37] These patients possibly account for a distinct HCV-infected subgroup characterized by an additional pathogenetic role played by LKM-1 antibodies. Anti-LKM-1 antibodies are detected against different epitopes displayed on cythochrome P450 II D6. Indeed, overlapping but distinct specificities have been reported in HCV-positive or type 2 AIH patients.[38] LKM-1 antibodies in HCV-positive patients occur at low titer, are present in older patients without female predominance, and are often associated with low titers of serum HCV RNA.[39] In terms of clinical response to interferon therapy, these patients do not differentiate from the LKM-1-negative HCV-positive group.

Anti-asialoglycoprotein receptor,[40] anti-liver membrane antigen,[41] anti-liver cytosol antigen,[42] anti-hepatocyte plasma membrane,[43] anti-thyroglobulin, anti-thyroid peroxidase,[44] anti-phospholipids,[45] and anti-neutrophil cytoplasmic autoantibodies[46] have also been described in anti-HCV-positive patients. However, both their pathogenic significance and the immunogenic stimulus for their production are unknown. Each antibody is directed against intracellular antigens released during cell death and freely presented to the immune system. The absence of any association between them, however, suggests that their appearance is not simply a consequence of cell necrosis. In each condition, a disease-specific intracellular antigen is perhaps presented on the hepatocyte membrane by molecules of the major histocompatibility complex, or alternatively, a disease-specific antigen is expressed on the plasma membrane with epitopes that cross-react with certain intracellular components. Because these antibodies are usually present at low titer, have relatively poor affinity for their corresponding antigens, and largely belong to the IgM class, they can be considered "natural" autoantibodies and hence an epiphenomenon with no definite clinical significance.

In terms of pathogenic potential, it can be emphasized that RFs represent a reliable biologic marker of the HCV infection, and in almost one third of HCV-infected patients they occur at high titers and are deposited in vascular structures of organ-localized autoimmune diseases such as skin and kidney.[47,48] Thus, RFs seem to assume a substantial pathogenetic role in extrahepatic autoimmune diseases associated with HCV infection.

LIVER AS A MAJOR SITE OF RHEUMATOID FACTOR PRODUCTION

In chronic hepatitis C, intraportal lymphoid nodules (IPLNs) are characterized by nodular lymphocytic aggregates, frequently with a germinal centerlike structure. The phenotype of the immunocompetent cells present in and around IPLNs suggests they are functional structures, in that activated B cells are surrounded by a follicular dendritic cell network. A T-cell zone comprising CD4-positive helper T cells and CD8-

positive suppressor/cytotoxic T cells is detected at the periphery of the nodules.[49] These structures resemble the so-called ectopic germinal centers found in nonlymphoid tissues or other abnormal sites in a variety of autoimmune and inflammatory diseases, including rheumatoid synovial membrane,[50] thyroid glands of patients with Hashimoto's thyroiditis,[51] the choroid in uveoretinitis,[52] and lung in cryptogenic fibrosing alveolitis.[53]

However, despite the use of different D (segment located between the variable and the J-constant region of the Igs) and J (a segment involved in joining V and C genes in heavy and light chains of the Igs) segments, the resulting amino acid sequences matched, suggesting the presence of a common selected antigen-translation of CDR3 sequences of lymphocyte clusters from liver tissues. Rearrangements usually occurred in the appropriate reading frame for the production of potentially functional proteins in that they were frequently proved to be very similar to a database IgM RF sequence, thus suggesting a possible RF activity of such clones.[54]

To better characterize the B-cell response in these patients, we cloned and sequenced rearranged IgV genes of IPLNs isolated by microdissection technique from sections of liver biopsies. All the clusters examined were hypermutated. Features and degree of mutations were usually different between lymphoid clusters in the same section. Hypermutated genes were not present in large numbers (not more than two representatives of each identical rearrangement). Two pairs of hypermutated genes differing by three to seven point mutations were probably derived from cells that divided within the cluster.[55]

The presence of multiple B-cell clusters suggests many explanations of their origin. We ruled out the possibility that they arise by aggregation of infiltrating polyclonal B cells by demonstrating a clonal B-cell expansion within the clusters. The second possibility is that a single B-cell clone proliferates to form a germinal center and B cells then migrate into the liver to seed other clusters. The third is that individual infiltrating B cells are stimulated independently by antigen-presenting cells at different locations to proliferate and produce separate clusters. Because none of the cells in any of the larger clusters expanded the same VDJ combination as cells in the neighboring cluster, it would appear that B-cell clones proliferate and mutate independently in IPLNs and do not migrate.

The cell origin from which the clone arises is not known, but the low number of mutations suggests that it arose from naive B cells, whereas the clones that were more heavily mutated probably arose from memory cells. This pattern is consistent with a chronic immune response against a persistent antigen stimulation. Memory B cells are possibly generated in a secondary lymphoid organ and subsequently migrate to the liver where they become activated and induced to proliferate.

The relationship between different compartments was studied in our laboratory. The results indicated that B-cell clonal expansions were demonstrable in the liver and in the bone marrow and in the peripheral blood lymphocytes (PBL). Sequence analysis of the dominant band confirmed the expansion of the same B-cell clone in liver, bone marrow, and PBL. DNA and CDR3 sequence analysis showed that in all patients, the human protein sequences were closely related to those encoded by the IgH variable region. In most cases, a closer homology to human RF was noticed within the antibody specificity database available.[56] The finding of multiple D segments in a high percentage of cases in HCV-infected livers provides further evidence of antigen-driven selection in the development of intrahepatic B-cell clonal expansion. It may be inferred that in the response to an antigen where a simple VDJ rearrangement does not provide a high-affinity antibody, a clone with an unusual D segment is able to produce antibodies of greater specificity. This increased ability to bind the antigen gives the B-cell clone a growth advantage over those that cannot respond or respond less efficiently. Hence, due to antigenic selection and clonal expansion, B-cell clones could become predominant in the response.[57] Similarly, due to perpetuation of antigenic stimulation provided by persistence of the virus in the liver, a B-cell clone may gain an advantage over the others and becomes prevalent.[58]

The production of RF in the liver may have many pathogenetic implications. It has been shown that RFs contain a spectrum of partially overlapping specificities among three members of the Ig gene superfamily (IgG, β_2-microglobulin, and class I molecules) that do not appear to be similarly increased in normal human sera. It could be that some RFs generated in the course of the immune response are directed to portions of class I antigen-binding pockets or clefts, and this results in a modulatory and protective role through peptide recognition by the cell-mediated response.[59] This may provide a plausible explanation for the so-called protective effect of RF on liver disease in HCV-infected cryoglobulinemic patients. Indeed, from the first clinical studies, it appeared that compared with noncryoglobulinemic HCV-infected patients, those with mixed cryoglobulinemia showed a more benign clinical course of liver disease.[60]

B-CELL EXPANSION: A KEY FEATURE OF MIXED CRYOGLOBULINEMIA

Soon after the discovery of HCV, a striking association was recognized between this virus and the so-called essential mixed cryoglobulinemia, a clinical syndrome in which circulating cryoglobulins induce systemic vasculitis, which mainly involves skin, kidney, and peripheral nerve fibers.[61,62] Cryoglobulins are single or mixed Igs that can reversibly precipitate in the cold. Mixed cryoglobulinemia is a major clinical picture among the extrahepatic features of chronic HCV infection. Its prevalence varies widely and ranges from 13 to 54%.[62–66] in selected HCV-infected patients, though these values suffer from the lack of standardized diagnostic criteria. The restricted monoclonal RF that characterizes type II mixed cryoglobulinemia is detected in almost two thirds of all mixed cryoglobulins. As compared with mixed cryoglobulinemia containing polyclonal RF (named type III mixed cryoglobulinemia), type II is more frequently associated with cutaneous vasculitis, membranoproliferative glomerulonephritis, and peripheral neuropathies. The pathogenetic activity of monoclonal IgM-RF is demonstrated by its deposition in the sites of damage, such as the skin and the kidney.[47,67,68]

Cryogenic IgM-RFs are derived from a limited set of germline genes.[69] It is likely that any alleged immunoregulatory role displayed by monoclonal IgM-RFs (10% of which are cryoglobulins) is germline encoded and not dependent on random somatic mutations of their genes. However, even in chronic viral infections, IgM antiglobulins may react with different antigens, including the $F(ab')_2$ fragment of both autologous (derived from the subject's body) and isologous (molecule of identical gene construction) IgG.[70,71] It has been shown that in HCV infection the reaction of IgM with the corresponding IgG is inhibited by the addition of HCV antigens, and this suggests that the antigen-binding site of the IgG is also reactive with IgM antiglobulins, thus showing the peculiar properties of anti-idiotypic antibodies.[10,48]

The levels of monoclonal or polyclonal RF activity, as well as of HCV-RNA, are consistently higher in the cryoprecipitating material than in the corresponding whole serum. This enrichment indicates that cryoprecipitation reflects specific interactions rather than a merely nonspecific precipitation of cold-insoluble proteins. Analysis of monoclonal IgM-RF in the cryoglobulins shows that more than 90% of unrelated patients have the same H and L chain cross-reactive idiotypes, named WA (so dubbed after the patient whose monoclonal RF was used to raise the original typing antiserum[69]) group, as recognized by G6 and 17.109 monoclonal antibodies, respectively.[72] These findings indicate that the antibody repertoire is restricted and that monoclonal RFs are encoded by the same germline genes, probably through stimulation by the same antigen(s).

Genes encoding RFs have been shown in normal people who exhibit remarkably abundant RF receptors on the plasma membrane of their lymphocytes.[73] This suggests an important physiologic role for RFs in the capture, processing, and presentation to T cells of anti-

gens trapped within immune complexes and may explain the sustained RF production in many autoimmune and lymphoproliferative diseases.[74] As stated above, immune complexes are a prominent biologic feature of acute and chronic HCV-infected patients. We used an antigen-specific immune complex assay to demonstrate that immune complexes comprise hepatitis C virions bound to IgG molecules with specific anti-HCV activity, which in turn are linked to IgM molecules bearing WACRI (IgG-IgM WACRI) immune complexes. These immune complexes appear in step with IgG anti-HCV seroconversion and remain detectable for a long period, irrespective of the clinical outcome. Interestingly, despite similar serum levels of IgM WACRI molecules, IgG-IgM WACRI immune complexes were not found in acute and chronic hepatitis B and acute hepatitis A infections. Thus, IgG–IgM WACRI immune complexes appear to be uniquely associated with HCV infection, supporting the view that they derive from an antigen-driven response closely related to the involved antigen.[10]

It can be postulated that immune complexes that enter lymphoid tissue via the afferent lymphatics often localize in the marginal and mantle zones, where RF precursor cells are abundant as demonstrated by the 17.109 probe.[75] The possibility that the major role of these cells is not related to antibody secretion but rather to the antigen-processing functions of mantle zone B lymphocytes is supported by a recent immunomorphologic analysis of the distribution of HCV-related proteins in lymph nodes from patients with type II mixed cryoglobulinemia.[76] In a sequential reconstruction from the capsule to hilar structures of lymph nodes, viral proteins were mainly detected in interfollicular areas, including the mantle zones of the follicles.

WACRI specificities highly associate with IgM RF molecules that often occur on fetal B cells. Therefore, coexpression of light (17.109) and heavy (G6) chain idiotypes usually indicates RF autoantibody activity and drives the early expansion of RF precursors.[77,78] However, IgM WACRI molecules demonstrated in immune complexes of HCV-infected patients do not possess RF activity, do not associate with systemic vasculitis, and do not lead to cryoprecipitating material or complement consumption.[9]

The nature of WA RF-producing cells has been questioned. Immunophenotypic analysis of cellular constituents of IPLNs in liver biopsies from HCV-positive cryoglobulinemic patients showed that they consist of a B-cell population expressing IgM and, to a certain extent, CD5 antigen.[79] However, though it is impossible to draw any firm conclusion based on CD5 expression of WA proliferating B cells, secretion of the expressed IgM molecules, and clinical evaluation, a pathogenetic model can be proposed in which HCV probably stimulates CD5+ B cells to produce polyspecific IgM molecules bearing WACRI. These molecules enter into soluble noncryoprecipitating immune complexes, whereas monospecific IgM WA are probably secreted by CD5⁻ B cells as a result of somatic diversification after preselection in germinal centers.

RF production in HCV-infected patients is associated with either oligoclonal or monoclonal intrahepatic B-cell expansions.[80] Different clones probably derive from different B cells within the polyclonal repertoire of liver-infiltrating B cells and different foci may contain unrelated B-cell clones. The frequency of oligoclonal B-cell expansion is consistent with this hypothesis, and such expansion may indeed be a key pathobiologic feature of HCV-associated nonmalignant B-cell lymphoproliferation.[79,80] The preferential expansion of one clone would in turn lead to a monoclonal pattern, which was observed only in patients with type II mixed cryoglobulinemia.[80]

It can be inferred that the initial response to HCV includes an IgM WACRI without antiglobulin reactivity that acquires RF activity as a consequence of somatic mutations, which accompany proliferation of WACRI-positive B cells and then progress to WACRI mono-

clonal RF with persistent infection. This implies that production of cryoglobulins may be directly related to the duration of HCV infection. It was indeed reported that cryoglobulins are more prevalent in patients with cirrhosis than in those without.[7] Because cirrhosis is obviously found in patients with a longer liver disease, it was concluded that length of HCV infection may have a role in the production of mixed cryoglobulinemia. Thus, it can be speculated that polyclonal RF developing with chronic stimulation of immune complexes leads first to type III and then to monoclonal RF and type II mixed cryoglobulinemia. However, this biologic event can rarely be assessed in the clinical follow-up even after decades. Cryoglobulins are rarely detected in patients presenting with acute hepatitis C progressing to chronicity and followed for many years. This suggests that cryoglobulin production is an independent effect of HCV infection that can take place specifically in a subgroup of patients whose mechanisms for the silencing of higher affinity, potentially pathologic, RF-expressing B cells have failed.[81]

An alternative hypothesis for the pathogenetic mechanisms underlying mixed cryoglobulinemia pro-

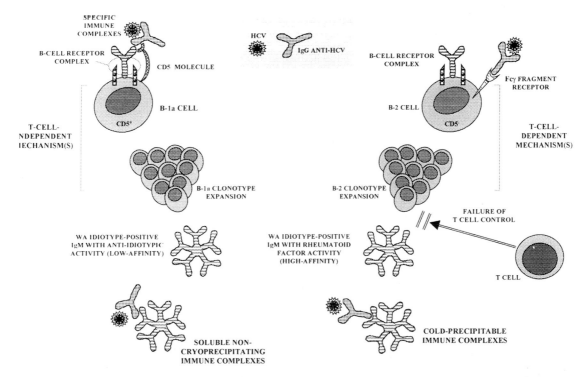

FIG. 1. Proposed model of B-cell pathway in the production of WA cross-reactive idiotype soluble and cryoprecipitating immune complexes. According to this model, the persistent signal needed for B-cell maintenance is provided by the interaction of surface Ig with CD5 molecule and endogenous antigens represented by the F(ab′)$_2$ fragment of IgG. Once HCV is provided, they differentiate into antibody-secreting cells, mainly IgM with anti-idiotypic activity. Restricted expression of unmutated V$_H$ and possibly L$_H$ genes would provide the structural correlate for the high degree of idiotypic cross-reactive (polyreactive) antibodies through a T-independent mechanism. Although molecules with RF activity are found among low-affinity antibodies, high-affinity potentially pathogenetic RFs were found to display a number of somatic mutations that cluster in CDR regions. This favors the view that they result from an antigen-driven process in that conventional B (CD5⁻) cells are implicated in their production. Persistence of higher affinity RFs underlies the failure of the mechanism capable of inactivating the corresponding RF B-cell clones likely induced by the lack of T-cell control required for cell differentiation.

duction could account for the specific nature of circulating immune complexes formed in HCV infection, as proposed in the model described in Figure 1. B cells can progress along two discrete differentiation pathways, B-1 or B-2, in response to different antigenic stimuli. Natural antibody-producing B-1 cells possibly undergo a process of clonal expansion and selection mediated by occupancy of the surface CD5–F(ab′)$_2$ region interaction for HCV by structures borne on self-components. Such HCV-dependent clonal selection would be consistent with the oligoclonality pattern detected by IgH VDJ rearrangement. The V$_H$, D, and J$_H$ gene sequence analysis suggests that natural polyreactive antibodies derived from human B-1 cells are produced by a selection assortment of clonotypes containing a load of R mutations comparable in distribution with that of V$_H$DJ$_H$ genes expressed by the nonreactive antibody-producing B-2 cells and consistent with positive clonal selection by antigen. Because B-1 cells are thought to be primarily involved in T-independent immune responses and not to participate in germinal center reaction, the small number of mutated V$_H$DJ$_H$ rearrangements could be the result of recurrent T-cell-independent stimulation outside germinal centers.[82]

RFs derived from chronic stimulation reveal extensive somatic mutations.[83–86] Persistence of HCV immune complexes activates B-2 cells through cross-linking of Fcγ receptors (receptors present on various cells for the Fc fragment of IgG) expressed on their surface. Under normal circumstances, these cells proliferate, and serum IgM RF levels may rise as a consequence. However, RF molecules, though revealing extensive somatic mutations, are transient in production and show no evidence of affinity maturation. This suggests the presence of efficient peripheral mechanisms for silencing of higher affinity potentially pathologic RF-expressing B cells that arise by mutation of lower affinity RF genes or by random somatic mutations on other antibody genes capable of generating antibodies cross-reactive with IgG. This mechanism, however, is not yet clarified. A peripheral control of RF clonal expansion is proposed with a Fas-independent mechanism, likely mediated by the lack of T-cell-derived helper factors through blocking of CD40 ligand–CD40 interaction.[87] This mechanism is possibly lacking in almost 20–30% of chronically HCV-infected patients, in whom somatic mutations generate higher affinity RFs and cryoprecipitating immune complexes.

The above-described autoimmune response interfaces with the specific anti-HCV immunity schematically outlined in Figure 2. Anti-HCV antibodies are directed against virtually every viral antigen. The earliest responses are thought to be IgM against core, envelope, and NS3 regions, with antibodies directed against NS4 and NS5 appearing later in the course of infection.

However, both the onset and the pattern of antibody responses are highly variable, and no specific feature has been identified. There is considerable controversy about whether natural infection with HCV results in induction of neutralizing antibodies and about what they may be directed against. Most infected persons develop chronic infection despite the presence of multiple HCV-specific antibodies suggesting that they do little to alter the course of infection.

In this context, production of anti-F(ab′)$_2$ and anti-Fc autoantibodies may exert a persistent challenge to the immune system. Idiotype- and isotype-directed interactions between Igs derived from CD5$^+$ or CD5$^-$ B cells represent an interacting network potentially contributing to establish HCV chronicity.

OVERT B-CELL MALIGNANCIES

In the light of the extremely high prevalence of HCV infection among patients with mixed cryoglobulinemia, the possible relationship of HCV-related cryoglobulinemia to malignant lymphoproliferative diseases should be emphasized. This issue is based on the following clinical and biologic aspects: an increased prevalence of HCV infection in patients with B-cell NHLs,[88–95] an increased primary localization of NHL in organs considered frequent targets of HCV infection,[93,96–100] an increased prevalence of B-cell NHLs in hepatopathic patients,[101–105] a relatively frequent occurrence of monoclonal gammopathies in patients with HCV infection,[106–110] the localization of HCV genomic sequences and viral proteins in neoplastic and nonneoplastic lymph nodes in HCV-infected patients,[76] and a decrease in B-cell lymphoproliferation after HCV eradication.[111,112]

Two subsets of B-cell NHL associated with HCV infection with distinct clinical and pathologic features have been identified: NHLs complicating the course of mixed cryoglobulinemia, which are usually of low-grade, involve the bone marrow and may possibly evolve into an aggressive phenotype and NHLs unrelated to mixed cryoglobulinemia, which frequently show an aggressive phenotype ab initio and often lack bone marrow involvement.[91,93]

When HCV-infected cryoglobulinemic patients were analyzed after a long-term observation, progression to NHL was documented in 5–10%. Their symptoms were usually mild, and an expanding spectrum of autoimmune phenomena was recorded, resulting in hemolytic anemia, thrombocytopenia, and granulocytopenia.[69]

The mechanism(s) of clonal expansion of B cells in determining the conversion to a lymphoproliferative disorder is unclear. It has been shown that after viral infection, viruses can persist in the host indefinitely

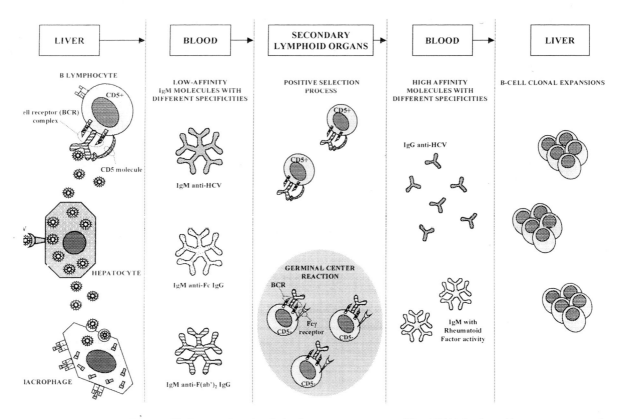

FIG. 2. Interactions of HCV-specific humoral and cellular immune responses. After HCV infection of hepatocytes, a variety of cellular and humoral responses occurs aimed at eliminating the virus. Virus particles released from infected cells are recruited mainly by phagocytosis into antigen-presenting cells (macrophages, monocytes, dendritic cells, and B lymphocytes). Once antigens/pathogens are localized within an organ, the passing naive B lymphocytes are retained and activated and undergo clonal expansion. In the proposed model, CD5+ (B-1) B cells are responsible for the primary response. IgM derived from CD5+ B cells bind with relatively low affinity either to the immunizing virus or to various self-antigens such as F(ab')$_2$ and Fc fragments of IgG. These polyreactive antibodies enhance the early recruitment of the virus to secondary lymphoid organs in that a specific protective response is generated. On the basis of established features in the marked difference of CD5⁻ (B-2) B cells to acquire somatic mutations and to undergo isotype switching, these cells are possibly stimulated to proliferate and differentiate into antibody-secreting cells within germinal centers. In addition to specific anti-HCV antibodies, high-affinity RF molecules are likely secreted by these cells.

through latency or continuous low level replication.[113] We recently approached this issue by studying B cells isolated from neoplastic lymph nodes of patients with type II mixed cryoglobulinemia.[56] We investigated HCV infection in NHL B cells by means of sensitive methods in two patients in whom a low-grade NHL developed over a period of almost 20 years after diagnosis of type II mixed cryoglobulinemia. Low-level HCV infection was detected in neoplastic B cells of both patients. HCV was demonstrated by an *in situ* reverse transcriptase polymerase chain reaction (RT-PCR) technique capable of detecting ~10 genomes/cell. In this selected population, HCV positivity was estimated to be in the range of 20–36% of NHL B cells. In these cells, viral genomic sequences were found in the absence of viral protein production, suggesting a latency status of the infection.

In the same study, we analyzed three further HCV-positive patients with high-grade NHL unrelated to

mixed cryoglobulinemia without a history of autoimmune disorders. We were unable to demonstrate HCV infection in their neoplastic B cells. Neither HCV RNA nor viral proteins were found. These data confirmed those obtained in a previous study in which HCV-related proteins were detected in lymphomatous lesions of only 3 of 12 patients (25%), associating type II mixed cryoglobulinemia and a low-grade disease.[76] This suggests that the expression of viral gene products is related to certain stages of cell differentiation and emphasizes that a frank malignant phenotype is not permissive to HCV replication.[114]

It is not known whether HCV is present in normal nonproliferating lymph nodes because they are rarely available for study. However, indirect information from other studies indicates that perihepatic lymphadenopathies are common in HCV-infected patients.[115] Interestingly, lymph node enlargement seems directly related to viral replication rather than to the severity or activity of liver disease. Furthermore, lymph nodes may represent a major site of extrahepatic active replication of HCV in that HCV negative-polarity strand (putative replicative intermediates) was demonstrated in more than 60% of lymph nodes from HCV-infected patients with acquired immunodeficiency syndrome, indicating the presence of productive infection in these sites.[116]

Demonstration of active replication of HCV in extrahepatic sites remains a crucial issue due to possible mispriming events during RT-PCR subsequent to excess of genomic strand. Indeed, different weights of negative and positive-polarity strands during virogenesis are a consistent feature of all Flavivirus members, and this supports the existence of a regulatory mechanism that favors the production of positive-polarity over negative-polarity stranded RNA.[117] Using optimized strand-specific assays, HCV replication was demonstrated in human lymphomonocytes[118] and in lymphocyte cell lines in vitro.[119] Some authors suggest the existence of HCV strains with particular affinity for immunocompetent cells.[120] Of substantial biologic interest was the evidence of HCV replication in hematopoietic cells in an in vivo model, namely mice with severe combined immunodeficiency that lack both humoral and cellular immunity caused by a deficit in the recombinase enzyme system.[121] Indeed, the evidence that hematopoietic cells support HCV replication is both biologically and clinically significant, because HCV may directly affect the function of immunocytes by interfering with their ability to eliminate HCV from infected cells and/or by modifying their property to activate in response to a suitable stimulation or to exert adequate effector functions.

As stated above, infection of circulating mononuclear cells seems to be strictly correlated with the progression of HCV carrier state. HCV was not detected in blood mononuclear cells during the incubation period of acute hepatitis C.[122] The demonstration that B, T, and monocyte/macrophage cell lines are susceptible to HCV infection supports its multilineage character. A likely explanation of this phenomenon is the recent finding of productive infection in CD34+ cells recovered from either bone marrow or peripheral blood.[123]

It was indeed shown that HCV-harboring CD34+ cells are present in more than 80% of HCV chronic carriers. CD34+ cells are stem cells with in vivo reconstituting capacity on virtually all colony-forming cells and on early myeloid and lymphoid precursors.[124] In view of their peculiar biologic characteristics, CD34+ cells could be the initial site of HCV infection, a continuous source of virus production and possibly an efficient mode for its dissemination. Interestingly, CD34+ cells have been recently identified in the adult human liver, where the expression of CD34 transcripts fluctuates and tends to decrease at the lowest levels after birth but increases during inflamed or neoplastic conditions.[125] The presence of CD34 reactivity in the liver demonstrates that this organ retains CD34+ cells and possibly acts as a hematopoietic microenvironment from the fetal period or as a reservoir of circulating CD34+ cells in the adult organ.

In view of the evidence that CD34 molecules may be involved in leukocyte adhesion and "homing" during inflammatory processes, the liver may be the localization site of progenitor hematopoietic cells infected with HCV. An intriguing question is whether established HCV infection in CD34+ cells transmits the infection directly through the multilineage differentiation of hematopoietic cells. Because infection of hematopoietic stem cells is maintained for several years (personal observations), it seems reasonable to assume that this is an effective way of inducing an established chronic carrier state of HCV infection. The next intriguing question is whether infection of CD34+ cells has a role in the induction of the host-specific tolerance for the virus. It is well known that antigen-presenting stromal cells derived from hematopoietic stem cells migrate to the thymus and present peptides on their MHC molecules to remove self-reactive T cells.[126] This process, called negative selection, may be responsible for induction of host-specific tolerance toward neutralizing epitopes of the virus and could explain why apparent immunocompetent individuals become unable to eradicate HCV infection.

Except for anecdotal reports, the studies published so far are inadequate to assess the long-term impact of HCV infection on patients with NHL not associated with mixed cryoglobulinemia. At present, indeed, the possible link is based on the high prevalence of HCV infection in NHL patients. Up to 42% of HCV-infected NHL patients have been described in some Mediterranean and Japanese studies,[95,127–131] whereas a very low prevalence not different from that in the general population has been assessed in studies from Northern Europe.[132–134] These findings may indeed reflect the geographically variable epidemiology of HCV infection and differences in ethnicity and possibly account for the results of a Northern American study in which 22% of lymphoma patients (mostly Hispanics) were HCV-infected compared with 4.5% of the controls.[94] An additional reason why the prevalence data should be taken with particular caution is that it is difficult to know whether HCV infection occurred before NHL was diagnosed or acquired in the course of the therapy through the transfusion of blood and blood derivatives. It is likely that immunosuppression that results from the lymphoma process and conditioning therapies may predispose to more frequent viral infections. Furthermore, in most of these studies the controls were not truly comparable in that they differed in many end points.

We studied patients with B-cell NHL of recent onset referred to a single oncologic center in Northeastern Italy,[93] where the incidence of HCV infection in the general population is less than 1%, as in Northern Europe. Out of 35 NHL patients, 17 (48.6%) had serologic evidence of HCV infection 1 to 4 years before the diagnosis of NHL. Abnormalities of liver function tests lasting for several years were demonstrable in most of the remaining 18 patients in whom tests for HCV were performed at the time of NHL onset. In this study control groups included 122 consecutive HCV-negative patients with B-cell NHL, 464 histopathologic cases referred over a period of 5 years, and 127 consecutive patients with HCV infection without overt lymphoma. Results indicated that HCV-infected patients frequently presented at onset an extranodal localization of B-cell NHL (especially in the liver and major salivary glands), a diffuse large cell histotype without any prior history of low-grade B-cell malignancy or bone marrow involvement, and a weak association with a full-blown predisposing autoimmune disease. Indeed, in this series, a definite clinical picture of autoimmune disease (i.e., mixed cryoglobulinemia or Sjögren's syndrome) preceded NHL onset in 14.7% and in 2.9%, respectively.

The virtual absence of HCV-positive lymphoid cells in neoplastic lymph nodes and the large number of HCV-carrying B cells detected in hyperplastic reactive lymphadenopathy suggest that viral infection contributes to the early steps in the development of malignancy.[76] The potential transforming activity of HCV has been suggested by *in vitro* studies in which the role of core protein on the transcriptional regulation of cellular proto-oncogenes that may affect the normal cell growth has been emphasized.[135] The transforming activities of HCV, however, are not needed in the later stages and may disappear, probably through negative selection. At these stages of lymphomagenesis, other factors are likely to contribute to the malignant process, including stimulation of cell proliferation and aberrant protein expression through cytogenetic abnormalities.

The wide heterogeneity of HCV-associated lymphoproliferation includes further distinct clinical pictures characterized by noncryoprecipitating monoclonal Igs. This biologic condition is defined monoclonal gammopathy of undetermined significance (MGUS) and underlies clonal expansion of plasma cells that produce a unique Ig, most frequently of IgG isotype. In HCV chronic carriers, MGUS ranges from 2 to 15%.[106-110] In our series its prevalence is 8% and appears highly significant when compared with an age-matched control population (1-2%).[128] MGUS in HCV-positive patients has an indolent clinical course and is not associated with

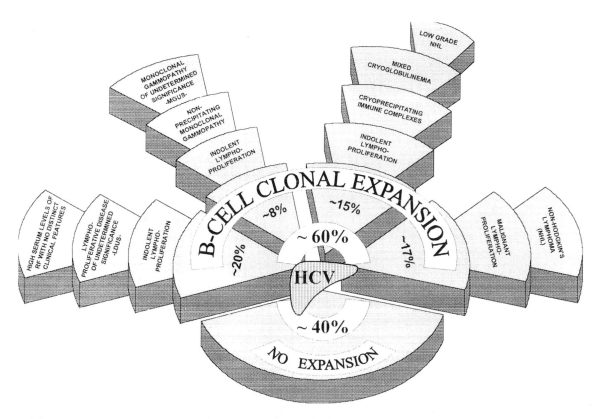

FIG. 3. Clinical variables associated with intrahepatic B-cell clonal expansion. Either polyclonal or monoclonal profiles of B-cell expansions may occur in the liver of almost 60% of patients with chronic hepatitis C. They show a large spectrum of clinical variables that include a clinically silent condition with higher levels of polyclonal RF molecules (tentatively dubbed lymphoproliferative disease of undetermined significance); monoclonal gammopathy, mostly IgG, mimicking the clinical picture of monoclonal gammopathy of undetermined significance; mixed cryoglobulinemia; and, finally, B-cell NHL. No distinct clinical or laboratory findings were found to characterize the remaining quota of patients who do not associate intrahepatic B-cell lymphoproliferation.

bone lytic lesions nor with plasmocytosis. The presence of a monoclonal protein does not modify the therapeutic response to interferons.

Finally, Figure 3 tentatively summarizes, on the basis of current evidence, the clinical spectrum associated with the presence of intrahepatic B-cell clonal expansion in chronic HCV-positive patients. At one end of the spectrum, there is the absence of clinical manifestations in patients (~20%) in whom the only biochemical marker is increased titers of serum polyclonal RFs without activation of the complement pathway; we have provisionally dubbed this situation "lymphoproliferative disease of undetermined significance." Next, there are noncryoprecipitating monoclonal proteins (~8%), that is, monoclonal gammopathies mainly of IgG isotype, clinically indistinguishable from MGUS; mixed cryoglobulinemia (~15%); and finally overt B-cell NHLs (~17%). These NHLs are possibly a pathobiologic entity different from NHLs emerging in the course of type II mixed cryoglobulinemia.

It is conceivable that a better understanding of the mode of HCV persistence and of the role that HCV plays in the malignant process will permit the development of new approaches aimed at the prevention and treatment of HCV-associated tumors.

ACKNOWLEDGMENTS. Supported in part by "Associazione Italiana per la Ricerca sul Cancro (AIRC)," by a grant from the Italian Ministry of University and Scientific and Technological Research for the Project "Mechanisms of Chronic Damage Induced by Hepatitis Viruses," and by a grant from the University of Bari. We thank Dr. Salvatore De Vita (University of Udine) and Dr. Valli De Re (CRO, Aviano) for critical discussion and biomolecular studies.

ABBREVIATIONS

AIH	autoimmune hepatitis
ANA	anti-nuclear autoantibodies
BCR	B-cell receptor
CDR	complementarity determining region
F(ab')$_2$	antigen-binding fragment
Fcγ	Fc fragment of IgG
FR	framework region
HCV	hepatitis C virus
Ig	immunoglobulin
IPLNs	intraportal lymphoid nodules
LKM	liver/kidney microsomal autoantibodies
MGUS	monoclonal gammopathy of undetermined significance
NHLs	non-Hodgkin's lymphomas
PBL	peripheral blood lymphocytes
PCR	polymerase chain reaction
RFs	rheumatoid factors
RT	reverse transcriptase
SMA	smooth muscle autoantibodies
VDJ	variable diversity joining region
V$_H$	heavy chain variable region

REFERENCES

1. Gumber SC, Chopra S. Hepatitis C. A multifaced disease. Review of extrahepatic manifestations. Ann Intern Med 1995;123:615–620
2. Agnello V, Chung RT, Kaplan LM. A role for hepatitis C virus infection in type II cryoglobulinemia. N Engl J Med 1992;327:1490–1495
3. Ferri C, La Civita L, Longombardo G, et al. Mixed cryoglobulinaemia: A cross-road between autoimmune and lymphoproliferative disorders. Lupus 1998;7:275–279
4. Krawitt EL. Autoimmune hepatitis. N Engl J Med 1996;334:897–903
5. Bianchi FB. Autoimmune hepatitis: The lesson of the discovery of hepatitis C virus. J Hepatol 1993;18:273–275
6. Clifford BD, Donahue D, Smith L, et al. High prevalence of serological markers of autoimmunity in patients with chronic hepatitis C. Hepatology 1995;21:613–619
7. Lunel F. Hepatitis C virus and autoimmunity: Fortuitous association or reality? Gastroenterology 1994;107:1550–1555
8. Dupin N, Chosidow O, Lunel F, et al. Essential mixed cryoglobulinemia. A comparative study of dermatologic manifestations in patients infected or noninfected with hepatitis C virus. Arch Dermatol 1995;131:1124–1127
9. Dammacco F, Sansonno D. Mixed Cryoglobulinemia as a model of systemic vasculitis. Clin Rev Allergy Immunol 1997;15:97–119
10. Sansonno D, Iacobelli AR, Cornacchiulo V, et al. Immunochemical and biomolecular studies of circulating immune complexes isolated from patients with acute and chronic hepatitis C virus infection. Eur J Clin Invest 1996;26:465–475
11. Stott DI, Hiepe F, Hummel M, et al. Antigen-driven clonal proliferation of B cells within the target tissue of an autoimmune disease. J Clin Invest 1998;102:938–946
12. Lam KP, Kuhn R, Rajewsky K. In vivo ablation of surface immunoglobulin on mature B cells by inducible gene targeting results in rapid cell death. Cell 1997;90:1073–1083
13. Neuberger MS. Antigen receptor signaling gives lymphocytes a long life. Cell 1997;90:971–973
14. Zouali M. B-cell superantigens: Implications for selection of the human antibody repertoire. Immunol Today 1995;16:399–405
15. Silverman GJ. B-cell superantigens. Immunol Today 1997;18:379–386
16. Pospisil R, Fitts MG, Mage RG. CD5 is a potential selecting ligand for B cell surface immunoglobulin framework region sequences. J Exp Med 1996;184:1279–1284
17. Pospisil R, Mage RG. Rabbit appendix: A site of the development and selection of the B cell repertoire. Curr Top Microbiol Immunol 1998;229:59–70
18. Schroeder HW Jr, Dighiero G. The pathogenesis of chronic lymphocytic leukemia: Analysis of the antibody repertoire. Immunol Today 1994;15:288–294
19. Pospisil R, Mage RG. CD5 and other superantigens as "ticklers" of the B-cell receptor. Immunol Today 1998;19:106–108
20. Dighiero G. CD5$^+$ B cells and autoimmunity. Semin Clin Immunol 1998;2:5–13

21. Stall AM, Wells SM, Lam K-P. B-1 cells: Unique origins and functions. Semin Immunol 1996;8:45–59

22. Tsiagbe VK, Inghirami G, Thorbecke GJ. The physiology of germinal centers. Crit Rev Immunol 1996;16:381–421

23. Crouzier R, Martin T, Pasquali JL. Monoclonal IgM rheumatoid factor secreted by CD5-negative B cells during mixed cryoglobulinemia. Evidence for somatic mutations and intraclonal diversity of the expresses V_H region gene. J Immunol 1995;154: 413–421

24. Soto-Gil RW, Olee T, Klink BK, et al. A systematic approach to defining the germline gene counterparts of a mutated autoantibody from a patient with rheumatoid arthritis. Arthritis Rheum 1992;35:356–363

25. Tran A, Benzaken S, Braun HB, et al. Anti-GOR and anti-thyroid auto-antibodies in patients with chronic hepatitis C. Clin Immunol Immunopathol 1995;77:127–130

26. Quiroga JA, Pardo M, Navas S, et al. Patterns of immune responses to the host-encoded GOR and hepatitis C virus core-derived epitopes with relation to hepatitis C viremia, genotypes and liver disease severity. J Infect Dis 1996;173:300–305

27. Michel G, Ritter A, Gerken G, et al. Anti-GOR and hepatitis C virus in autoimmune liver diseases. Lancet 1992;339: 267–269

28. Andersen P, Small JV, Andersen HK, Sobieszek A. Reactivity of smooth-muscle antibodies with F- and G-actin. Immunology 1979;37:705–709

29. Johnson PJ, McFarlane IG. Meeting report. International autoimmune hepatitis group. Hepatology 1993;18:998–1005

30. Fried MW, Draguesku JO, Shindo M, et al. Clinical and serological differentiation of autoimmune and hepatitis C virus-related chronic hepatitis. Dig Dis Sci 1993;38:631–636

31. Reichlin M. ANAs and antibodies to DNA: Their use in clinical diagnosis. Bull Rheum Dis 1993;42:3–5

32. Van Venroij WJ, Maini RN. Manual of Biological Markers of Disease. The Netherlands: Kluwer Academic Publishers, 1994, pp 1–28

33. Rizzetto M, Swana G, Doniach D. Microsomal antibodies in active chronic hepatitis and other disorders. Clin Exp Immunol 1973;15:331–334

34. Homberg J-C, Abuaf N, Bernard O, et al. Chronic active hepatitis associated with antiliver/kidney microsome antibody type 1: A second type of "autoimmune" hepatitis. Hepatology 1987; 7:1333–1339

35. Homberg J-C, Andre C, Abuaf N. A new anti-liver-kidney microsome antibody (anti-LKM2) in tienilic acid-induced hepatitis. Clin Exp Immunol 1984;55:561–570

36. Crivelli O, Lavarini C, Chiaberge E, et al. Microsomal autoantibodies in chronic infection with HBsAg associated δ (delta) agent. Clin Exp Immunol 1983;54:232–238

37. Bortolotti F, Vairo P, Balli F, et al. Non-organ specific autoantibodies in children with chronic hepatitis C. J Hepatol 1996;25: 614–620

38. Klein R, Zanger UM, Berg T, et al. Overlapping but distinct specificities of anti-liver-kidney microsome antibodies in autoimmune hepatitis type II and hepatitis C revealed by recombinant native CYP2D6 and novel peptide epitopes. Clin Exp Immunol 1999;118:290–297

39. Lunel F, Abuaf N, Frangeul L, et al. Liver/kidney microsome antibody type 1 and hepatitis C virus infection. Hepatology 1992; 16:630–636

40. Koskinas J, McFarlane M, Kayhan T, et al. Cellular and humoral immune reactions against autoantigens and hepatitis C viral antigens in chronic hepatitis C. Gastroenterology 1994;107: 1436–1442

41. Takase S, Tsutsumi M, Kawahara H, et al. The alcohol-altered liver membrane antibody and hepatitis C virus infection in the progression of alcoholic liver disease. Hepatology 1993;17:9–13

42. Abuaf N, Johanet C, Chretien P, et al. Characterization of the liver cytosol antigen type 1 reacting with autoantibodies in chronic active hepatitis. Hepatology 1992;16:892–898

43. Swanson NR, Reed WD, Yarred LJ, et al. Autoantibodies to isolated human hepatocyte plasma membranes in chronic active hepatitis. II. Specificity of antibodies. Hepatology 1990;11: 613–621

44. Tran A, Quaranta J-F, Benzaken S, et al. High prevalence of thyroid autoantibodies in a prospective series of patients with chronic hepatitis C before interferon therapy. Hepatology 1993; 18:253–257

45. Prieto J, Yuste JR, Beloqui O, et al. Anticardiolipin antibodies in chronic hepatitis C: Implication of hepatitis C virus as the cause of the antiphospholipid syndrome. Hepatology 1996;23: 199–204

46. Mulder L, Horst G, Haagsma E, et al. Prevalence and characterization of neutrophil cytoplasmic antibodies in autoimmune liver diseases. Hepatology 1993;17:411–417

47. Sansonno D, Cornacchiulo V, Iacobelli AR, et al. Localization of hepatitis C virus antigens in liver and skin tissues of chronic hepatitis C virus-infected patients with mixed cryoglobulinemia. Hepatology 1995;21:305–312

48. Khella SL, Frost S, Hermann GA, et al. Hepatitis C infection, cryoglobulinemia, and vasculitic neuropathy. Treatment with interferon alfa: Case report and literature review. Neurology 1995;45:407–411

49. Mosnier JF, Degott C, Marcellin P, et al. The intraportal lymphoid nodule and its environment in chronic hepatitis C: An immunohistochemical study. Hepatology 1993;17:366–371

50. Young CL, Adamson TC, Vaughan JH, Fox RI. Immunohistologic characterization of synovial membrane lymphocytes in rheumatoid arthritis. Arthritis Rheum 1984;27:32–39

51. Knecht H, Saremaslani P, Hedinger C. Immunohistological findings in Hashimoto's thyroiditis, focal lymphocytic thyroiditis and thyroiditis de Quervain. Comparative study. Virchows Arch Abteil Pathol Anat 1981;393:215–231

52. Liversidge J, Dick A, Cheng Y-F, et al. Retinal antigen specific lymphocytes, TCR-gamma delta T cells and CD5+ B cells cultured from the vitreous in acute sympathetic ophthalmitis. Autoimmunity 1993;15:257–266

53. Wallace WAH, Howie SEM, Krajewski AS, Lamb D. The immunological architecture of B-lymphocyte aggregates in cryptogenic fibrosing alveolitis. J Pathol 1996;178:323–329

54. De Vita S, De Re V, Sansonno D, et al. Gastric mucosa as an additional extrahepatic localization of hepatitis C virus: Viral detection in gastric low-grade lymphoma associated with autoimmune disease and in chronic gastritis. Hepatology 2000;31: 182–189

55. Sansonno D, De Vita S, Dammacco F, et al. Molecular analysis of intraportal lymphoid nodules isolated by microsection technique from liver biopsies of HCV chronically-infected patients (Submitted)

56. De Vita S, De Re V, Sansonno D, et al. Latent infection of neoplastic B cells by HCV in a patient with low-grade non-Hodgkin's lymphoma and mixed cryoglobulinemia (Submitted).

57. Ikematsu W, Kobarg J, Ikematsu H, et al. Clonal analysis of a human antibody response. III. Nucleotide sequences of monoclonal IgM, IgG, and IgA to rabies virus reveal restricted Vκ gene utilization, junctional VκJκ and VλJλ diversity, and somatic hypermutation. J Immunol 1998;161:2895–2905

58. Murakami J, Shimizu Y, Kashii Y, et al. Functional B-cell response in intrahepatic lymphoid follicles in chronic hepatitis C. Hepatology 1999;30:143–150

59. Williams RC Jr, Malone CC, Kao K-J. IgM rheumatoid factors react with human class I HLA molecules. J Immunol 1996; 156:1684–1694

60. Dammacco F, Sansonno D. Antibodies to hepatitis C virus in essential mixed cryoglobulinemia. Clin Exp Immunol 1992; 87:352–356

61. Agnello V. Hepatitis C virus infection and type II cryoglobulinemia: An immunological perspective. Hepatology 1997;26: 1375–1379

62. Dammacco F, Sansonno D, Cornacchiulo V, et al. Hepatitis C virus infection and mixed cryoglobulinemia: A striking association. Int J Clin Lab Res 1993;23:45–49

63. Pascual M, Perrin L, Giostra E, Schifferli JA. Hepatitis C virus in patients with cryoglobulinemia type II. J Infect Dis 1990;162:569–570

64. Ferri C, Greco F, Longombardo G, et al. Association between hepatitis C virus and mixed cryoglobulinemia. Clin Exp Rheumatol 1991;9:621–624

65. Cacoub P, Lunel Fabiani F, Musset L, et al. Mixed cryoglobulinemia and hepatitis C virus. Am J Med 1994;96:124–132

66. Pawlotsky JM, Roudot-Thoraval F, Simmonds P, et al. Extrahepatic immunologic manifestations in chronic hepatitis C and hepatitis C virus serotypes. Ann Intern Med 1995;122:169–173

67. Feiner HD. Relationship of tissue deposits of cryoglobulin to clinical features of mixed cryoglobulinemia. Hum Pathol 1983; 14:710–715

68. Sansonno D, Gesualdo L, Manno C, et al. Hepatitis C virus-related proteins in kidney tissue from hepatitis C virus-infected patients with cryoglobulinemic membranoproliferative glomerulonephritis. Hepatology 1997;25:1237–1244

69. Gorevic PD, Frangione B. Mixed cryoglobulinemia cross-reactive idiotypes: Implications for the relationship of MC to rheumatic and lymphoproliferative diseases. Semin Hematol 1991;28:79–94

70. Geltner D, Franklin EC, Frangione B. Antiidiotypic activity in the IgM fractions of mixed cryoglobulins. J Immunol 1980;125: 1530–1535

71. Bona CA, Victor-Kobrin C, Manheimer AJ, et al. Regulatory arms of the immune network. Immunol Rev 1984;79:25–44

72. Knight GB, Agnello V, Bonagura V, et al. Human rheumatoid factor cross-idiotypes. IV. Studies on WA XId-positive IgM without rheumatoid factor activity provide evidence that the WA XId is not unique to rheumatoid factors and is distinct from the 17.109 and G6 XIds. J Exp Med 1993;178:1903–1911

73. Stewart JJ, Agosto H, Litwin S, et al. A solution to the rheumatoid factor paradox. Pathologic rheumatoids factors can be tolerized by competition with natural rheumatoid factors. J Immunol 1997;159:1728–1738

74. Wykes M, Pombo A, Jenkins C, MacPherson GG. Dendritic cells interact directly with naive B lymphocytes to transfer antigen and initiate class switching in a primary T-dependent response. J Immunol 1998;161:1313–1319

75. Carson DA, Chen PP, Kipps TJ. New roles for rheumatoid factor. J Clin Invest 1991;87:379–383

76. Sansonno D, De Vita S, Cornacchiulo V, et al. Detection and distribution of hepatitis C virus-related proteins in lymph nodes of patients with type II mixed cryoglobulinemia and neoplastic or non-neoplastic lymphoproliferation. Blood 1996;88:4638–4645

77. Newkirk MM, Mageed RA, Jefferis R, et al. Complete amino acid sequences of variable regions of two human IgM rheumatoid factors, BOR and KAS of the Wa idiotypic family, reveal restricted use of heavy and light chain variable and joining region gene segments. J Exp Med 1987;166:550–564

78. Martin T, Duffy SF, Carson DA, Kipps TJ. Evidence for somatic selection of natural autoantibodies. J Exp Med 1992;175: 983–991

79. Monteverde A, Sabattini E, Poggi S, et al. Bone marrow findings further support the hypothesis that essential mixed cryoglobulinemia type II is characterized by a monoclonal B-cell proliferation. Leuk Lymph 1995;20:119–124

80. Sansonno D, De Vita S, Iacobelli AR, et al. Clonal analysis of intrahepatic B cells from HCV-infected patients with and without mixed cryoglobulinemia. J Immunol 1998;160:3594–3601

81. Tighe H, Warnatz K, Brinson D, et al. Peripheral deletion of rheumatoid factor B cells after abortive activation by IgG. Proc Natl Acad Sci USA 1997;94:646–651

82. Schettino EW, Chai SK, Kasaian MT, et al. V_HDJ_H gene sequences and antigen reactivity of monoclonal antibodies produced by human B-1 cells. Evidence for somatic selection. J Immunol 1997;158:2477–2489

83. Zhang M, Majid A, Bardwell P, et al. Rheumatoid factor specificity of a VH3-encoded antibody is dependent on the heavy chain CDR3 region and is independent of protein A binding. J Immunol 1998;161:2284–2289

84. Mannik MF, Nardella A, Sasso EH. Rheumatoid factors in immune complexes of patients with rheumatoid arthritis. Springer Semin Immunopathol 1988;10:215–230

85. Youngblood K, Fruchter L, Ding G, et al. Rheumatoid factors from the peripheral blood of two patients with rheumatoid arthritis are genetically heterogeneous and somatically mutated. J Clin Invest 1994;93:852–861

86. De Vita S, Boiocchi M, Sorrentino D, et al. Characterization of prelymphomatous stages of B cell lymphoproliferation in Sjögren's syndrome. Arthritis Rheum 1997;40:318–331

87. Kyburz D, Corr M, Brinson DC, et al. Human rheumatoid factor production is dependent on CD40 signaling and autoantigen. J Immunol 1999;163:3116–3122

88. Ferri C, Caracciolo F, Zignego AL, et al. Hepatitis C virus infection in patients with non-Hodgkin's lymphoma. Br J Haematol 1994;88:392–394

89. Pozzato G, Mazzaro C, Crovatto M, et al. Low-grade malignant lymphoma, hepatitis C virus infection, and mixed cryoglobulinemia. Blood 1994;84:3047–3053

90. Mazzaro C, Zagonel V, Monfardini S, et al. Hepatitis C virus and non-Hodgkin's lymphomas. Br J Haematol 1996;94:544–550

91. Silvestri F, Pipan C, Barillari G, et al. Prevalence of hepatitis C virus infection in patients with lymphoproliferative disorders. Blood 1996;87:4296–4301

92. De Rosa G, Gobbo ML, De Renzo A, et al. High prevalence of hepatitis C virus infection in patients with B-cell lymphoproliferative disorders in Italy. Am J Hematol 1997;55:77–82

93. De Vita S, Sacco C, Sansonno D, et al. Characterization of overt B-cell lymphomas in patients with hepatitis C virus infection. Blood 1997;90:776–782

94. Zuckerman E, Zuckerman T, Levine AM, et al. Hepatitis C virus infection in patients with B-cell non-Hodgkin lymphoma. Ann Intern Med 1997;127:423–428

95. Vallisa D, Bertè R, Rocca A, et al. Association between hepatitis C virus and non-Hodgkin's lymphoma, and effects of viral infection on histologic subtype and clinical course. Am J Med 1999;106:556–560

96. Ryan J, Wallace S, Jones P, et al. Primary hepatic lymphoma in a patient with chronic hepatitis C. J Gastroenterol Hepatol 1994;9:308–310

97. Borgonovo G, d'Oiron R, Amato A, et al. Primary lymphoplasmacytic lymphoma of the liver associated with a serum monoclonal peak of IgG κ. Am J Gastroenterol 1995;90:137–140

98. De Vita S, Sansonno D, Dolcetti R, et al. Hepatitis C virus within a malignant lymphoma lesion in the course of type II mixed cryoglobulinemia. Blood 1995;86:1887–1892

99. Satoh T, Yamada T, Nakano S, et al. The relationship between primary splenic malignant lymphoma and chronic liver disease associated with hepatitis C virus infection. Cancer 1997;80: 1981–1988

100. De Vita S, Zagonel V, Russo A, et al. Hepatitis C virus, non-Hodgkin's lymphomas and hepatocellular carcinoma. Br J Cancer 1998;77:2032–2035

101. Lombardo L, Rota Scalabrini D, Vineis P, De La Pierre M. Malignant lymphoproliferative disorders in liver cirrhosis. Ann Oncol 1993;4:245–250
102. Di Stasi M, Sbolli G, Fornari F, et al. Hepatocellular carcinoma and B-cell tumors. J Hepatol 1994;21:1146–1147
103. Clarke G, MacMathuna P, Fenlon H, et al. Primary hepatic lymphoma in a man with chronic hepatitis C. Eur J Gastroenterol Hepatol 1997;9:87–90
104. Möhler M, Gutzler F, Kallinowsky B, et al. Primary hepatic high-grade non-Hodgkin's lymphoma and chronic hepatitis C infection. Dig Dis Sci 1997;42:2241–2245
105. Rasul I, Sheperd FA, Kamel-Reid S, et al. Detection of occult low-grade B-cell non-Hodgkin's lymphoma in patients with chronic hepatitis C infection and mixed cryoglobulinemia. Hepatology 1999;29:543–547
106. Viala JJ, Trepo C, Creyssel R, et al. Gammapathie monoclonale apparemment non myélomateuse associé à l'antigène de l'hépatite non-A non-B. Nouv Presse Med 1982;11:52
107. Heer M, Joller-Jemelka H, Fontana A, et al. Monoclonal gammopathy in chronic active hepatitis. Liver 1984;4:255–263
108. Mussini C, Ghini M, Mascia MT, et al. HCV and monoclonal gammopathies. Clin Exp Rheumatol 1995;13(Suppl 13):S45–49
109. Mangia A, Clemente R, Musto P, et al. Hepatitis C virus infection and monoclonal gammopathies not associated with cryoglobulinemia. Leukemia 1996;10:1209–1213
110. Andreone P, Zignego AL, Cursaro C, et al. Prevalence of monoclonal gammopathies in patients with hepatitis C virus infection. Ann Intern Med 1998;129:294–298
111. Misiani R, Bellavita P, Fenili D, et al. Interferon alfa-2a therapy in cryoglobulinemia associated with hepatitis C virus. N Engl J Med 1994;330:751–756
112. Mazzaro C, Franzin F, Tulissi P, et al. Regression of monoclonal B-cell expansion in patients affected by mixed cryoglobulinemia responsive to α-interferon therapy. Cancer 1996;77:2604–2613
113. Zur Hausen H. Viruses in human cancers. Science 1991;254:1167–1173
114. Sansonno D, Cornacchiulo V, Racanelli V, Dammacco F. In situ simultaneous detection of hepatitis C virus RNA and hepatitis C virus-related antigens in hepatocellular carcinoma. Cancer 1997;80:22–26
115. Dietrich CF, Lee J-H, Herrmann G, et al. Enlargement of perihepatic lymph nodes in relation to liver histology and viremia in patients with chronic hepatitis C. Hepatology 1997;26:467–472
116. Laskus T, Radkowski M, Wang L-F, et al. Search for hepatitis C virus extrahepatic replication sites in patients with acquired immunodeficiency syndrome: Specific detection of negative-strand viral RNA in various tissues. Hepatology 1998;28:1398–1401
117. Stollar V, Schlesinger RW, Stevens TM. Studies on the nature of Dengue virus. III. RNA synthesis in cells infected with type 2 Dengue virus. Virology 1967;33:650–658
118. Lerat H, Rumin S, Habersetzer F, et al. In vivo tropism of hepatitis C virus genomic sequences in hematopoietic cells: Influence of viral load, viral genotype, and cell phenotype. Blood 1998;91:3841–3849
119. Shimizu YK, Yoshikura H. Multicycle infection of hepatitis C virus in cell culture and inhibition by alpha and beta interferons. J Virol 1994;68:8406–8408
120. Nakajima N, Hijikata M, Yoshikura H, Shimizu YK. Characterization of long-term cultures of hepatitis C virus. J Virol 1996;70:3325–3329
121. Bronowicki J-P, Loriot M-A, Thiers V, et al. Hepatitis C virus persistence in human hematopoietic cells injected into SCID mice. Hepatology 1998;28:211–218
122. Chang T-T, Young K-C, Yang Y-J, et al. Hepatitis C virus RNA in peripheral blood mononuclear cells: Comparing acute and chronic hepatitis C virus infection. Hepatology 1996;23:977–981
123. Sansonno D, Lotesoriere C, Cornacchiulo V, et al. Hepatitis C virus infection involves CD34+ hematopoietic progenitor cells in hepatitis C virus chronic carriers. Blood 1998;92:3328–3337
124. Krause DS, Fackler MJ, Civin CI, Stratford May W. CD34: Structure, biology, and clinical utility. Blood 1996;87:1–13
125. Crosbie OM, Reynolds M, McEntee G, et al. In vitro evidence for the presence of hematopoietic stem cells in the adult human liver. Hepatology 1999;29:1193–1198
126. Taniguchi H, Toyoshima T, Fukao K, Nakauchi H. Presence of hematopoietic stem cells in the adult liver. Nat Med 1996;2:198–203
127. Satoh T, Yamada T, Nakano S, et al. The relationship between primary splenic malignant lymphoma and chronic liver disease associated with hepatitis C virus infection. Cancer 1997;80:1981–1988
128. Dammacco F, Gatti P, Sansonno D. Hepatitis C virus infection, mixed cryoglobulinemia, and non-Hodgkin's lymphoma: An emerging picture. Leuk Lymph 1998;31:463–476
129. Ascoli V, Lo Coco F, Artini M, et al. Extranodal lymphomas associated with hepatitis C virus infection. Am J Clin Pathol 1998;109:600–609
130. Ohsawa M, Shingu N, Miwa H, et al. Risk of non-Hodgkin's lymphoma in patients with hepatitis C virus infection. Int J Cancer 1999;80:237–239
131. Rubbia-Brandt L, Bründler M-A, Kerl K, et al. Primary hepatic diffuse large B-cell lymphoma in a patient with chronic hepatitis C. Am J Surg Pathol 1999;23:1124–1130
132. McColl MD, Singer IO, Tait RC, et al. The role of hepatitis C virus in the aetiology of non-Hodgkin's lymphoma. A regional association? Leuk Lymph 1997;26:127–130
133. Germanidis G, Haioun C, Pourquier J, et al. Hepatitis C virus infection in patients with overt B-cell non-Hodgkin's lymphoma in a French center. Blood 1999;93:1778–1779
134. Collier JD, Zanke B, Moore M, et al. No association between hepatitis C and B-cell lymphoma. Hepatology 1999;29:1259–1261
135. Ray RB, Martin Lagging L, Meyer K, Ray R. Hepatitis C virus core protein cooperates with ras and transforms primary rat embryo fibroblasts to tumorigenic phenotype. J Virol 1996;70:4438–4443

Diagnostic Testing for Hepatitis C

ROBERT L. CARITHERS, JR., M.D., ANTHONY MARQUARDT, and DAVID R. GRETCH, M.D., Ph.D.

ABSTRACT: *Diagnostic tests for hepatitis C virus have improved dramatically over the past decade. Highly accurate tests are now available for screening patients for possible hepatitis C infections and confirming the presence of active viral infection. HCV RNA levels and genotype are very useful in assessing the likelihood of response to antiviral therapy and in guiding the optimum duration of treatment. Absence of detectable HCV RNA using PCR methodology has become the gold standard of successful treatment of patients with chronic hepatitis C. The various tests for hepatitis C are expensive and have their limitations. However, selective use of these assays has greatly improved the care of patients with chronic hepatitis C.*

KEY WORDS: hepatitis C virus, diagnostic tests, HCV genotypes, HCV RNA, anti-viral therapy

There have been remarkable advances in diagnostic testing for hepatitis C virus (HCV) over the past decade. This has included progressive improvement in both the sensitivity and specificity of tests for antibodies to HCV (anti-HCV). These tests now provide rapid and inexpensive means of identifying individuals who have been infected with hepatitis C. Qualitative and quantitative tests for HCV RNA provide a molecular basis for determining the presence of viremia. Qualitative tests for HCV RNA have become the gold standard of successful antiviral therapy. Finally, determining the HCV genotype and viral load has become increasingly important in guiding the duration of combination therapy with interferon and ribavirin.[1,2] As a result, HCV testing has become the mainstay of both diagnosis and management of patients with hepatitis C.

Objectives
Upon completion of this article, the reader should be able to accurately and efficiently use serologic tests for hepatitis C.

Accreditation
The Indiana University School of Medicine is accredited by the Accreditation Council for Continuing Medical Education to provide continuing medical education for physicians.

Credit
The Indiana University School of Medicine designates this educational activity for a maximum of 1.0 hours credit toward the AMA Physicians Recognition Award in category one. Each physician should claim only those hours of credit that he/she actually spent in the educational activity.

Disclosure
Statements have been obtained regarding the authors' relationships with financial supporters of this activity. There is no apparent conflict of interest related to the context of participation of the author of this article.

University of Washington, Seattle, Washington

Reprint requests: Dr. Carithers, University of Washington, 1959 NE Pacific Street, Box 35614, Seattle, WA 98195-6174. E-mail: doctorc@u.washington.edu

The goals of this chapter are to review the currently available diagnostic tests for hepatitis C, to emphasize limitations of the various assays, and to suggest the most efficient means of using these tests in clinical practice.

SCREENING ASSAYS FOR ANTI-HCV

The most commonly used assay for anti-HCV is the enzyme immunoassay (EIA) in which viral antigens are imbedded in the wells of a microtiter plate. Antibodies directed against any of these antigens in patients' sera will adhere to the well. Rapid detection of antibodies is facilitated by adding anti-immunoglobulins containing a colorometric marker (Fig. 1). The advantages of this technique include ease of automation, highly reproducible results, and low cost.

Three generations of EIA for anti-HCV have been developed over the past decade. The first EIA (EIA-1), initially used clinically in 1990, contained a single recombinant antigen from the NS4 region of the HCV genome. This assay represented a major breakthrough in screening blood donors for hepatitis C and in clarifying the diagnosis of most patients with non-A, non-B hepatitis. However, it became quickly apparent that this test had a number of serious limitations. There were numerous false-positive reactions, particularly among groups such as blood donors, where the prevalence of hepatitis C is low. In retrospect, only one third to one half of blood donors with a positive EIA-1 test for anti-HCV actually had hepatitis C (Table 1). In addition, there were occasional nonspecific false-positive reactions in patients with various autoimmune disorders. Furthermore, the test was insensitive. As many as 30% of high-

TABLE 1. Sensitivity and Positive Predictive Value of EIA for Anti-HCV

Assay	Sensitivity* (%)	Positive Predictive Value† (%)	
		Low Prevalence	High Prevalence
EIA-1	70–80	30–50	70–85
EIA-2	92–95	50–61	88–95
EIA-3	97	25	Unknown

*Based on detection of HCV RNA by PCR.
†Compared with RIBA.
From ref. 3, with permission.

risk individuals subsequently found to have hepatitis C had negative reactions to this test (Table 1). Finally, there was a considerable delay between acute HCV infection and the first evidence of anti-HCV (Fig. 2). Two complementary approaches were taken to overcome these limitations: development of newer EIA tests with better sensitivity and specificity and supplemental tests to augment EIAs for anti-HCV.

Many limitations of the first-generation EIA were overcome by the second EIA for anti-HCV (EIA-2). This assay, the clinical standard since 1992, contains antigens from the core and nonstructural three (NS3) and four (NS4) regions of the HCV genome. This test is both more sensitive and specific than the first-generation EIA assay. Use of the second-generation assay further reduced the risk of posttransfusion hepatitis C and false-positive reactions among blood donors (Table 1). Furthermore, it has proved to be quite effective as a screening test in high-risk individuals for chronic hepatitis C. Approximately 92–95% of patients in whom chronic hepatitis C is suspected can be detected using this second-generation EIA (Table 1). Finally, the

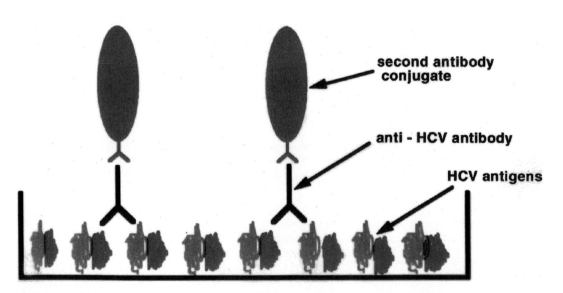

FIG. 1. EIA technique for anti-HCV. The first-generation EIA (EIA-1) contained only one HCV antigen. Subsequent tests (EIA-2 and EIA-3) contain additional viral antigens. These additions have improved both the sensitivity and specificity of the test.

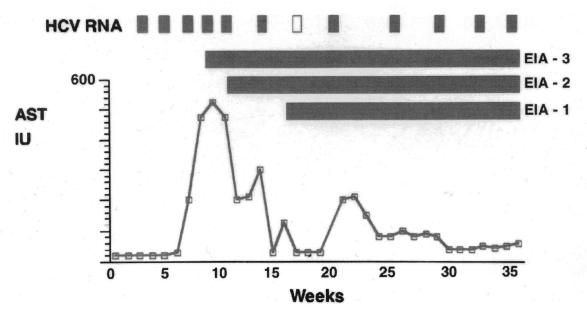

FIG. 2. First detection of HCV RNA and anti-HCV by various assays after acute HCV infection. With each successive EIA, the "window" between the onset of viremia and initial detection of anti-HCV has decreased. Despite these advances, the average window after HCV infection remains over 80 days. (From Ref. 23.)

use of this test shortens the window from blood transfusion to the first detection of anti-HCV to approximately 10 weeks compared with an average of 16 weeks with the first-generation EIA (Fig. 2).[3] False-positive reactions with the EIA-2 assay are primarily limited to low-risk populations such as blood donors. False-negative tests are seen most commonly among immunosuppressed individuals such as transplant recipients and patients coinfected with HIV.[4] EIA-2 coninues to be the test routinely used by most clinical laboratories.

A third-generation EIA (EIA-3) has been approved for screening blood donors in the United States. This assay contains reconfigured core and NS3 antigens and an additional antigen from the NS5 region of the HCV genome.[3] This test offers a slight improvement in sensitivity over the EIA-2 test, particularly in low-risk settings such as a blood bank (Table 1).[5] The time from infection to anti-HCV seroconversion is shortened to 7–8 weeks in approximately 30% of patients (Fig. 2).[6,7] Although this test is used by some clinical laboratories for routine screening of high-risk populations for hepatitis C, the positive predictive value of the EIA-3 assay is not well defined.[8] As a result, the benefit of replacing EIA-2 with EIA-3 assays for routine testing in clinical laboratories is unclear.

SUPPLEMENTAL TESTS FOR ANTI-HCV

Because of the high false-positive rate of EIA assays, particularly in low prevalence settings such as blood banks, supplemental tests for anti-HCV were developed. These tests contain the same antigens as the corresponding EIA assay. However, in the commonly used recombinant immunoblot assays (RIBA, Chiron Corporation, Emeryville, CA), individual HCV antigens are displayed on a nitrocellulose strip (Fig. 3). As a result, antibodies against specific HCV antigens can be identified. A positive RIBA assay requires at least two reactive bands. Tests with only one reactive band are considered indeterminate. Individuals with only c-100-3 or 5-1-1 positive antigens rarely, if ever, have circulating HCV RNA.[3] Therefore, we would argue that single reactive band at c-100-3 or 5-11 should be considered a negative rather than indeterminate RIBA result. RIBA tests are no more sensitive than corresponding EIA tests.[9] However, RIBA tests can be used to distinguish false-positive EIA results from prior exposure to HCV. Patients with false-positive EIA tests usually have negative RIBA assays. In contrast, patients previously exposed to hepatitis C typically have positive or indeterminate (C22 or C33) RIBA results.[9]

The RIBA 2.0 assay, which contains the same antigens as the EIA-2 assay, has been the most commonly used supplemental assay for anti-HCV. In the low prevalence blood bank setting, 40–50% of EIA-2 positive test results are RIBA 2.0 negative, indicating a false-positive result (Table 1).[3,10] A RIBA 3.0 assay has been approved for use by blood banks as a supplemental test for EIA-3-positive test results. This test has the advantage over the RIBA-2 assay of fewer indeterminate results and a better correlation with the presence of viremia.[11,12] Other supplemental assays are under evaluation.[13]

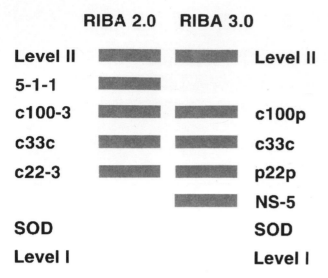

FIG. 3. RIBA assays for anti-HCV. Each strip is precoated with specific HCV antigens. HCV antibodies against these antigens in the patient's serum react with the corresponding strip. The strips are then overlaid with anti-human IgG bound to peroxidase. This allows colorimetric detection of the specific antigens.[13] Internal controls include two levels of human IgG (level I, weak positive; level II, moderate positive) and superoxide dismutase (SOD).[13] A result is considered positive if two or more HCV bands have an intensity at least as strong as the level I control. A single reactive band is considered indeterminate. In this RIBA assay four positive bands to the HCV antigens in the RIBA 2.0 and RIBA 3.0 assays are illustrated, indicating strongly positive results and high probability of active HCV infection.

RIBAs are standardized and reproducible. However, they are more difficult to perform than EIAs, time consuming, and relatively expensive. Their primary utility has been in excluding false-positive results in blood banks. They have limited if any usefulness among patients clinically suspected of harboring a chronic HCV infection. Fewer than 1% of EIA-2- or EIA-3-positive specimens from such high-risk individuals are RIBA negative.[3,14] Furthermore, over 90% of EIA-2-positive specimens from such patients are HCV RNA positive (Table 1).[3,14] Thus, it is more efficient to confirm the presence of active infection in these patients using qualitative or quantitative tests for circulating HCV RNA.

QUALITATIVE TESTS FOR HCV RNA

Detection of HCV RNA in a patient's blood confirms the presence of active infection. The most sensitive laboratory method of doing so is the reverse transcription polymerase chain reaction (RT-PCR).[9,15] Under optimal conditions, the sensitivity of RT-PCR for HCV RNA is 100 molecules/mL of serum or less.

To achieve these conditions, serum or plasma should be separated from whole blood within 4 hours of venipuncture, followed by rapid storage of specimens at −70°C. Failure to follow these procedures can result in false-negative results for circulating HCV RNA.[9,16,17]

In the laboratory, viral RNA must be isolated and converted into complementary DNA. This is usually accomplished by using oligonucleotide primers specific to the 5′untranslated region of the HCV genome. The DNA product is then amplified using a bacterial DNA polymerase. In some laboratories, this first-round PCR is followed by a second PCR reaction using additional primers. The advantage of this nested-set PCR is the ease of visualizing the amplified DNA products using routine agarose gel electrophoresis.[18] The potential disadvantage is an increased risk of sample contamination and false-positive results.[18]

An alternative approach is to combine a single-stage PCR with a more sensitive DNA detection system. One example is to hybridize the DNA amplification products with a radiolabeled oligonucleotide (Fig. 4). This hybridized radioactive product can then be detected using acrylamide gel electrophoresis.[18] This method is as sensitive as nested-set PCR but avoids excess sample handling with potential contamination and false-positive results.[19]

Whatever technique is used, extreme care and high standards must be maintained to avoid false-positive or -negative results.[20] Technologists must be well trained, and all runs require negative controls and multiple low and high copy standards to achieve maximum sensitivity and specificity of test results.[9] Initial proficiency tests using blinded specimens indicated abysmally low rates of error-free detection of HCV RNA by PCR in many laboratories.[21,22] However, more recent surveys suggest improved performance.[9] Development of uniform reference specimens and standardization of virologic testing of blood and blood products should continue to improve the accuracy of qualitative testing for HCV RNA.[23]

In addition to improved quality of the multiple "home brew" PCR assays, progress has been made to develop commercially available tests for detection of HCV RNA. An example of this is the Roche Amplicor test (Roche Molecular Systems, subsidiary of Hoffman-La Roche, Inc., Brandenburg, NJ).[24–26] The second-generation Amplicor test has a sensitivity of approximately 100 copies/mL of serum.[9] A semiautomated version of this assay (COBAS, Roche Molecular Systems), which has comparable sensitivity and specificity with the manual Amplicor assay, is undergoing extensive clinical investigation.[9,27] Some laboratories have reported that the use of whole blood rather than serum improves the sensitivity of qualitative testing for HCV RNA using the Roche Amplicor assay and RT-PCR.[28,29] These interesting observations need confirmation. Using the Roche Amplicor assay for HCV RNA in our clinical laboratory, we have found a slight better sensitivity using serum

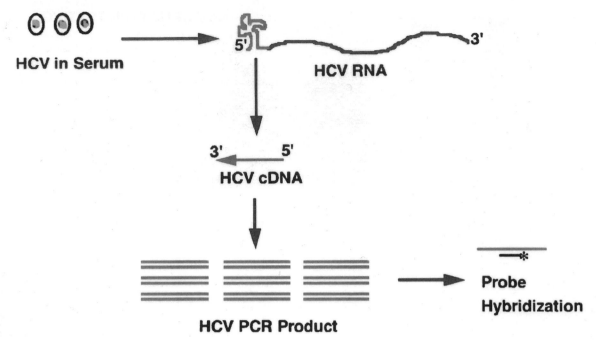

FIG. 4. HCV RNA testing using single-step PCR. RNA is first isolated from the patient's serum. Complementary DNA is produced using oligonucleotide primers specific to the 5′ untranslated region of the HCV genome. The DNA product is amplified and then hybridized with a radiolabeled oligonucleotide. The radioactive product can be detected using acrylamide gel electrophoresis.

compared with whole blood as a source of HCV RNA (D.R. Gretch, unpublished observations, 2000).

QUANTITATIVE TESTS FOR HCV RNA

A variety of methods are available for assessing the quantity of circulating HCV RNA in patients with chronic hepatitis C. The most commonly used techniques of determining viral load involve extraction of HCV RNA from serum or plasma, followed by amplification of the target (PCR-based methods) or the signal (branched DNA [bDNA] methods).[9]

PCR-based Quantitative Assays

The amount of circulating HCV RNA can be determined by a variety of PCR-based assays. Clinical samples can be serially diluted followed by PCR amplification of each dilution, with the quantity of HCV RNA estimated from the last dilution at which the PCR product can be detected. Quantitative competitive PCR is a more elegant approach to determining the quantity of HCV RNA in clinical specimens. Competitor DNA or RNA is constructed that contains sequences at the 5′ and 3′ ends complementary to the primers used in the PCR. However, these constructs differ from HCV RNA in molecular weight or contain restriction enzyme sites, which allow the competitor and native HCV RNA to be

distinguished.[9] Although extremely accurate in some laboratories, each method is tedious, expensive, and difficult to replicate from laboratory to laboratory.

The Roche Monitor assay (Amplicor HCV Monitor, Roche Molecular Systems, Nutley, NJ) is the most extensively tested commercial PCR-based assay used for quantitation of HCV RNA. Advantages are standardization and high throughput in the clinical laboratory. The lower limit of sensitivity of this assay is approximately 1,000 copies/mL, 10-fold less than qualitative PCR tests for HCV RNA (Fig. 5).[9,30] A disadvantage reported with the first generation of this assay is underestimation of HCV RNA levels in patients with genotypes 2 and 3 compared with those with genotype 1.[9,30–33]

bDNA Assay

An alternative approach to determining viral load in patients with chronic hepatitis C is the bDNA assay (Bayer Diagnostics, Emeryville, CA). In this assay, HCV RNA is captured in a microtiter well by hybridization to synthetic oligonucleotide probes complementary in sequence to the 5′-noncoding region and core of the HCV genome. Additional target probes bind the HCV RNA to bDNA molecules, which are amplified and labeled with a chemiluminescent probe.[9,15,34] This assay is well standardized, has a high level of precision, and is quite reproducible from laboratory to laboratory. Its major limitation is a relative lack of sensitivity, with a

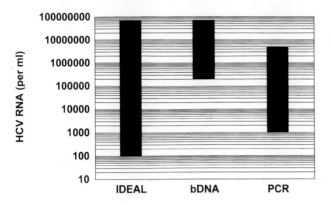

FIG. 5. Dynamic ranges of the ideal test for quantitating HCV RNA compared with the most commonly used commercial assays. The ideal assay has a dynamic range of 100 to 10^8 copies of HCV RNA. The bDNA assay (bDNA HCV 2.0, Bayer Diagnostics, Emeryville, CA) has a range of 200,000 to 10^8. In comparison, the most commonly used PCR based assay (Roche Amplicor Monitor, Roche Diagnostics, Nutley, NJ) has a reported range of 1,000 to 5×10^6.

lower limit of approximately 200,000 equivalents of HCV RNA/mL of serum (Fig. 5).

Comparison of PCR and bDNA Methods

The Roche Monitor and Bayer bDNA assays have been extensively evaluated by a number of investigators. Results from the bDNA assay are quite reproducible, with lower intraassay and kit-to-kit variation than the Monitor assay.[9,30,35] The bDNA assay more accurately reflects HCV RNA levels in patients with genotype 2 and 3 infection and has better linearity in patients with high viral loads (Fig. 5).[9,30,36] In contrast, the Monitor assay has a lower detection limit than the bDNA assay (Fig. 5). Although this would suggest much higher sensitivity for the Monitor assay, when the two assays have been directly compared in patients with clinical features of chronic hepatitis C, the sensitivity of each is virtually identical.[30,32] For example, in one study of 100 patients with chronic hepatitis C evaluated before treatment, the sensitivity of the Monitor was 98% compared with 97% for the bDNA assay.[32] These finding underscore the infrequency in which untreated patients with chronic hepatitis C have HCV RNA values between 1,000 and 200,000 copies/mL, the lower detection limits of these two assays. Another clinically important observation is that values obtained with each of the two assays are not interchangeable because different internal standards are used.[9] Results from the bDNA tst are generally a log higher than those obtained with the Monitor assay.[30–33] Therefore, these tests cannot be used interchangeably to follow patients. Nevertheless, changes in viral load that occur over time can be consistently measured using either assay.[33,37]

HCV GENOTYPE TESTING

Hepatitis C is a heterogeneous virus with at least six genotypes and numerous subtypes identified from isolates collected throughout the world.[38,39] Although considerable controversy surrounds the natural history of disease is patients with different genotypes, there is consensus that the HCV genotype is one of the most important predictors of response to antiviral therapy. A variety of methods has been developed to determine the genotype of a specific HCV infection. These can be broadly separated into two categories: (1) gold standard tests using nucleotide sequencing and (2) phylogenetic analysis of specific HCV genes, and screening tests that detect point mutations within the HCV genome.[34]

Genotype Analysis by Nucleotide Sequencing and Phylogenetic Analysis

The most accurate methods of determining the genotype of any isolate of HCV include determining the sequence of specific areas within the HCV genome and comparing the sequence obtained to phylogenetic maps of known genotypes. The envelope (E1) and NS5B genes have been studied most extensively in this regard.[39–41] Although these methods offer the most precise means of determining the HCV genotype, they are labor intensive and prohibitively expensive, especially for routine clinical use.

Screening Tests for HCV Genotypes

A number of methods have been developed to rapidly and less expensively determine the genotype of HCV specimens in clinical laboratories. Three of these methods apply innovative uses of PCR for hepatitis C. One technique uses PCR using primers constructed with sequences unique to specific genotypes.[42,43] Only HCV specimens that contain these genotype-specific sequences are amplified. Genotype-specific primers for both the core and NS5B regions have been used in this manner.[42,43] The core method was optimized for use in Japan and performs less accurately with the most common U.S. genotypes.[34]

Another approach relies on the knowledge that the nucleotides of most HCV genotypes have unique restriction sites. The HCV genotype can be deduced by digesting amplified PCR products with specific restriction enzymes and determining the differential migration of the resulting nucleic acid fragments using agarose gel electrophoresis.[15,44–47] This technique, referred to as restriction fragment length polymorphism (RFLP), has proved to be one of the most accurate screening tests for HCV genotype.

A final creative screening test for HCV genotype uses genotype-specific probes, which are embedded on a nitrocellulose strip. Amplified PCR products from the 5′ noncoding region of the HCV genome differentially hybridize to the nitrocellulose strip only when the amplified sequence is complementary to the sequence of an embedded genotype-specific probe. This assay, referred to as the line probe or reverse dot-blot hybridization assay, is now commercially available for HCV genotyping in clinical laboratories (INNO-LiPA, Immunogenetics, Belgium). Reliability and concordance between the RFLP and line probe assays is quite good.[48,49] However, these methods of determining HCV genotype remain relatively expensive.

The genotype of HCV infection also can be determined by detecting genotype-specific antibodies. These antibodies are distinguished by reacting patient sera with genotype-specific antigens presented in an immunoblot format. The HCV NS4 region appears to be the best candidate for serotyping assays because this gene encodes specific epitopes that can be used to distinguish HCV genotypes 1 through 3.[9,50] Although their concordance with other genotyping methods is quite good, serotyping methods may not be as sensitive as PCR-based methods[48,49,51,52] In addition, serotyping currently cannot be used to differentiate HCV subtypes, such as genotypes 1a and 1b.[9] However, the low cost and ease of testing of serotyping make them attractive candidates for continued research and development.

CLINICAL APPLICATIONS OF HCV TESTING

The dramatic improvement in HCV testing over the past decade has provided clinicians with a variety of powerful tools for evaluating patients with hepatitis C. However, these tests are expensive (Table 2). Therefore, virologic tests for hepatitis C should be used judiciously, based on the specific clinical setting.

Diagnosis of Acute Hepatitis C

The diagnosis of acute hepatitis C can be quite difficult. Fewer that half of patients develop jaundice and many have few if any obvious symptoms of hepatitis.[53,54] Specific IgM antibodies, which are so useful in the diagnosis of acute hepatitis A and B, have not been found to reliable in the diagnosis of acute hepatitis C. The diagnostic difficulties are compounded by considerable delay between HCV infection and detection of antibodies to the virus in patients' sera.[13] This was particularly true for the first-generation EIA test for anti-HCV in which the average lag between infection and seroconversion was 16 weeks.[3] This window has been progressively

TABLE 2.   Current Cost of Various HCV Tests

Assay	Price
Anti-HCV (EIA)	$ 57.15
Anti-HCV (RIBA)	$140.00
Qualitative HCV RNA	$131.75
Quantitative HCV RNA	$197.75
HCV genotype	$236.30

From the University of Washington Hepatitis Virology Laboratory.

shortened with each generation of EIA testing. For example, the average time from infection to seroconversion is 10 weeks with EIA-2 and is shortened in some patients by an additional 2–3 weeks with the EIA-3 assay.[3,6] However, even with the EIA-3 assay, the "window period" between HCV infection and seroconversion is at least 6 to 8 weeks. In contrast, HCV RNA usually can be detected in the patient's serum within 10–14 days after infection (Fig. 2). Thus, if there is a strong clinical suspicion of acute hepatitis C, such as recent drug abuse or marked elevation of aminotransferases but anti-HCV cannot be detected, qualitative testing for HCV RNA can be used to confirm the diagnosis.

Diagnosis of Chronic Hepatitis C

It is estimated that 85% of individuals exposed the hepatitis C develop persistent viremia, presumably for life.[54–56] However, many patients with chronic HCV infection have minimal symptoms until late in the course of disease. As a consequence, most individuals with chronic hepatitis C are unaware of their condition. The most effective means of screening patients clinically suspected of harboring chronic hepatitis C virus infection is with EIA testing for anti-HCV. In this setting, RIBA confirmation is not necessary because HCV RNA can be detected in more than 90% of anti-HCV-positive sera.[8,9] Qualitative HCV RNA testing can be useful to distinguish individuals with prior infection who have cleared the virus from those with persistent HCV infection. However, because some patients with chronic hepatitis C may be only intermittently viremic, repeated qualitative testing for HCV RNA by PCR may be necessary to exclude ongoing infection.

HCV Testing Before, During, and After Treatment

Successful medical treatment of patients with chronic hepatitis C has increased fourfold over the past decade. Interferon remains the mainstay of therapy, but more aggressive treatment schedules and addition of ribavirin have steadily improved the chance of durable responses to treatment.

HCV Testing Before Treatment

The HCV genotype and circulating viral load have emerged as two of the best predictors of response to antiviral therapy for chronic hepatitis C.[1,2,57–59] Patients with genotype 1 infection are far less likely to respond to interferon therapy than patients with genotype 2 or 3 infection. High levels of circulating HCV RNA further reduce the chance of achieving sustained response to either interferon or combination therapy with interferon and ribavirin. The differences can be quite striking. For example, sustained response to 6 months of 3 MU interferon tiw is more than 25 times higher among patients with genotype 2 or 3 and <2 million copies of HCV RNA than in genotype 1 patients with >2 million copies of virus per mL of serum (Table 3). Differential response rates to combination therapy with interferon and ribavirin also are quite impressive. Patients with genotype 2 or 3 are six times more likely to achieve a sustained response to 6 months of treatment with combination therapy than patients with genotype 1 infection and >2 million copies of HCV RNA per mL of serum (Table 3).[1,2,57]

Genotype and HCV RNA level are also quite useful in determining the optimum duration of combination therapy with interferon and ribavirin. Sustained response rates are almost three times as high among patients with genotype 1 infection and >2 million copies of virus who receive 12 months of combination therapy compared with those who receive only 6 months of treatment. In contrast, patients with genotype 2 or 3 infections or those who have <2 million copies of HCV RNA per mL of serum do not benefit from more than 6 months of treatment with interferon and ribavirin (Table 3).

Thus, assessment of genotype and quantity of circulating HCV RNA provide essential information for counseling and determining the duration of therapy in patients with chronic hepatitis C. In this setting, quantitative measurement of HCV RNA is quite useful, because 90–97% of samples are HCV RNA positive by either PCR or bDNA methods.[30,32,36]

HCV Testing During and After Treatment

Well-defined and standardized criteria for response to antiviral therapy have been established.[60] These include biochemical virologic, and histologic responses both at the end of treatment and 6 months after completion of therapy. Virologic end points have proven to be more accurate than biochemical measures in predicting sustained clearance of virus.[61] For example, patients who have normal aminotransferases but detectable HCV RNA at the end of treatment are more likely to relapse after completion of therapy than patients with abnormal aminotransferases and absence of circulating HCV RNA.[61,62]

Sustained virologic response, defined as continued absence of circulating HCV RNA for at least 6 months after completion of therapy using an assay with detection limits <100 copies/mL of serum, has become the gold standard of successful treatment (Fig. 6). Because of their relative insensitivity, quantitative tests for HCV RNA are inadequate measures of end of treatment or sustained virologic response in patients with chronic hepatitis C. Long-term studies of sustained virologic responders to interferon therapy are quite encouraging. Over the ensuing 5–10 years, circulating HCV RNA has recurred in fewer than 10% of patients in most follow-up studies (Table 4).[63–66] A striking exception was reported by Vento et al.[67] (Table 4). In most studies, histologic injury has continued to improve over time in sustained virologic responders to antiviral therapy.[63–66]

Patients who achieve a sustained response to interferon monotherapy 3 MU tiw often clear circulating virus quite early in the course of treatment (Fig. 6). Very few, if any, patients who have detectable HCV RNA after 3 months of treatment develop a sustained response. For this reason, it has been suggested that therapy should be discontinued in patients who have detectable HCV RNA after 3 months of treatment.[68] However, as many as 20% of sustained responders to combination therapy with interferon plus ribavirin first clear circulating HCV RNA between 3 and 6 months after initiating treatment.[1,2,57] Thus, a minimum of 6 months of treatment is recommended in patients who receive combination therapy. The rate of viral clearance has not been well established in other more aggressive regimens of interferon or combination therapy.

Measurement of circulating HCV RNA at the end of antiviral treatment can also be quite useful in predicting response to subsequent courses of therapy.[69–71] For

TABLE 3. Response to Therapy by Genotype and HCV RNA Level

	Intron A (24 weeks)	Intron A (48 weeks)	IFN + Ribavirin (24 weeks)	INF + Ribavirin (48 weeks)
Genotype 1 and HCV RNA >2 million copies/mL	0.8%	3%	10%	27%
Genotype 1 and HCV RNA <2 million copies/mL	4%	25%	32%	33%
Genotype 2/3 and HCV RNA >2 million copies/mL	11%	26%	62%	60%
Genotype 2/3 and HCV RNA <2 million copies/mL	25%	36%	61%	64%

Adapted from ref. 4, with permission.

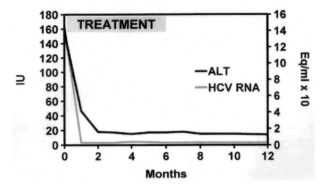

FIG. 6. Sustained response to treatment in a patient with chronic hepatitis C. The patient was treated for 6 months and had monthly assessment of ALT and HCV RNA for an additional 6 months.

TABLE 4. Long-term Follow-up of Sustained Virologic Responders

Author	Number	Follow-up (yr)*	SR (%)
Marcellin et al.[63]	75	4.0 ± 2.0	72 (96%)
Lau et al.[64]	5	10.4 ± 0.6	5 (100%)
Reichard et al.[66]	25	5.4 ± 1.6	24 (96%)
Larghi et al.[65]	23	3.3	23 (100%)
Vento et al.[67]	29	7	0

*Values are means ± SD.
SR: sustained virologic response (absence of circulating HCV RNA at end of follow-up using qualitative HCV RNA testing).

example, patients with no detectable HCV RNA at the end of a first course of treatment with interferon therapy have sustained response rates greater than 50% to retreatment with more aggressive interferon therapy or treatment with interferon and ribavirin.[72–74] In contrast, patients who have detectable HCV RNA at the end of the first course of treatment have sustained response rates to retreatment less than 15%.[74,75]

Screening for HCV in Blood Banks and Among Organ Donors

The risk of acquiring hepatitis C from blood products or donor organs has decreased dramatically over the past decade.[76] Because of increased sensitivity, each subsequent generation of anti-HCV tests has reduced the possibility that transfused products may harbor HCV.[13] The third-generation EIA and RIBA assays have reportedly reduced the number of false-negative, false-positive, and indeterminate results.[6,77]

The two primary challenges facing blood banks are to eliminate transfused blood products as a source of HCV infection and to determine whether anti-HCV-positive donors actually have HCV infection. One of the major limitations of EIA assays for anti-HCV is the delay from onset of infection to development of detectable antibodies to hepatitis C. Currently available assays can detect antibodies as soon as 40 to 60 days after infection and 30 to 40 days after first appearance of circulating HCV RNA (Fig. 2). However, the average delay between infection and first appearance of detectable antibodies remains more than 80 days.[23] For this reason, many blood banks are exploring the feasibility of testing all potential donors with qualitative assays for HCV RNA. This approach has the dual advantage of eliminating donors who are in the "window period" of early infection and clarifying the clinical status of donors positive for anti-HCV by EIA.

Use of HCV Testing in Special Situations

The evaluation of patients with potential HCV infection can be confusing in certain clinical settings. This is particularly true in patients with chronic renal failure, immunosuppressed patients, and in infants with HCV. Selective use of HCV tests can be extremely useful in clarifying the clinical status of these patients.

Hemodialysis Units

Approximately 10% of chronic hemodialysis patients in the United States have chronic hepatitis C.[78–80] However, the prevalence of infection varies widely from center to center.[76,80] Because of the high risk of infection in hemodialysis units, the Centers for Disease Control and Prevention recommends routine testing of patients who have not been previously evaluated for the possibility of HCV infection.[81]

Most chronic renal failure patients with HCV infection have normal serum aminotransferase values.[82,83] Thus, screening for hepatitis C in these patients requires sensitive and specific serologic testing.[82] The EIA-1 test for anti-HCV had extremely poor sensitivity in this patient population. As many as half of HCV-infected patients tested negative using this assay.[76,79,82] However, the EIA-2-assay is far more sensitive and specific for detecting HCV infection in hemodialysis patients. Over 90% of EIA-2-positive patients have detectable HCV RNA, and false-positive results are uncommon.[82,84] EIA-3 testing does not appear to add substantially to either the sensitivity or specificity of HCV screening in patients with chronic renal failure.[84]

Organ Transplant Recipients and Other Immunosuppressed Populations

Chronic HCV infection is quite common in solid organ and bone marrow transplant recipients. Virtually all patients with infection before transplantation have persistent viremia after transplantation.[4,85] In fact, viral levels often increase by a log or more within a few weeks after these operations. HCV infection also can be acquired at the time of transplantation from the use of infected donor organs or blood products. This was particularly true before universal anti-HCV screening of blood products and organ donors was initiated in 1992. Cirrhosis secondary to chronic hepatitis C has emerged as a major concern, particularly in renal and marrow transplant recipients.[78,86]

The diagnosis of chronic hepatitis C in potential transplant recipients is straightforward. EIA-2 or EIA-3 assays for anti-HCV are quite effective in identifying most patients with prior exposure to the virus. Active infection can be differentiated from patients with previous HCV infection by qualitative testing for HCV RNA. However, after transplantation, antibody tests are inadequate for the diagnosis of hepatitis C because of depression of antibody titers and prolonged delay in seroconversion after de novo infection.[87–89] The only means of accurately assessing the presence of hepatitis C in transplant recipients is with direct measurement of serum HCV RNA.[4,90]

The diagnosis of chronic hepatitis C also can be challenging in other immunosuppressed patients, particularly those coinfected with HIV. Some HIV patients with chronic hepatitis C lose anti-HCV antibodies over time.[91] For this reason, it is prudent to consider direct measurement of HCV RNA in HIV patients with negative anti-HCV in whom there is a strong clinical suspicion of chronic hepatitis C infection.[9]

HCV Infection in Children

The two primary modes of infection in children are transfusion of blood products and perinatal transmission. Spontaneous clearance of active HCV infection after blood transfusions appears to be much higher in children than adults. In one recent study, only 55% of children with anti-HCV after blood transfusions had detectable HCV RNA on long-term follow-up, far lower than the 85% of patients with persistent HCV infection reported in adults.[92] Documenting resolution of HCV infection with qualitative measurements of HCV RNA may be reassuring to both these children and their parents.

The risk of perinatal transmission of hepatitis C from viremic mothers to their infants is approximately 5% to 10%.[93,94] Despite the concern about perinatal transmission, it is prudent to delay anti-HCV testing in these infants for 12 to 15 months to allow clearance of maternal antibodies.[95] Qualitative HCV RNA testing is the best method to evaluate newborns with elevated aminotransfeases and suspected hepatitis C in the perinatal period.

SUMMARY

Currently available tests provide powerful tools for the management of patients with chronic hepatitis C. They can be used to inexpensively screen patients for possible HCV infection and to confirm or exclude the presence of active infection. In addition, they have proven extremely useful in the management of patients undergoing antiviral therapy for chronic hepatitis C.

ABBREVIATIONS

HCV	hepatitis C virus
anti-HCV	antibodies to HCV
EIA	enzyme immunoassay
RIBA	recombinant immunoblot assay
RT-PCR	reverse transcriptase polymerase chain reaction
bDNA	branched DNA
RFLP	restriction fragment length polymorphism

REFERENCES

1. McHutchison JG, Gordon SC, Schiff ER, et al. Interferon alfa-2b alone or in combination with ribavirin as initial treatment for chronic hepatitis C. N Engl J Med 1998;339:1485–1492
2. Poynard T, Marcellin P, Lee SS, et al. Randomised trial of interferon alpha2b plus ribavirin for 48 weeks or for 24 weeks versus interferon alpha2b plus placebo for 48 weeks for treatment of chronic infection with hepatitis C virus. International Hepatitis Interventional Therapy Group (IHIT). Lancet 1998;352:1426–1432
3. Gretch DR. Diagnostic tests for hepatitis C. Hepatology 1997;26(Suppl 1):43S–47S
4. Gretch DR, Bacchi CE, Corey L, et al. Persistent hepatitis C virus infection after liver transplantation: Clinical and virological features. Hepatology 1995;22:1–9
5. Kao J-H, Lai M-Y, Hwang Y-T, et al. Chronic hepatitis C without anti-hepatitis C antibodies by second-generation assay. A clinicopathologic study and demonstration of the usefulness of a third-generation assay. Dig Dis Sci 1996;41:161–165
6. Uyttendaele S, Claeys H, Mertens W, Verhaert H, Vermylen C. Evaluation of third-generation screening and confirmatory assays for HCV antibodies. Vox Sang 1994;66:122–129
7. Barrera J, Prancis B, Ercilla G, et al. Improved detection of anti-HCV in post-transfusion hepatitis by a third-generation ELISA. Vox Sang 1995;68:15–18
8. Pawlotsky JM, Lonjon I, Hezode C, et al. What strategy should be used for diagnosis of hepatitis C virus infection in clinical laboratories? Hepatology 1998;27:1700–1702
9. Morishima C, Gretch DR. Clinical use of hepatitis C virus tests for diagnosis and monitoring during therapy. In: Keefe EB, ed. Treatment of Chronic Hepatitis C. Philadelphia: W.B. Saunders, 1999, pp 717–740
10. Atrah HI, Hutchinson F, Gough D, Ala FA. Hepatitis C seroconversion rate in established blood donors. J Med Virol 1995;46:329–333
11. Pawlotsky JM, Bastie A, Pellet C, et al. Significance of indeterminate third-generation hepatitis C virus recombinant immunoblot assay. J Clin Microbiol 1996;34:80–83

12. Damen M, Zaaijer HL, Cuypers HT, et al. Reliability of the third-generation recombinant immunoblot assay for hepatitis C virus. Transfusion 1995;35:745–749

13. Younossi ZM, McHutchison JG. Serological tests for HCV infection. Viral Hepatol Rev 1996;2:161–173

14. Pawlotsky JM, Bastie A, Lonjon I, et al. What technique should be used for routine detection and quantification of HBV DNA in clinical samples? J Virol Methods 1997;65:245–253

15. Fried MW. Clinical application of hepatitis C virus genotyping and quantitation. In: Davis GL, ed. Clinics in Liver Disease. Philadelphia: W.B. Saunders, 1997, pp 631–645

16. Busch MP, Wilber JC, Johnson P, Tobler L, Evans CS. Impact of speciman handling and storage on detection of hepatitis C virus RNA. Transfusion 1992;32:420–425

17. Davis GL, Lau JY, Urdea MS, et al. et al. Quantitative detection of hepatitis C virus RNA with a solid-phase signal amplification method: Definition of optimal conditions for specimen collection and clinical application in interferon-treated patients. Hepatology 1994;19:1337–1341

18. Polyak SJ, Gretch DR. Molecular diagnostic testing for viral hepatitis: Methods and applications. In: Willson RA, ed. Viral Hepatitis. New York: Marcel Dekker, 1997, pp 1–33

19. Gretch DR, Wilson JJ, Carithers RL Jr, dela Rosa C, Han JH, Corey L. Detection of hepatitis C virus RNA: Comparison of one-stage polymerase chain reaction (PCR) with nested-set PCR. J Clin Microbiol 1993;31:289–291

20. Kwok S, Higuchi R. Avoid false positives with PCR. Nature 1989;339:237–238

21. Zaaijer HL, Cuypers HT, Reesink HW, Winkel IN, Gerken G, Lelie PN. Reliability of polymerase chain reaction for detection of hepatitis C virus. Lancet 1993;341:722–724

22. Damen M, Cuypers HT, Zaaijer HL, et al. International collaborative study on the second Eurohep HCV RNA reference panel. J Virol Methods 1996;58:175–185

23. Saldanha J. Standardization, quantification and quality control of assays for HCV RNA. Viral Hepatol Rev 1999;5:1–11

24. Nolte FS, Thurmond C, Fried MW. Preclinical evaluation of AMPLICOR hepatitis C virus test for detection of hepatitis C virus RNA. J Clin Microbiol 1995;33:1775–1778

25. Young KK, Archer JJ, Yokosuka O, Omata M, Resnick RM. Detection of hepatitis C virus RNA by a combined reverse transcription PCR assay: Comparison with nested amplification and antibody testing. J Clin Microbiol 1995;33:654–657

26. Zeuzem S, Ruster B, Roth WK. Clinical evaluation of a new polymerase chain reaction assay (Amplicor™ HCV) for detection of hepatitis C virus. Z Gastroenterol 1994;32:342–347

27. Albadalejo J, Alonso R, Antinozzi R, et al. Multicenter evaluation of the COBAS AMPLICOR HCV assay, an integrated PCR system for rapid detection of hepatitis C in the diagnostic laboratory. J Clin Microbiol 1998;36:862–865

28. Stapleton JT, Klinzman D, Schmidt WN, et al. Prospective comparison of whole-blood- and plasma-based hepatitis C virus RNA detection systems: Improved detection using whole blood as the source of viral RNA. J Clin Microbiol 1999;37:484–489

29. Schmidt WN, Wu P, Brashear D, et al. Effect of interferon therapy on hepatitis C virus RNA in whole blood, plasma, and peripheral blood mononuclear cells. Hepatology 1999;28:1110–1116

30. Lunel F, Cresta P, Vitour D, et al. Comparative evaluation of hepatitis C virus RNA quantitation by branched DNA, NASBA, and monitor assays. Hepatology 1999;29:528–535

31. Hawkins A, Davidson F, Simmonds P. Comparison of plasma virus loads among individuals infected with hepatitis C virus (HCV) genotypes 1, 2, and 3 by quantiplex HCV RNA assay versions 1 and 2, Roche monitor assay, and an in-house limiting dilution method. J Clin Microbiol 1997;35:187–192

32. Reichard O, Norkrans G, Fryden A, Braconier JH, Sonnerborg A, Weiland O. Comparison of 3 quantitative HCV RNA assays—accuracy of baseline viral load to predict treatment outcome in chronic hepatitis C. Scand J Infect Dis 1998;30:441–446

33. Tong CY, Hollingsworth RC, Williams H, Irving WL, Gilmore IT. Effect of genotypes on the quantification of hepatitis C virus (HCV) RNA in clinical samples using the Amplicor HCV Monitor test and the Quantiplex HCV RNA 2.0 assay (bDNA). J Med Virol 1998;55:191–196

34. Gretch DR. Use and interpretation of HCV diagnostic tests in the clinical setting. In: Davis GL, ed. Clinic in Liver Disease. Philadelphia: W.B. Saunders, 1997, pp 543–557

35. Gretch DR, dela Rosa C, Carithers RL Jr, Willson RA, Williams B, Corey L. Assessment of hepatitis C viremia using molecular amplification technologies: Correlations and clinical implications. Ann Intern Med 1995;123:321–329

36. Pawlotsky JM, Martinot-Peignoux M, Poveda JD, et al. et al. Quantification of hepatitis C virus RNA in serum by branched DNA-based signal amplification assays. J Virol Methods 1999;79:227–235

37. Trabaud MA, Bailly F, Si-Ahmed SN, et al. Comparison of HCV RNA assays for the detection and quantification of hepatitis C virus RNA levels in serum of patients with chronic hepatitis C treated with interferon. J Med Virol 1997;52:105–112

38. Bukh J, Miller RH, Purcell RH. Genetic heterogeneity of hepatitis C virus: Quasispecies and genotypes. Semin Liver Dis 1995;15:41–63

39. Simmonds P, Holmes EC, Cha TA, et al. Classification of hepatitis C virus into six major genotypes and a series of subtypes by phylogenetic analysis of the NS-5 region. J Gen Virol 1993;74:2391–2399

40. Bukh J, Purcell RH, Miller RH. At least 12 genotypes of hepatitis C virus predicted by sequence analysis of the putative E1 gene of isolates collected worldwide. Proc Natl Acad Sci USA 1993;90:8234–8238

41. Stuyver L, Van Arnhem W, Wyseur A, Hernandez F, Delaporte E, Maertens G. Classification of hepatitis C viruses based on phylogenetic analysis of the envelope 1 and nonstructural 5B regions and identification of 5 additional subtypes. Proc Natl Acad Sci USA 1994;91:10134–10138

42. Okamoto H, Sugiyama Y, Okada S, et al. Typing hepatitis C virus by polymerase chain reaction with type specific primers: Application to clinical surveys and tracing infectious sources. J Gen Virol 1992;73:673–679

43. Chayama K, Tsubota A, Arase Y, et al. Genotype subtyping of hepatitis C virus. J Gastroenterol Hepatol 1993;8:150–156

44. Nakao T, Enomoto N, Takada N, Takada A, Date T. Typing of hepatitis C virus genomes by restriction fragment length polymorphism. J Gen Virol 1991;72:2105–2112

45. Simmonds P, McOmish F, Yap PL, et al. Sequence variability in the 5′ non-coding region of hepatitis C virus: Identification of a new virus type and restrictions on sequence diversity. J Gen Virol 1993;74:661–668

46. Davidson F, Simmonds P, Ferguson JC, et al. Survey of major genotypes and subtypes of hepatitis C virus using RFLP of sequences amplified from the 5′-non-coding region. J Gen Virol 1995;76:1197–1204

47. Mahaney K, Tedeschi V, Maertens G, et al. Genotypic analysis of hepatitis C virus in American patients. Hepatology 1994;20:1405–1411

48. Lau JY, Mizokami M, Kolberg JA, et al. Application of six hepatitis C genotyping systems to sera from chronic hepatitis C patients in the United States. J Infect Dis 1995;171:281–289

49. Lau JYN, Davis GL, Prescott LE, et al. Distribution of hepatitis C virus genotypes determined by line probe assay in patients with chronic hepatitis C seen at tertiary referral centers in the United States. Ann Intern Med 1996;124:868–876

50. Simmonds P, Rose KA, Graham S, et al. Mapping of serotype-specific, immunodominant epitopes in the NS-4 region of hepatitis C virus (HCV): Use of type-specific peptides to serologically differentiate infections with HCV types 1, 2, and 3. J Clin Microbiol 1993;31:1493–1503

51. Pawlotsky JM, Prescott L, Simmonds P, et al. Serological determination of hepatitis C virus genotype: Comparison with a standardized genotyping assay. J Clin Microbiol 1997;35: 1734–1739

52. Prescott LE, Berger A, Pawlotsky JM, Conjeevaram P, Pike I, Simmonds P. Sequence analysis of hepatitis C virus variants producing discrepant results with two different genotyping assays. J Med Virol 1997;53:237–244

53. Hoofnagle JH. Hepatitis C: The clinical spectrum of disease. Hepatology 1997;26(Suppl 1):15S–20S

54. Alter MJ, Margolis HS, Krawczynski K, et al. The natural history of community-acquired hepatitis C in the United States. The Sentinel Counties Chronic Non-A, Non-B Hepatitis Study Team. N Engl J Med 1992;327:1899–1905

55. Farci P, Alter HJ, Wong D, et al. A long-term study of hepatitis C virus replication in non-A, non-B hepatitis. N Engl J Med 1991;325:98–104

56. Alter HJ. Descartes before the horse: I clone, therefore I am. The hepatitis C virus in current perspective. Ann Intern Med 1991;115:644–649

57. McHutchison JG, Poynard T. Combination therapy with interferon plus ribavirin for the initial treatment of chronic hepatitis C. Semin Liver Dis 1999;19(Suppl 1):57–65

58. Davis GL, Lau JY. Factors predictive of a beneficial response to therapy of hepatitis C. Hepatology 1997;26(Suppl 1):122S–127S

59. Barnes E, Webster G, Whalley S, Dusheiko G. Predictors of a favorable response to alpha interferon therapy for hepatitis C. In: Keefe EB, ed. Clinics in Liver Disease. Philadelphia: W.B. Saunders, 1999, pp 775–791

60. Lindsay KL. Therapy of hepatitis C: Overview. Hepatology 1997;26(Suppl 1):71S–77S

61. Tong MJ, Blatt LM, McHutchison JG, Co RL, Conrad A. Prediction of response during interferon alfa 2b therapy in chronic hepatitis C patients using viral and biochemical characteristics: A comparison. Hepatology 1997;26:1640–1645

62. Chemello L, Cavalleto L, Casarin C, et al. Persistent hepatitis C viremia predicts late relapse after sustained response to interferon-alpha in chronic hepatitis C. Ann Intern Med 1996; 124:1058–1060

63. Marcellin P, Boyer N, Gervais A, et al. Long-term histologic improvement and loss of detectable intrahepatic HCV RNA in patients with chronic hepatitis C and sustained response to interferon-alpha therapy. Ann Intern Med 1997;127:875–881

64. Lau D-TY, Kleiner DE, Ghany MG, Park Y, Schmid P, Hoofnagle JH. 10-Year follow-up after interferon-alpha therapy for chronic hepatitis C. Hepatology 1998;28:1121–1127

65. Larghi A, Tagger A, Crosignani A, et al. Clinical significance of hepatic HCV RNA in patients with chronic hepatitis C demonstrating long-term sustained response to interferon-alpha therapy. J Med Virol 1998;55:7–11

66. Reichard O, Glaumann H, Fryden A, Norkrans G, Wejstal R, Weiland O. Long-term follow-up of chronic hepatitis C patients with sustained virological response to alpha-interferon. J Hepatol 1999;30:783–787

67. Vento S, Concia E, Ferraro T. Lack of sustained efficacy of interferon in patients with chronic hepatitis C. N Engl J Med 1996;334:1479–1480

68. National Institutes of Health Consensus Development Conference Panel statement. Management of hepatitis C. Hepatology 1997;26(Suppl 1):2S–10S

69. Alberti A, Chemello L, Noventa F, Cavalletto L, De SG. Therapy of hepatitis C: Retreatment with alpha interferon. Hepatology 1997;26(Suppl 1):137S–142S

70. Chemello L, Cavalletto L, Donada C, et al. Efficacy of a second cycle of interferon therapy in patients with chronic hepatitis C. Gastroenterology 1997;113:1654–1659

71. Camma C, Giunta M, Chemello L, et al. Chronic hepatitis C: Interferon retreatment of relapsers. A meta-analysis of individual patient data. Hepatology 1999;30:801–807

72. Davis GL, Esteban-Mur R, Rustgi V, et al. Interferon alfa-2b alone or in combination with ribavirin for the treatment of relapse of chronic hepatitis C. International Hepatitis Interventional Therapy Group. N Engl J Med 1998;339:1493–1499

73. Davis GL. Combination therapy with interferon alfa and ribavirin as retreatment of interferon relapse in chronic hepatitis C. Semin Liver Dis 1999;19(Suppl 1):49–55

74. Heathcote EJ, Keeffe EB, Lee SS, et al. et al. Retreatment of chronic hepatitis C with consensus interferon. Hepatology 1998;27:1136–1143

75. Barbaro G, Di Lorenzo G, Belloni G, et al. Interferon alpha-2B and ribavirin in combination for patients with chronic hepatitis C who failed to respond to, or relapsed after, interferon alpha therapy: A randomized trial. Am J Med 1999;107:112–118

76. Schreiber GB, Busch MP, Kleinman SH, Korelitz JJ. The risk of transfusion-transmitted viral infections. N Engl J Med 1996; 334:1685–1690

77. Vrielink H, Zaaijer HL, Reesink HW, van der Poel CL, Cuypers HT, Lelie PN. Sensitivity and specificity of three third-generation anti-hepatitis C virus ELISAs. Vox Sang 1995;69: 14–17

78. Terrault NA, Wright TL, Pereira BJG. Hepatitis C infection in the transplant recipient. Infect Dis Clin North Am 1995;9: 943–964

79. Roth D. Hepatitis C virus: The nephrologist's view. Am J Kidney Dis 1995;25:3–16

80. Tokars JI, Alter MJ, Favero MS, Moyer LA, Miller E, Bland LA. National surveillance of dialysis associated diseases in the United States, 1993. ASAIO J 1996;42:219–229

81. Recommendations for prevention and control of hepatitis C virus (HCV) infection and HCV-related chronic disease. MMWR Morb Mortal Wkly Rep 1998;47:1–39

82. Chan TM, Lok ASF, Cheng IKP, Chan RT. Prevalence of hepatitis C virus infection in hemodialysis patients: A longitudinal study comparing the results of RNA and antibody assays. Hepatology 1993;17:5–8

83. Fabrizi F, Lunghi G, Andrulli S, et al. Influence of hepatitis C virus (HCV) viraemia upon serum aminotransferase activity in chronic dialysis patients. Nephrol Dial Transplant 1997;12: 1394–1398

84. Couroucé AM, Bouchardeau F, Chauveau P, et al. Hepatitis C virus (HCV) infection in haemodialysed patients: HCV-RNA and anti-HCV antibodies (third-generation assays). Nephrol Dial Transplant 1995;10:234–239

85. Strasser SI, Myerson D, Spurgeon CL, et al. Hepatitis C virus infection and bone marrow transplantation: A cohort study with 10-year follow-up. Hepatology 1999;29:1893–1899

86. Strasser SI, Sullivan KM, Myerson D, et al. Cirrhosis of the liver in long-term marrow transplant survivors. Blood 1999;93: 3259–3266

87. Hsu HH, Wright TL, Tsao SC, et al. Antibody response to hepatitis C virus after liver transplantation. Am J Gastroenterol 1994;89:1169–1174

88. Lok AS, Chien D, Choo QL, et al. Antibody response to core, envelope and nonstructural hepatitis C virus antigens: Comparison of immunocompetent and immunosuppressed patients. Hepatology 1993;18:497–502

89. Feray C, Gigou M, Samuel D, et al. The course of hepatitis C virus infection after liver transplantation. Hepatology 1994;20:1137–1143

90. Wright TL, Donegan E, Hsu HH, et al. Recurrent and acquired hepatitis C viral infection in liver transplant recipients. Gastroenterology 1992;102:317–322

91. Chamot E, Hirschel B, Wintsch J, et al. Loss of antibodies against hepatitis C virus in HIV-seropositive intravenous drug users. AIDS 1990;4:1275–1277

92. Vogt M, Lang T, Frosner G, et al. Prevalence and clinical outcome of hepatitis C infection in children who underwent cardiac surgery before the implementation of blood-donor screening. N Engl J Med 1999;341:866–870

93. Ohto H, Terazawa S, Sasaki N, et al. Transmission of hepatitis C virus from mothers to infants. The Vertical Transmission of Hepatitis C Virus Collaborative Study Group. N Engl J Med 1994;330:744–750

94. Giacchino R, Tasso L, Timitilli A, et al. Vertical transmission of hepatitis C virus infection: Usefulness of viremia detection in HIV-seronegative hepatitis C virus-seropositive mothers. J Pediatr 1998;132:167–169

95. Jonas MM. Hepatitis C infection in children. N Engl J Med 1999;341:912–913

SEMINARS IN LIVER DISEASE—VOL. 20, NO. 2, 2000

Hepatitis C Kinetics: Mathematical Modeling of Viral Response to Therapy

THOMAS J. LAYDEN, M.D., BRIAN MIKA, B.Sc., and THELMA E. WILEY, M.D.

ABSTRACT: *Mathematical models have been used to study the dynamics of HIV. Using these same principles, the dynamics of hepatitis C virus (HCV) are reviewed during interferon (IFN) therapy. After initiating IFN treatment, there is an IFN dose-dependent exponential decline in viral RNA levels within the first 48 hours. This rapid 1.0 to 2.0 log decline was best explained by an effect of IFN in inhibiting viral production with a varying degree of effectiveness. By applying mathematical principles, viral serum half-life was estimated to be 3.0 hours and viral production rate was calculated to be 1.0×10^{12} virions per day. After this rapid first-phase decline there was a slower second phase decline in viral levels that was highly variable between subjects. This phase was dependent on the rate of elimination of HCV-infected liver cells. The rapidity of the second phase proved to be the best predictor of early viral clearance. The use of these models to understand the life cycle of viruses and their response to therapy is reviewed.*

KEY WORDS: hepatitis C virus, interferon, ribavirin

The hepatitis C virus (HCV) infects 1–3% of people in the United States, and in certain ethnic populations, 3–5% of subjects are infected with the virus.[1] Symptoms of viral infection are unusual, and the disease may progress in an indolent manner to cirrhosis, liver failure, and hepatocellular carcinoma (HCC). Patients who develop cirrhosis clinically decompensate at a rate of 2 to 5% per year, and HCC develops in 3 to 5% of patients per year.[2,3] This progression is hastened when patients drink alcohol, even in moderation.[1,4,5] HCV with or without concomitant alcohol ingestion is now the leading cause for hepatic transplantation. It has been estimated that unless therapy is dramatically improved, hepatic failure, HCC, and hepatic transplantation will increase five- to sevenfold in the next two decades even though the number of new HCV infections has decreased compared with a decade ago.[6] These epidemiologic results indicate that effective therapy is

---

Objectives
Upon completion of this article, the reader should be able to understand 1) how the kinetics of viral decline can help mold therapy, and 2) the two phases of HCV decline following IFN treatment.

Accreditation
The Indiana University School of Medicine is accredited by the Accreditation Council for Continuing Medical Education to provide continuing medical education for physicians.

Credit
The Indiana University School of Medicine designates this educational activity for a maximum of 1.0 hours credit toward the AMA Physicians Recognition Award in category one. Each physician should claim only those hours of credit that he/she actually spent in the educational activity.

Disclosure
Statements have been obtained regarding the authors' relationships with financial supporters of this activity. There is no apparent conflict of interest related to the context of participation of the author of this article.

University of Illinois at Chicago, Section of Digestive and Liver Diseases, Chicago, Illinois.

Reprint requests: Thomas J. Layden, M.D., Professor of Medicine and Chief, Section of Digestive and Liver Diseases m/c 787; 840 S. Wood Street, Chicago, IL 60612-7323.

needed to eradicate the virus and prevent disease progression.

Currently, interferon-α (IFN-α) is the mainstay of therapy, although recently the addition of ribavirin to IFN therapy has dramatically improved sustained viral response rates (SVR) (i.e., loss of virus in serum 6 months after stopping therapy). IFN-α has been used in patients infected with HCV for over a decade, and results of therapy have slowly improved with modifications of IFN dose, duration of treatment, and most importantly the addition of ribavirin.[7–9] Sustained clearance of virus occurs in 35 to 40% of patients treated with combination therapy for 12 months, whereas IFN-α monotherapy leads to clearance rates of only 10 to 15%. However, in patients infected with genotype 1 virus, sustained viral clearance occurs in only 25% of patients treated with combination therapy, indicating that 75% of patients infected with the most common HCV viral genotype (65 to 75%) do not develop sustained virologic clearance. This problem is magnified further in the African-American community, where >90% of HCV-infected patients have genotype 1 virus.[10] Nonresponders to combination therapy or IFN monotherapy are even less likely to respond to further therapy, even with high-dose IFN, for reasons that may be related to either viral or host factors or both. These results indicate that new treatment strategies, using existing drugs or new therapeutic agents, are required to improve both end of treatment response and particularly sustained virologic response. There are many problems with improving existing treatment strategies. First, we do not have an HCV culture system that would allow study of new drugs that could block viral entry, decrease viral replication, prevent viral release, enhance viral clearance, or accelerate infected cell death rate. In any drug trial it takes at least 2 years before one determines whether a new treatment strategy or new drug improves sustained viral clearance. Also, decisions regarding effective doses of IFN or dosing patterns of IFN are not and have not been based on careful analysis of HCV RNA levels both early in therapy or as therapy progresses. It is apparent from a number of studies using IFN alone that the earlier a patient clears HCV RNA from serum during treatment, the more likely SVR develops.[11–13] This relationship is not quite as clear with combination therapy because patients have developed SVR even when they clear virus from serum after 3 to 6 months of therapy.[8,9,14] Nevertheless, most studies highlight the importance of early virologic clearance in the ultimate development of SVR. However, the early kinetic parameters that follow initiation of therapy have not been studied in great detail until the last few years.

Recently, a number of studies have begun to carefully analyze the kinetics of HCV in response to IFN or combination therapy.[15–21] These studies have used and expanded on mathematical models of viral infection developed to study the kinetics and dynamics of HIV in response to protease and reverse transcriptase inhibitors.[22–24] Similar mathematical principles have also been exploited to study the kinetics of hepatitis B virus (HBV) after initiation of therapy with lamuvidine and adefovir dipivoxil.[25,26] These mathematical principles have greatly improved our fundamental understanding of the dynamics and life cycle of HIV and HBV and have given insight into the rationale for therapy. The mathematical principles used to study viral kinetics are relatively similar whether one is examining the HIV, HBV, or HCV life cycle and are summarized in the next section.

KINETICS OF VIRAL INFECTION AND THE RESPONSE TO THERAPY

Mathematical Models of Viral Infection

The dynamics of a viral infection can be defined using standard models of viral infection described by Ho et al.,[22] Perelson et al.,[23,24] and Neumann et al.[16]

$$dT/dt = s - dT - (1 - \eta)\beta VT \qquad (1)$$

$$dI/dt = (1 - \eta)\beta VT - \delta I \qquad (2)$$

$$dV/dt = (1 - \varepsilon)\rho I - cV \qquad (3)$$

These equations relate the dynamic relationship between uninfected target cells (T), infected cells (I), and free virions (V). The dynamics of these equations are graphically depicted in Figure 1. New target cells (T) are produced at a rate of s and die at a rate of d. Target cells become infected (new infection) at a rate constant of β, thereby becoming virus-producing infected cells (I). Infected cells die at a rate of δ presumably by either immune-mediated cell necrosis and/or apoptosis or directly by viral injury. The virus is released into the circulation and is cleared (c, intrinsic viral clearance) either by humoral mechanisms, phagocytic engulfment, or by serum RNAse. Free virus can also infect target cells, thereby producing infected cells. The virus is produced (p) at a certain rate per day in the infected cell. Viral persistence comes about when the rate of viral production (p), de novo infection of target cells (β), and production of T cells (s) exceeds the rate to which the virus is cleared from the circulation (c), infected cells die (δ), and new target cells die (d). This state of viral persistence occurs when there is a weak immune response to the virus or virus-infected cells and/or the virus has developed strategies to escape immune recognition. At some point, a steady-state serum level develops, and at this viral set point production equals clearance. At this steady state, it is not possible to assess

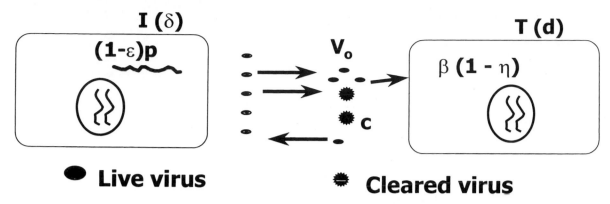

FIG. 1. **The dynamics of HCV, where *I* refers to infected cells and *T* refers to uninfected target T cells.** Infected cells die at a variable rate δ depending on immune recognition. Virus is produced (p) at a given rate, released into the circulation, and cleared [intrinsic viral clearance (c)]. Target cells become infected at a given rate constant (β) and become infected cells (I). A drug could reduce serum viral levels by preventing new infections with a given efficacy $(1 - \eta)$. A drug could also inhibit viral production with a given rate of effectiveness $(1 - \varepsilon)$. As is discussed, if IFN acts by blocking de novo infection, HCV production and clearance would continue at the pretreatment level and viral levels would decline as infected cells are cleared. In this case, the first phase of viral decline would be slow, which is not what we observed with IFN (see Fig. 4).

whether a virus is being produced slowly or rapidly. To accomplish this, antiviral therapy needs to be initiated. Treatment then can perturb the steady-state viral dynamics and decrease serum viral load either by blocking new target cell infection by a fraction $(1 - \eta)$ or by inhibiting viral production by a fraction $(1 - \varepsilon)$. Both actions can occur with treatment, as will be seen for treatment of HBV. This change in the steady state creates the opportunity to calculate the serum clearance of the virus, the production rate, and the death rate or half-life of viral infected cells. The effectiveness (ε) of an antiviral agent in blocking viral production can also be calculated. How these equations describe HBV dynamics under treatment is briefly outlined in the following section.

HBV Dynamics: Mathematical Modeling

HBV dynamics have been studied after therapy with lamuvidine[25] and adefovir dipivoxil.[26] These agents theoretically could reduce HBV serum viral levels by both inhibition of viral production and/or by preventing new infection of target cells (Fig. 1).[25,26] Treatment could lower viral levels by inhibiting the synthesis of new HBV DNA from pregenomic mRNA template.[25,26] This action would effectively block viral production by a fraction $(1 - \varepsilon)$ referred to as drug effectiveness. They can also block new infections by a fraction $(1 - \eta)$ by inhibiting the formation of double-stranded circular DNA before it migrates to the nucleus.[25,26] Although this is not discussed in detail, lamivudine and adefovir dipivoxil would both be more effective in inhibiting new infections but would have a variable effectiveness in inhibiting viral production $(1 - \varepsilon)$.[26] So what is observed when therapy is initi-

ated and the steady state perturbed? After therapy is started, there is a relatively rapid exponential 2.0 to 3.0 logs decline in serum viral DNA levels that eventually plateaus after 12 to 20 days (Fig. 2). This first phase of viral decline is followed by a slower second phase of viral DNA decline. As opposed to the first phase, the rate of the second phase proved to be highly variable between patients (Fig. 2). When these results were fit to the mathematical models (Eqs. 1 to 3). Tsiang et al.[26] were able to estimate drug effectiveness of adefovir dipivoxil in blocking viral production, intrinsic viral clearance (c), and infected cell half-life (δ). The mean value for drug effectiveness was 0.993 ± 0.008, implying that only 0.7% of viral production persisted during therapy. This estimate was greater than the 97% effectiveness reported by Nowak et al.[25] for lamuvidine. If either agent were 100% effective in inhibiting viral production, serum viral DNA would be undetectable within 25 to 30 days and the decline would reflect the intrinsic viral clearance (i.e., serum half-life of HBV) (Fig. 2). Calculations of HBV viral half-life revealed values ranging from 22 to 26 hours with either antiviral agent. The second phase of viral decline is determined by the rate of removal of HBV-infected liver cells (δ) and was estimated to be 18 ± 7 days by Tsiang et al.[26] and 10 to 100 days by Nowak et al.[25] The variability in HBV-infected cell death determines the rate of decline of the second phase. In summary, antiviral therapy for HBV perturbed the steady state and two distinct phases of viral decline were observed. The first phase, which lasted 15 to 20 days, was dependent on drug effectiveness and intrinsic viral clearance, whereas the second phase was dependent on the death rate of infected liver cells. So how do these kinetic results compare with HCV kinetics after IFN?

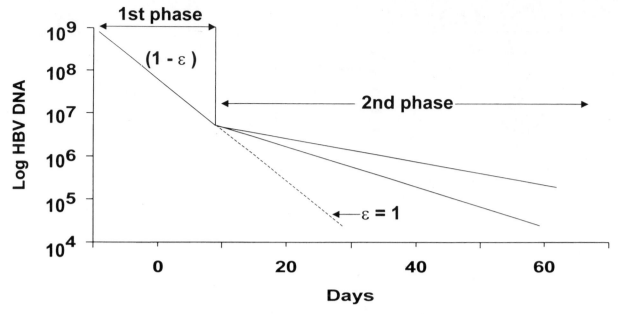

FIG. 2.   **The first and second phase of HBV DNA decline after therapy with adefovir dipivoxil at 30 mg.** The first-phase decline over 20 days accounts for a 2.5 to 3.0 log decline in DNA levels and in both the result of drug effectiveness (ε) in blocking viral production and the intrinsic viral clearance (half-life) of virus (24 hours). If the drug was 100% effective (ε = dashed line) in blocking viral production, viral DNA would be undetectable at day 30 to 40 and the viral DNA decline would not be biphasic. After the rapid phase there is a variable second-phase decline. Declines of two separate patients are depicted. (From Ref. 26.)

HCV Viral Kinetics Impact of IFN

We and others have examined in a series of studies the kinetics of HCV in response to IFN and IFN in combination with ribavirin.[15–21] In our first study, we assessed the impact of different single doses of IFN-α2b on serum HCV RNA levels over a 24- to 48-hour period of time.[15] These studies were designed to assess whether IFN effects on HCV RNA levels were dose dependent and to determine what happened to serum viral levels over a 48-hour period of time, which simulates tiw dosing. These initial studies were only performed in geno-

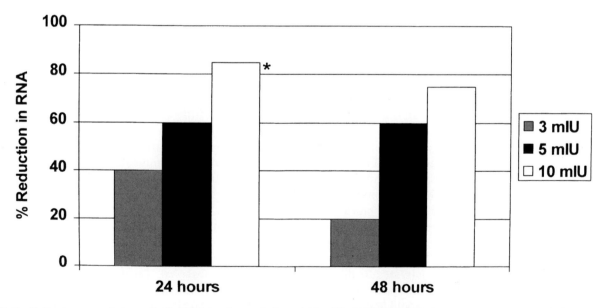

FIG. 3.   **Patients were given a single IFN injection at 3, 5, and 10 mIU of IFN-α2b and viral RNA levels were measured at 24 and 48 hours.** There was dose-dependent percent reduction in HCV RNA levels (3 < 5 < 10 mIU) in the first 24 hours (*$p < 0.001$ ANOVA). In the 3-mIU group there was a significant increase in HCV RNA levels at 48 hours from 24-hour values after the single injection. Viral RNA levels also increased in the 5- and 10-mIU dose but not to the same extent as seen with 3 mIU at 48 hours.

type 1a- or 1b-infected subjects. We found that there was a dose-dependent decline with 3, 5, and 10 mIU of IFN-α2b, giving a 41%, 64%, and 86% decline, respectively, in HCV RNA levels over the first 24 hours (Fig. 3).

Although it is discussed in greater detail, the rapid and dose-dependent lowering of HCV RNA levels is best explained by an effect of IFN in inhibiting viral production and not by inhibiting new viral infections. After the nadir in viral levels at 24 hours, there was an increase in serum viral RNA levels over the next 24 hours (Fig. 3). This rise in HCV RNA levels was most dramatic in the 3-mIU dose, which was and is the current recommended dose of IFN-α2b. An increase in viral levels at 48 hours was also seen in preliminary findings examining the effects of Infergen alfacon-1 (cIFN) and 9 and 15 μg over 48 hours.[21] Intriguingly, viral rebound coincided with the loss of measurable IFN in the peripheral blood.

This sawtooth pattern of HCV RNA levels was also observed over a 6-month period of time when IFN was used at 3 mIU tiw in genotype 1-infected patients.[27] HCV RNA levels 48 hours after the first 3 mIU dose were no different than values 48 hours after a dose of 3 mIU IFN at months 1, 3, or 6.[27] These viral kinetic findings indicate that in genotype 1-infected patients, standard doses and dosing patterns currently used to treat

this viral strain are insufficient when given as monotherapy. Indeed, large-scale studies have shown that with either IFN-α2b or cIFN given as monotherapy, sustained virologic responses occurred in only 5 to 13% of patients infected with genotype 1 virus.[7,9,28]

Many limitations with our initial study led us to perform additional studies where more frequent viral levels were measured over a longer period of time where higher daily doses of IFN-α2b were used. In these studies, the mathematical models that have been described earlier were used to calculate viral dynamics and drug effectiveness. In this subsequent study, we administered IFN-α2b daily at 5, 10, and 15 mIU for 14 days. After 14 days patients received IFN daily at 5 mIU for 3 to 12 months. Serum viral levels were measured frequently (every 4 hours) in the first 48 hours and then every other day for the first 14 days of treatment. Independent of IFN dose, there was an 8- to 10-hour pharmacologic delay before viral RNA levels began to decline. A similar pharmacologic delay of 8–10 hours was also noted in a kinetic study using cIFN at varying doses.[21] Viral levels then declined rapidly in an exponential manner for 48 hours with a viral decline slope of 3.0 ± 0.7, 6.1 ± 2.5, and 5.0 ± 0.5 day^{-1} for the 5-, 10-, and 15-mIU dose, respectively (Fig. 4). Both the 10- and 15-mIU dose produced a similar viral decline rate that was significantly greater than the 5-mIU dose.[16]

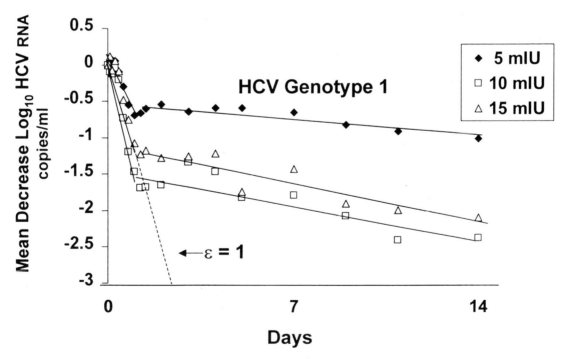

FIG. 4. **Viral RNA levels over a 14-day period in patients receiving 5, 10, and 15 mIU of IFN-α2b daily.** In the first 48 hours there was a rapid and dose-dependent 1.0 to 2.0 log drop in viral levels. This rapid decline is best explained by a variable effect of IFN in inhibiting viral production $(1 - \varepsilon)$. If IFN was 100% effective $(\varepsilon = 1)$, virus decline would be determined by the intrinsic viral clearance (—-). After this rapid decline, viral loss slowed and was not IFN dose dependent. This phase of viral decline is determined in part by the death of infected liver cells. Although not shown, there was a very significant variability in the rate of decline with some patients showing no decline where others demonstrated a very fast decline with viral serum clearance within 1 month. The rate of decline in the second phase was a highly significant determinant of early viral eradication. (From Ref. 16.)

When compared with results after HBV therapy (Fig. 2), the first phase of HCV viral decline was over within 48 hours of initiating IFN therapy (Fig. 4). After the first 48 hours, viral decline slowed over the next 12 days of high-dose daily IFN treatment (Fig. 4). The decay slopes over 2 to 14 days were 0.11 ± 0.14, 0.16 ± 0.23, and 0.28 ± 0.23 day^{-1} for the 5-, 10-, and 15-mIU dose, respectively. Note that the onset of the second phase started at day 2, whereas it started at day 15 to 20 during therapy with adefovir dipivol (Fig. 2). There were no statistical differences in the second phase slope between the three doses, suggesting that the second phase was not IFN dose dependent. However, the number of subjects was small, and significant differences may have resulted if larger numbers of patients were used. Indeed, Beckering et al.,[29] in preliminary studies, showed that the second-phase viral decline could be enhanced by higher doses of IFN-α.

First-Phase HCV Decline

What are the potential explanations for this rapid decline in viral levels, its dose dependency, and its eventual plateauing after 48 hours? Standard models of viral infection as described previously were used to analyze these results. IFN could reduce HCV RNA levels by inhibiting viral production by a fraction $(1 - \varepsilon)$ or by inhibiting new viral infections by a fraction $(1 - n)$. If we propose that IFN acts solely by blocking new infection, viral production and intrinsic viral clearance would remain the same after initiating therapy and the first-phase decline would be slow, which is not what we observed.[16] This mechanism of action would not account for the rapid 1.0 to 2.0 log decline seen within 48 hours nor could it account for the dose-dependent effects of IFN. Instead, the findings in this study and preliminary results from another study[21] are best explained by an effect of IFN in blocking viral production by infected cells with a varying degree of effectiveness $(1 - \varepsilon)$. If ε is 1 (100% effective in blocking production), viral levels would continue to decline in an exponential manner dependent on intrinsic viral clearance rate (Fig. 3). If ε is <1, viral RNA levels will plateau at a new steady level, which is consistent with the biphasic decline seen in this and other studies.[19,21] The initial decline would be then governed by the effectiveness of IFN in blocking production and the intrinsic viral clearance.

By using nonlinear regression analysis to fit the kinetics of RNA decline from day 0 and to day 2, we estimated the intrinsic viral clearance and drug effectiveness using the following equation. This equation represents the solution of Eq. 3 in the first 2 days of therapy.

$$V(t) = V_o [1 - \varepsilon + \varepsilon \exp (-c (t - t_o))] t > t_o \qquad (4)$$

We assume that during these first 2 days of treatment, infected cell mass (I) remains the same. Viral decay is measured from t_o, which corresponds to the pharmacologic delay (8 to 10 hours). The initial exponential decay slope is $c\varepsilon$ and $V(t)$ approaches the constant value $(1 - \varepsilon)V_o + \gg 1/c$. The mean intrinsic clearance rate was $c = 6.2 \pm 1.8$ days^{-1}, giving a viral half-life of 2.7 hours (1.5 to 4.6 hours). These results are similar to other estimates of viral clearance.[19] Intrinsic viral clearance rate was not dependent on IFN dose. Drug effectiveness (ε) demonstrated strong dose dependency with $\varepsilon = 0.81 \pm 0.06$, $\varepsilon = 0.95 \pm 0.04$, and $\varepsilon = 0.96 \pm 0.04$ for 5-, 10, and 15-mIU doses. Effectiveness was significantly less with the 5-mIU but the 10- or 15-mIU dose was similarly effective in inhibiting viral production and/or release. Thus, with maximum doses of IFN-α2b (10 to 15 mIU), 95% of viral production can be blocked. The effectiveness of other IFN products needs to be determined.

As baseline HCV RNA levels are relatively constant before therapy, viral production must equal viral clearance (i.e., cV_o times a factor for extracellular fluid volume). Production was calculated to be 1.3×10^{12} virions per day. As seen in Table 1, this production rate is greater than the estimates for HIV and is equivalent to that of HBV. Note that HCV has a faster clearance (shorter half-life) than HIV and an eightfold faster turnover than HBV. This in part accounts for why the first-phase decline is terminated within 48 hours, whereas >15 to 18 days to plateau for HBV during therapy despite a similar or greater degree of drug effectiveness in blocking HBV production.

TABLE 1.   Comparative Dynamics among Three Viruses

	HBV Adefovir[26]	HBV Lamivudine[25]	HIV Ritonavir[23]	HCV IFN-α[15,16]
Plasma Virus				
Half-life	26.4 hr	24 hr	5.8 hr	2.7–7.2 hr
Daily production (plasma)	2.1×10^{12}	10^{11}	10^{10}	$(1.1 - 12.7) \times 10^{11}$
Infected Cells				
Half-life	11–30 days	10–100 days	1.6 days	2.4–4.9 days

Cellular Mechanisms to Reduce Viral Production by IFN

What IFN-induced cellular mechanisms account for this inhibition of viral production? IFN-αhas many actions that could effect the dynamics of HCV. First, it has significant immunomodulatory actions that could enhance the eradication of infected liver cells. Certainly, it is well recognized in HBV infection that IFN enhances the immune response to HBV-infected liver cells, giving rise to an increase in alanine transferase (ALT) levels, which reflects immune destruction of infected liver cells.[30,31] On occasion, this immune response can be too vigorous, causing hepatic failure. In hepatitis C-infected patients, serum transaminases decline during successful IFN therapy, and it is very unusual to observe an increase unless the patient has concomitant autoimmune liver disease. Patients undergoing treatment with lamuvidine and adefovir dipivoxil for HBV also have a decline in ALT values, which generally parallels the fall in HBV DNA levels. However, it has been noted that patients who clear HBV DNA during therapy and seroconvert HBe Ag to anti-HBe generally have higher pretreatment ALT values than those patients who do not clear virus.[30,31] Also, patients who have higher HAI values generally clear HBV more readily. This suggests that patients who respond better to HBV antiviral therapy have preexisting immune recognition of HBV-infected liver cells. We observed similar results in patients infected with HCV (i.e., patients with higher pretreatment ALT values generally had higher calculated hepatocyte death rates, faster second phase viral declines, and earlier viral clearance).[16] However, it is unlikely that this mechanism could account for the rapid fall in viral levels within 24 to 48 hours. We would instead anticipate that this mechanism would enhance the second phase of viral decline.

At the cellular level, IFN exerts its antiviral effect by binding to receptors on the outside membrane of cells and in the liver it binds to type 1 IFN receptors. Binding activates a diverse number of intercellular signals that leads to an upregulation of a number of antiviral proteins including 2′5′ oligoadenylate synthetase, RNAse L, and PKR protein kinase. These IFN-effector proteins block viral gene expression at several different sites.[32,33] PKR protein kinase has undergone extensive study, and an interesting interaction between PKR and the HCV viral genome has recently been described. PKR is activated by binding to double-stranded RNA, including viral RNAs. It then phosphorylates the α subunit of a translation initiation factor referred to as eIF-2α.[32] Activation of this product results in an inhibition of protein synthesis and a block of viral replication (Fig. 5). This cellular action would lower viral production and serum viral levels. As therapy with IFN alone only leads to a long-term clearance of virus in 10% of treated

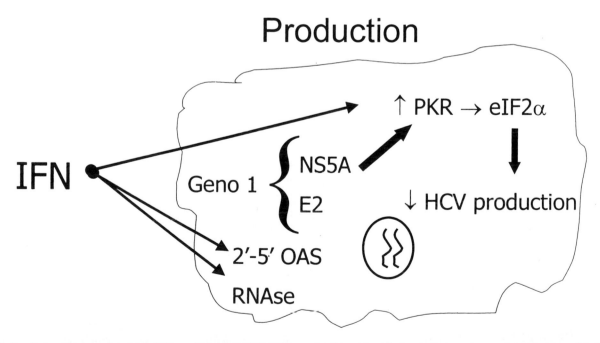

FIG. 5.   Potential ways in which IFN could inhibit HCV RNA production. After binding to its type 1 receptor of the liver cell, it activates a number of intercellular pathways that have been shown to inhibit viral production. When PKR is activated, it phosphorylates a translation-initiating factor (eIF-2α) that causes an inhibition of viral production. Intriguingly, a portion of the NS5A region and the E2 region of the genotype 1 viral genome can interact with PKR, preventing its activation and inhibition of viral production. A greater number of mutations in these regions prevent this interaction.

patients, it is apparent that the virus has developed strategies to counteract these inhibitory cellular pathways. In the last several years, some of these interesting viral strategies have been described. The NS5A region of the viral genome in genotype 1b virus has an IFN-sensitive region between codon 2209 and 2248. Enomoto et al.[34,35] reported that patients with the wild-type virus (HJV), having three or less mutations in this region, tend not to respond to IFN, whereas patients with three or more mutations respond to IFN with sustained virologic clearance.

It has been shown that the NS5A region can interact with PKR interfering with its catalytic domain thereby attenuating its effect on viral production.[32] In contrast, mutations in this region prevent this interaction. Although results from Japan strongly implicate the importance of this region in IFN response, results from other countries, including the United States, have not seen this strong association between sustained viral response and NS5A mutation frequency.[36–40] The reasons for these discrepant results are unclear but may relate to geographic differences, IFN dosing differences, or other host factors. However, if we assume that activation of PKR primary results in a reduction in viral production, the relationship between mutation frequency and viral response may only be applicable early in treatment when IFN demonstrates its strong effect on viral production. Sustained viral clearance is also a function of eradication of the infected cells, which probably has no relationship to mutations in the NS5A region.

It appears that the genotype 1 virus has developed a double strategy to impair IFN's effect on inhibiting viral production. Although the E2 region of the viral genome is relatively heterogeneous, a relatively conserved 12 amino acid region has been described that can interact with PKR and interfere with its action.[41] Mutations in this region prevent this interaction. In genotype 2-infected patients, this genomic region has many mutations, thereby preventing interaction with PKR in vitro.[41] Thus, the greater and faster early viral decline seen in genotype 2-infected patients with IFN treatment may relate to the finding that the E2 region of the viral genome is not able to interact with PKR. This in turn would lead to greater inhibition of viral production or greater IFN effectiveness (ε), which is what we observed (see section on genotype 2). In summary, (IFN induces several cellular mechanisms that can lead to a rapid and dose-dependent inhibition of viral production and a rapid lowering of serum viral levels as seen with therapy.

Second-Phase HCV Clearance

The rate of viral RNA decline in the second phase was highly variable between subjects, which was accounted for by the variability in the half-life of infected liver cells.[16] Some patients had a very rapid decline in viral RNA levels and cleared the virus within 14 to 30 days, whereas other patients had no further decline in viral levels after 48 hours. Others developed viral rebound despite daily and high doses of IFN.[16] Calculations of the half-life of infected cells revealed a variation from 1.7 to >70 days. Hepatocyte death rates could not be calculated in all patients because viral RNA levels actually increased during therapy in some patients. We also observed significant patient variability in the second phase of viral decline in a preliminary study examining viral kinetics after the use of Infergen.[21]

If IFN is greater than 95% effective in blocking HCV viral production, then clearance of HCV RNA from serum and ultimately from the cell reservoirs will depend on the death rate of virally infected liver cells. In fact, we have shown that the best predictor of early HCV clearance is the rate of second phase viral decline,[16,42] which is determined by the clearance of HCV-infected liver cells. There was no correlation between the rate of the first-phase decline and early viral clearance. Our calculated death rates of HBV-infected liver cells are similar to those calculated during therapy with lamivudine and adefovir dipivoxil.[25,26] Nowak et al.[25] demonstrated that infected cell death rate calculation correlated with baseline ALT values (i.e., the higher the ALT, the faster the calculated turnover of infected cells). Infected cell death rate was shown in our studies to also directly correlate with baseline ALT and inversely with initial viral RNA loads. The faster the second-phase viral decline in the 12 days of induction therapy, the more likely the patients were to clear the virus at month 3.[16,42] In preliminary studies, we have shown that the second-phase viral decline slope from day 2 to 14 correlated with the histologic activity index of Knodell[43] (Fig. 6). In particular, it was shown to correlate with the degree of periportal piecemeal necrosis. Of special note, the patients who had positive viral RNA slopes (i.e., increased serum RNA levels during the second phase) actually had little or no histologic activity on biopsy. Results of these histologic findings and the correlation between the ALT value and the calculated death rate supports the concept that the second-phase viral decline is determined by the hosts response to HCV-infected liver cells. Indeed, a number of observations have shown that response to IFN is better in patients who have greater CTL recognition of viral proteins.[44–49] HLA class I-restricted CD8+ CTL detected in the liver tissue of HCV-infected subjects and the level of their CTL response to viral antigens have been shown to indirectly correlate with the initial viral load and directly with the histologic activity and response to antiviral therapy.[44–49] These composite results support the hypothesis that the second phase of viral clearance is secondary to immune recognition of HCV infected liver cells.

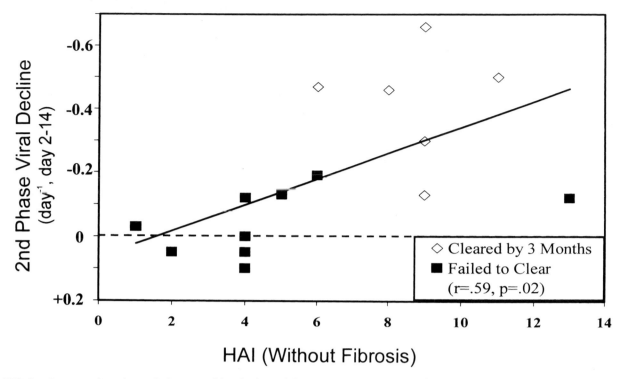

FIG. 6. A comparison is made between histologic activity using the Knodell scoring system and the rate of second-phase viral decline. Note that there is a significant correlation between second-phase viral decline and the extent of histologic activity. Patients with little or no activity in biopsy specimens had increases in HCV RNA levels over days 2 to 14. (From Ref. 43.)

In summary, during IFN-α therapy there is an initial rapid reduction (48 hours) in viral levels that can be explained by the effectiveness of IFN in blocking viral production and the intrinsic clearance of HCV. This rapid first phase is followed by a slower phase of viral clearance that is highly variable and is the result of a variable immune response to infected liver cells. The rate of decline of the second phase is the best predictor of early viral clearance. Whether the rate of second-phase slope can also be used as a predictor of sustained viral clearance will require further study.

Viral Kinetics with Other HCV Genotypes

It is very apparent from a number of studies that patients with genotype 2 or 3 virus have three- to fourfold greater likelihood of developing sustained virologic response with either IFN monotherapy or combination therapy. Although some of this may be secondary to a slightly lower baseline HCV RNA levels in genotype 2 or 3 infection, this certainly cannot explain such a dramatic difference in treatment response. Kohara et al.[50] have shown that patients with genotype 2 virus clear virus within 20 days of initiating IFN therapy and some even in less than 10 days. Sustained virologic response also occurred at lower total doses of IFN than needed to clear HCV genotype 1. In preliminary studies, we have

shown that IFN-α2b administered 10 mIU/day also causes a biphasic decline in HCV RNA levels similarly to what has been seen with therapy in genotype 1-infected patients.[51] However, both the rates of the first and second phase decline were significantly faster in genotype 2-infected patients. The faster first phase reflected both a significantly greater degree of drug effectiveness (99% versus 95%) and faster intrinsic viral clearance (i.e., serum viral half-life).[51] The faster turnover of the virus may relate to a greater humoral response, leading to faster serum viral clearance.[52,53] However, the second phase viral decline was also significantly faster, which presumably reflects a greater CTL response to infected liver cells.[54] These preliminary results provide the first evidence for a difference in treatment response between different strains of the same virus.

Kinetics of HCV in Nonresponders

The kinetics of HCV in response to IFN in patients who have been IFN nonresponders in the past have not been detailed to any great extent, except for the work of Beckering et al.[19] His group has shown that first-phase decline is seemingly the same as in IFN-naive patients. However, the second phase proved very flat with poor or no viral decline despite high doses of IFN. If verified, this would support the concept that IFN nonresponders do not have CTL recognition of virally infected liver cells. Alternatively, therapy may have selected a clone of the virus that is inherently resistant to IFN. Clearly, a detailed comparison of the first- and second-phase viral decline in responders and nonresponders is required to make rational decisions regarding the usefulness of continuing treatment.

Impact of Ribavirin on IFN Kinetics

Zeuzem et al.[18] studied the effect of the addition of ribavirin to HCV kinetics in patients taking 3 or 6 mIU or IFN. Their method of performing mathematical modeling was different than described by our group. They found that the higher doses of IFN actually enhanced early viral clearance and ribavirin had no impact on HCV kinetics after IFN. From a clinical point of view, this does not explain the well-known effect of ribavirin in enhancing IFN's sustained virologic response rates. Although studies have not shown an effect of ribavirin in decreasing viral levels by itself, it could either enhance second-phase viral response and/or it could reduce new viral infection of target cells. In preliminary results, Neumann et al.[55] demonstrated that ribavirin's effect wsa best explained by an effect on inhibiting new infections and not by increasing the death rate of HCV-infected liver cells. These results were produced from the large multisite Rebetron trials. A potential drawback of these studies is that frequent and early viral measurements were not made so that an effect on second-phase clearance could have been missed. Clearly, more studies are required to assess how, from a mathematical point of view, ribavirin enhances viral clearance.

SUMMARY

Mathematical modeling of viral response to antiviral therapy can be used to understand the dynamics of chronic viral infection. Differences in kinetic patterns between subjects or groups of patients can give important information and insight into why patients do or do not respond to therapy. Early viral dynamics after initiation of therapy may prove very useful in assessing early in therapy who is likely to have end of treatment and SVR. Viral kinetic studies may shed important light why African-Americans may not respond as well to therapy or why women respond better than men to antiviral therapy.[8] Application of these models could also prove to be very helpful when new drugs or modification of existing drugs are being tested such as pegylated IFN.

ACKNOWLEDGMENT. We thank Patricia Randle for typing the manuscript.

ABBREVIATIONS

HCV hepatitis C virus
HCC hepatocellular carcinoma
IFN interferon
SVR sustained viral response
HBV hepatitis B virus
CIFN Interfergen alfacon-1
ALT alanine transferase

REFERENCES

1. Alter MJ. Epidemiology of hepatitis C. Hepatology 1997; 26(Suppl 1):62S–65S
2. Tong MJ, El-Farra NS, Reikes AR, Co RL. Clinical outcomes after transfusion-associated hepatitis C. N Engl J Med 1995;332: 1463–1466
3. Liaw YF, Tsai SL. Pathogenesis and clinical significance of acute exacerbations and remissions in patients with chronic hepatitis B virus infection. Vital Hep Rev 1997;3:143–154
4. Wiley TE, McCarthy M, Breidi L, et al. Impact of alcohol on the histological and clinical progression of hepatitis C infection. Hepatology 1998;28:805–809
5. Poynard T, Bedossa P, Opolon P. Natural history of liver fibrosis progression in patients with chronic hepatitis C. Lancet 1997; 349:825–832
6. Davis GL, Albright JE, Cook SF, Rosenberg DM. Projecting the future healthcare burden from hepatitis C in the United States. Hepatology 1998;28:99A
7. Poynard T, Marcellin P, Lee SS, et al. Randomized trial of interferon alpha-2b plus ribavirin for 48 weeks or for 24 weeks versus interferon alpha-2b plus placebo for 48 weeks for treatment of chronic infection with hepatitis C virus. International Hepatitis Interventional Therapy Group (IHIT). Lancet 1998;352:1426–1432
8. McHutchinson JG, Gordon SC, Schiff ER, et al. Interferon alpha-2b alone or in combination with ribavirin as initial treatment for chronic hepatitis C. N Engl J Med 1998;339:1485–1492
9. Poynard T, Leroy V, Cohard M, et al. Meta-analysis of interferon randomized trials in the treatment of viral hepatitis C: Effects of dose and duration. Hepatology 1996;24:778–789
10. Reddy KR, Hoofnagle JH, Tong MJ, et al. Racial differences in responses to therapy with interferon in chronic hepatitis C. Hepatology 1999;30:787–793
11. Orito E, Mizokami M, Suzuki K, et al. Loss of serum HCV RNA at week 4 of interferon alpha therapy is associated with more favorable long-term response in patients with chronic hepatitis. J Med Virol 1995;46:109–115
12. Karino Y, Toyota J, Sugawara M, et al. Early loss of serum hepatitis C virus RNA can predict a sustained response to interferon therapy in patients with chronic hepatitis C. Am J Gastroenterol 1997;92:61–65
13. Matsumoto A, Tanaka E, Suzuki T, et al. Viral and host factors that contribute to efficacy of interferon alpha 2a therapy in patients with chronic hepatitis C. Dig Dis Sci 1994;39:1273–1280
14. Davis GL, Esteban-Mur R, Rustgi V, et al. Interferon alfa-2b alone or in combination with ribavirin for the treatment of relapse of chronic hepatitis C. N Engl J Med 1998;339:1493–1499
15. Lam NP, Neumann AU, Gretch DR, et al. Dose-dependent acute clearance of hepatitis C genotype 1 virus with interferon alpha. Hepatology 1997;26:226–231

16. Neumann AU, Lam NP, Dahari H, et al. Hepatitis C viral dynamics in vivo and the antiviral efficacy of interferon-α therapy. Science 1998;282:103–107

17. Zeuzem S, Schmidt JM, Lee J-H, et al. Effect of interferon alpha on the dynamics of hepatitis C virus turnover in vivo. Hepatology 1996;23:366–371

18. Zeuzem S, Schmidt JM, Lee J-H, et al. Hepatitis C virus dynamics in vivo: Effect of ribavirin and interferon alfa on viral turnover. Hepatology 1998;28:245–252

19. Beckering FC, Brouwer JT, Leroux-Roels G, et al. Ultrarapid hepatitis C virus clearance by daily high-dose interferon in non-responders to standard therapy. J Hepatol 1998;28:960–964

20. Yasui K, Okanoue T, Murakami Y, et al. Dynamics of hepatitis C viremia following interferon-alpha administration. J Infect Dis 1998;177:1475–1479

21. Layden TJ, Reddy R, et al. Effects of interferon alfacon-1 (Infergen) on the viral kinetics of hepatitis C. Hepatology 1999;30:823

22. Ho DD, Neumann AU, Perelson AS, et al. Rapid turnover of plasma virions and CD4 lymphocytes in HIV-1 infection. Nature 1995;373:123–126

23. Perelson AS, Neumann AU, Markowitz M, et al. HIV-1 dynamics in vivo: Virion clearance rate, infected cell life-span, and viral generation time. Science 1996;271:1582–1586

24. Perelson AS, Essunger P, Cao Y, et al. Decay characteristics of HIV-1 infected compartments during combination therapy. Nature 1997;386:188–191

25. Nowak MA, Banhoeffer S, Hill AM, Boehme R, Thomas HC, McDade H. Viral dynamics in hepatitis B infection. Proc Natl Acad Sci USA 1996;93:4398–4402

26. Tsiang M, Rooney JF, Toole JJ, et al. Biphasic clearance kinetics of hepatitis B virus from patients during adefovir dipivoxil therapy. Hepatology 1999;29:1863–1869

27. Wiley TE, Briedi L, Lam N, et al. Early HCV RNA values after interferon predicts response. Dig Dis Sci 1998;43:2169–2172

28. Tong MJ, Reddy KR, Lee WM, et al. Treatment of chronic hepatitis C with consensus interferon: A multicenter, randomized, controlled trial. Consensus Interferon Study Group. Hepatology 1997;26:747–754

29. Bekkering FC, Brouwer JT, Niesters HGM, et al. Viral kinetics in HCV genotype 1:L is the second phase of viral decline interferon dose dependent? Hepatology 1999;30:124

30. Chen R-N, Liaw Y-F, Atkins M, et al. Pretherapy alanine transaminas level as a determinant for hepatitis Be Antigen seroconversion during lamivudine therapy in patients with chronic hepatitis B. Hepatology 1999;30:770–774

31. Lok ASF, Chang MG, Watson G, et al. Predictive value of aminotransferase and hepatitis B virus DNA levels on response to interferon therapy for chronic hepatitis B. J Viral Hepat 1998;5:171–178

32. Gale MJ, Korth MJ, Tang NM, et al. Evidence that hepatitis C virus resistance to interferon is mediated through repression of the PKR protein kinase by the nonstructural 5A protein. Virology 1997;230:217–227

33. Sen GC, Lengyel P. The interferon system: A bird's eye view of its biochemistry. J Biol Chem 1992;267:5017–5020

34. Enomoto N, Sakuma I, Asahina Y, et al. Comparison of full-length sequences of interferon-sensitive and resistant hepatitis C virus 1b. Sensitivity to interferon is conferred by amino acid substitutions in the NS5A region. J Clin Invest 1995;96:224–230

35. Enomoto N, Sakuma I, Asahina Y, et al. Mutations in the nonstructural protein 5A gene and response to interferon in patients with chronic hepatitis C virus 1b infection. N Engl J Med 1996;334:77–81

36. Khorsi H, Castelain S, Wyseu A, et al. Mutations of hepatitis C virus 1b NS5A 2209-2248 amino acid sequence do not predict the response to recombinant interferon-alfa therapy in French patients. J Hepatol 1997;27:72–77

37. Duverlie G, Khorsi H, Castelain, et al. Sequence analysis of the NS5A protein of European hepatitis C virus 1b isolates and relation to interferon sensitivity. J Gen Virol 1998;79:1373–1381

38. Squardrito J, Leon F, Sartori M, et al. Mutations in the nonstructural 5A region of hepatitis C virus and response of chronic hepatitis C to interferon alfa. Gastroenterology 1997;113:567–572

39. Franguel L, Cresta P, Perrin M, et al. Mutations in NS5A region of hepatitis C virus genome correlate with presence of NS5A antibodies and response to interferon therapy for most common European hepatitis C virus genotypes. Hepatology 1998;28:1674–1679

40. Paterson M, Laxton CD, Thomas HC, et al. Hepatitis C virus NS5A protein inhibits interferon antiviral activity, but the effects do not correlate with clinical response. Gastroenterology 1999;117:1187–1197

41. Taylor DR, Shi ST, Romano PR, et al. Inhibition of the interferon inducible protein kinase PKR by HCV E2 protein. Science 1999;285:107–110

42. Lam NP, Neumann AU, Dahari H, et al. Early viral decline slopes during daily high dose interferon (IFN) are predictive markers of subsequent virologic response. Hepatology 1998;28:397A

43. Mika BB, Lam NP, McCarthy ME, et al. Pretreatment histological activity index (HAI) is an indicator of early HCV viral clearance with IFN therapy. Accepted for oral presentation to the American association for the study of liver diseases. Gastroenterology 1999;116:A1246

44. Nelson DR, Marousis CG, Ohno T, et al. Intrahepatic hepatitis C virus specific cytotoxic t lymphocyte activity and response to interferon alfa therapy in chronic hepatitis C. Hepatology 1998;28:225–230

45. Nelson DR, Marousis CG, Davis GL, et al. The role of hepatitis C virus-specific cytotoxic t lymphocytes in chronic hepatitis C. J Immunol 1997;158:1473–1481

46. Koziel MJ, Dudley D, Afdhal N, et al. Hepatitis C virus (HCV) specific cytotoxic T lymphocyte recognize epitopes in the core and envelope proteins of HCV. J Virol 1993;67:7522–7532

47. Koziel MJ, Dudley D, Wong JT, et al. Intrahepatic cytotoxic T lymphocytes specific for hepatitis C virus in persons with chronic hepatitis. J Immunol 1992;149:3339–3344

48. Cerny A, Chisari FV. Pathogenesis of chronic hepatitis C: Immunological features of hepatic injury and viral persistence. Hepatology 1999;30:595–601

49. Lau JYN. Mechanisms of hepatic toxicity IV. Pathogenetic mechanisms involved in hepatitis C virus-induced liver diseases. Pathogene Hepat C 1998;G1217–G1220

50. Kohara M, Tanaka T, Tsukiyama-Kohara K, et al. Hepatitis C virus genotypes 1 and 2 respond to interferon-α with different virologic kinetics. JID 1995;172:934–938

51. Neumann AU, Lam NP, Davidian M, et al. Differences in hepatitis C virus (HCV) dynamics between HCV of genotype 1 and genotype 2. Hepatology 1999;30:121

52. Hattori M, Yoshioka K, Aiyama T, et al. Broadly reactive antibodies to hypervariable region 1 in hepatitis C virus-infected patient sera: Relation to viral loads and response to interferon. Hepatology 1998;27:1703–1710

53. Mondelli MU, Cerino A, Brambilla S, et al. Antibody responses to hepatitis C virus hypervariable region 1: Evidence for cross-reactivity and immune-mediated sequence variation. Hepatology 1999;3:537–545

54. Missale G, Cariani E, Lamonaca V, et al. Effects of interferon treatment on the antiviral T-cell response in hepatitis C virus genotype 1b and genotype 2c infected patients. Hepatology 1997;26:792–797

55. Neumann AU, Dahari H, Conrad A, et al. Early prediction and mechanism of the ribavirin/IFN-α dual therapy effect on chronic hepatitis C virus (HCV) infection. Hepatology 1999;30:595

Antiviral Therapy for Patients with Chronic Hepatitis C

JENNY HEATHCOTE, M.B., B.S., M.D., F.R.C.P., F.R.C.P.(C)

ABSTRACT: *Several large, randomized, controlled treatment trials in persons with hepatitis C and ongoing hepatitis have been reported recently. These have shown that, in patients without other comorbid conditions, treatment for from 6 to 12 months with a combination of interferon-α2b, 3 MU three times a week (ttw), plus ribavirin, 1,000–1,200 mg daily, results in a higher incidence of sustained virologic response than does treatment with interferon -α2b monotherapy, 3 MU ttw, given for similar durations. Patients who have relapsed after interferon monotherapy may achieve a sustained virologic response when retreated with interferon plus ribavirin for 6 months or when given a higher dose of interferon for a longer duration than the initial treatment. By contrast, patients who had no virologic response to prior interferon monotherapy have only a small chance of achieving a sustained response when similarly retreated. Although the efficacy of treatment for hepatitis C has improved steadily over the last decade, current interferon-based therapies still achieve a sustained virologic response in fewer than half of patients who initiate therapy, are associated with appreciable side effects, and are expensive. Furthermore, the natural history of chronic hepatitis C suggests that even in the absence of therapy, most patients with chronic hepatitis C infection may experience little morbidity or mortality for decades. Finally, published therapeutic trials stem largely from tertiary referral centers, where an especially high level of commitment is expected from both the patients and the team in charge of therapy. Typically, such trials have also excluded patients with comorbid diseases, thus reducing their "generalizability." This review focuses on two fundamental questions about the currently available treatments for this disease: Who should be treated with them? And when should they be treated? Critical analysis suggests that the answers to these questions are not as clear as they may superficially appear.*

KEY WORDS: interferon, chronic hepatitis C, monotherapy, combination therapies

Acceptance of a physician's recommendation to undergo therapy for chronic hepatitis C (CHC) with one of the currently available interferon-based regimens commits a patient to a prolonged period of treatment that is expensive, sometimes unpleasant, and, in the individual patient, of uncertain efficacy. For these reasons, a number of factors need to be considered before initiating such treatment. First, as reviewed by Alter and Seeff in

---

Objectives
Upon completion of this article, the reader will be able to highlight the points that need to be taken into consideration when treatment is discussed with a patient who has chronic hepatitis C.

Accreditation
The Indiana University School of Medicine is accredited by the Accreditation Council for Continuing Medical Education to provide continuing medical education for physicians.

Credit
The Indiana University School of Medicine designates this educational activity for a maximum of 1.0 hours credit toward the AMA Physicians Recognition Award in category one. Each physician should claim only those hours of credit that he/she actually spent in the educational activity.

Disclosure
Statements have been obtained regarding the author's relationships with financial supporters of this activity. Dr. Heathcote is the recipient of a research grant from MRC/Industry (Schering, Canada) and has received funds for clinical trials from Hoffman La Roche and Amgen.

University of Toronto, University Health Network: Toronto Western Hospital, Toronto, Ontario, Canada

Reprint requests: Dr. Heathcote, University of Toronto, University Health Network: Toronto Western Hospital, 399 Bathurst St. WW4–828, Toronto, ON M5T 2S8, Canada.

Copyright © 2000 by Thieme Medical Publishers, Inc., 333 Seventh Avenue, New York, NY 10001, USA. Tel.: +1(212) 584-4662.

0272-8087,p;2000,20,02,185,198,ftx,en;sld00056x

the prior issue of *Seminars* (volume 20, number 1), the natural history of untreated hepatitis C, which has important implications for the need for therapy, is imperfectly defined. As the overall success of current therapy is still only ~40%, it is reasonable for a patient whose liver histology shows no evidence of progressive disease to opt to delay therapy until more efficient less toxic treatments are available. In particular, the efficacy of current treatment regimens in patients with comorbid conditions (e.g., cryoglobulinemia, co-infection with HIV/hepatitis B virus, chronic renal failure, and in patients with hepatitis C after liver transplantation) remains unknown. Second, the patient needs to understand that the costs of such treatment include not only the financial cost of the drugs and of the frequent blood tests and access to medical personnel required for monitoring, but also the personal costs resulting from the side effects of therapy. These lead 20% or more of patients to withdraw from treatment before completing planned 48-week regimens with interferon α2b plus ribavirin. Although these personal costs of undergoing antiviral therapy may be considerable, they have not been critically assessed in any of the trials of therapy or cost effectiveness analyses published to date. Third, there is even uncertainty about the proper benchmarks for the assessment of treatment efficacy. Early data suggest that histologic improvement **may** be seen even in the absence of a virologic response. However, the durability of this histologic response upon cessation of therapy remains unknown. By contrast, the durability of a sustained virologic response, which is **always** accompanied by histologic improvement, is greater than 95% for up to 10 years. Finally, the effect of therapy on symptomatology (e.g., fatigue) is even more unpredictable; hence such nonspecific symptoms alone are not an indication for antiviral therapy.

The issues to be considered are therefore complex. Accordingly, although interferon-based regimens represent currently standard therapies, patients considering a course of antiviral treatment for hepatitis C deserve the same level of education that would be given before requesting informed consent from a patient considering participation in a clinical trial. Such patients need to be made fully aware of their chance of benefit, and the costs and risks of current treatment strategies and then allowed to decide for themselves whether they wish to be treated. It could even be argued that fully informed consent requires that the patient have access to the results of a recent liver biopsy, which gives the best currently available indication of the likely natural history of their infection over the next several years, if left untreated.

Thus, it is wise that when therapy is being considered outside the setting of a clinical trial, it is tailored to the individual patient. Patients need to participate in the decision-making process in that they need to decide whether the risk–to–benefit and cost–to–benefit ratios

of therapy are acceptable for them. Although there are many questions that require discussion with the patient when antiviral therapy for CHC is being contemplated, many, unfortunately, are unanswered. These treatment "dilemmas" are the subject of this article.

SHOULD ALL SUBJECTS CHRONICALLY INFECTED WITH HEPATITIS C UNDERGO THERAPY?

Although indications for treatment may be debated in some patients, there are situations in which treatment with current regimens is contraindicated. Recognition of such contraindications can be very important for the patients involved.

Absolute Contraindications

The recognized absolute contraindications to therapy with currently licensed agents, that is, interferon-alfa (IFN) alone or combined with oral ribavirin, are shown in Table 1.

Pregnancy

Some side effects are common to both IFN-alfa and ribavirin, such as the potential to damage the unborn child, so that patients and their partners are required to avoid pregnancy during therapy and, in the case of ribavirin, for 6 months after cessation of treatment. Animal data indicate that ribavirin is teratogenic, and the outcome in humans who have reported accidental pregnancy during "combination" therapy indicates that fetal mortality is high.[1] These "accidents" have sometimes taken place during the conduct of formal therapeutic trials despite patients being reminded on a monthly basis to avoid conception. It is reasonable to assume that less careful monitoring may result in a higher rate of such accidents of nature.

Use in Patients with Psychiatric Disorders

Interferon-alfa therapy, alone or in combination with Ribavirin, induces malaise, fatigue and irritability

TABLE 1.   Absolute Contraindications to IFN-alfa-2b Plus Ribavirin Therapy

Pregnancy—during and for 6 months after cessation of therapy
Psychosis/suicidal ideation
Myocardial infarction/cardiac arrhythmias
Renal insufficiency (creatinine clearance < 50 mL/min)

and sometimes depression, symptoms that may be troublesome in some subjects with hepatitis C even before starting any therapy. It cannot be predicted which subjects are more or less likely to develop these symptoms during treatment. The symptoms described above are likely caused by a direct effect of IFN on the central nervous system.[2] Therapy with IFN tends to enhance the premorbid personality of the patient. Hence INFs should not be used in persons with severe psychiatric disorders (e.g., psychoses or suicidal ideation) although it is probably safe to use IFNs in patients with controlled depression/anxiety disorders or a controlled seizure disorder. It may be advisable to discuss this with the patient's psychiatrist or neurologist before the initiation of IFN therapy.

Cardiovascular Disease

Ribavirin accumulates in red blood cells[3] and may cause hemolysis, thus rendering the patient anemic. Worsening malaise and fatigue can be acute and profound when there is a sudden large fall (>2 − 3 g/L) in hemoglobin. Because of the potential for treatment with IFN-alfa 2b plus ribavirin to cause a sudden fall in hemoglobin, combination therapy should not be given to those who have a past history of myocardial infarction or cardiac arrhythmia. Treatment with combination therapy is only a relative contraindication in patients who are at increased risk of ischemic heart disease, such as patients with systemic hypertension, dyslipidemia and/or diabetes.

Renal Insufficiency

Ribavirin has a very large volume of distribution, a long cumulative half-life, and is excreted by the kidneys.[3] Hence if given to patients with renal failure prolonged uncontrollable hemolysis may occur. Ribavirin cannot be removed by hemodialysis. Hence no one with a creatinine clearance of less than 50 mL/min should receive ribavirin.

Relative Contraindications Due to Common Side Effects of Antiviral Therapy

Hematologic Side Effects

As the alfa-INFs have a depressive effect on bone marrow function, a minimum baseline hemoglobin of >12 g/L, an absolute neutrophil count of 1.5×10^9/L, and a platelet count of 75×10^9/L are required before treatment can be used. Patients with compensated cirrhosis but with marked hypersplenism may not be able to tolerate treatment safely. Very careful monitoring of the complete blood count is required throughout therapy. The toxic effect of alfa IFNs on bone marrow function is maximal during the first month of therapy, whereas the hemolytic effect of ribavirin persists throughout therapy. An immune thrombocytopenia is occasionally associated with untreated hepatitis C infection, and some patients give a prior history of "idiopathic thrombocytopenic purpura." Such patients may experience a marked fall in platelet count upon the introduction of IFN therapy. Hence, the patient needs to understand that they will be required to attend regular monitoring and make themselves available to discuss the blood test results. Sometimes timing the start of treatment needs to be tailored to the patients' vacation times/work schedule, thus ensuring their availability for frequent monitoring.

Other Potentially Troublesome Side Effects

Other less predictable but nevertheless common side effects resulting from treatment with alfa IFNs with or without the addition of ribavirin need to be discussed with all patients and their families when treatment is being considered.

Irritability is frequent and may persist for the duration of treatment, although the patient may often underplay this side effect. It is important that the spouse and/or household members feel free to report when treatment appears to have precipitated intolerable friction at home, as dose modification may be of benefit. Weight loss during treatment is almost universal, thinning of hair is common, and diarrhea may complicate IFN therapy. All are reversible upon the cessation of treatment. Thyroiditis occurs sufficiently often during IFN-alfa therapy that it is advisable to monitor the thyroid-stimulating hormone during therapy (every 3 months is probably sufficient in asymptomatic patients). Therapy for thyroid dysfunction may be required during treatment, often becoming unnecessary once therapy is completed. Control of diabetes is worsened by IFN-alfa therapy and some patients may become glucose intolerant for the first time during therapy with IFN-alfa. Patients given combination therapy may develop anorexia, nausea, and occasionally vomiting, insomnia, dyspnea, pruritus, and skin rashes are reported more often than when IFN-alfa is given alone. Frequent small meals may relieve some of the gastrointestinal side effects. Consumption of adequate quantities of water (e.g., 2–3 litres daily) reduces the dermatologic side effects. Lichen planus, a skin lesion associated with hepatitis C infection, often worsens during therapy and if present in the mouth may make eating very uncomfortable.

CURRENTLY LICENSED THERAPIES FOR HEPATITIS C

At present, three IFN products and the combination of IFN-alfa-2b with ribavirin have been licensed for use in the treatment of hepatitis C. These products, their suggested doses, and retail costs are listed in Table 2.

Factors to Consider in Deciding if All CHC Patients Without Absolute Contraindications to Current Therapies Should be Treated

Who Has Been Shown to Benefit from Antiviral Therapy?

The evidence we have to date (based on the results of randomized trials of therapy) is that IFN-alfa, alone or combined with ribavirin, may induce sustained viral clearance from serum when given to patients with ongoing infection associated with persistent elevation of serum aminotransferase levels, in the absence of coinfection with other viruses, ongoing alcohol ingestion, and/or illicit drug use, or any other co-morbidities. Antiviral therapy also reduces the severity of inflammation and the rate of development of fibrosis seen on liver histology in patients who have a sustained viral response. Some aspects of patient quality of life may be improved after successful therapy, but not all. However, the trials reporting these results recruited a very select population of patients. Most recruited few patients with cirrhosis, so that the patients included in these trials do not represent the population at large with CHC.

What is Currently the Best Licensed Therapy for CHC?

It has been the conclusion of consensus meetings in both Canada[4] and in Europe[5] that treatment with a combination of IFN alfa-2b and ribavirin is more effective than treatment with interferon alfa-2b alone; hence, in the absence of absolute contraindications to ribavirin, combination therapy is the current standard of care.

However, the overall efficacy of this therapy as judged by sustained loss of detectable HCV RNA in serum given to naive patients under ideal circumstances is only 38[6] to 42%[7] when 12 months of treatment is administered (Table 3). A number of factors may help to predict a good or poor response to such therapy. A recent more detailed analysis of the combined data from two major trials comparing IFN alfa-2b monotherapy with IFN alfa-2b plus ribavirin indicate that the "favorable" factors are genotype 2 and 3, viral load < 3.5 million copies/mL, no or minimal fibrosis, female gender, and age less than 40 years.[8]

What Is the Gold Standard for Measuring Treatment Success?

Sustained undetectability of HCV RNA in serum tested by sensitive polymerase chain reaction 24 weeks after cessation of therapy has been the gold standard of efficacy in all the most recent therapeutic trials. Long term follow-up studies have indicated that loss of detectable HCV RNA in serum is associated with improved or lack of progression of liver disease.[9–11] There are reports that treatment of hepatitis C improves survival,[12] but such reports do not stem from long term follow-up of randomized controlled trials—rather a comparison of outcome in subjects treated or not treated, thus selection bias cannot be avoided.

The durability of a sustained viral response observed 6 months or more after the cessation of IFN-alfa monotherapy[9–11,13,14] or combination therapy[15] (fewer years of follow-up for combination therapy) appears to be greater than 95% for up to 10 years. Some data suggest that testing whole blood rather than plasma/serum may be a more reliable marker of viral loss and may be more helpful in predicting which patients will relapse after cessation of therapy in those whose serum HCV RNA is undetectable at the end of treatment.[16]

The literature suggests that the risk of hepatocellular carcinoma (HCC) may be reduced in patients with cirrhosis due to hepatitis C who have received treatment with IFN.[17–20] It is logical to assume that eradication of the prime cause for the liver disease, namely hepatic C virus (HCV) infection, might reduce the chance of de-

TABLE 2. Currently Licensed Therapies for the Treatment of Hepatitis C

Alfa-IFNs	Brand Name	Suggested Dose	Cost per Month
Alfa-2b	Intron-A	3 Mu ttw/sc	U.S.$ 297
Alfa-2a	Roferon-A	3 Mu ttw/sc	U.S.$ 349.68
Alfa-con-1	Infergen	9 mg ttw/sc	U.S.$ 342.71
Combination therapy			
Alfa-2b + ribavirin	Rebetron	3 Mu ttw/sc + ribavirin 1,000 1,200 qd po	U.S.$ 1,200 >75 kg U.S.$ 1,086 <75 kg

TABLE 3. Percent of Sustained Virologic Response: IFN-a-2b + Ribavirin vs. IFN-a-2b Monotherapy—European Study[7]

Genotype	Viral Load	Combination Therapy for 48 Weeks	Combination Therapy for 24 Weeks	IFN for 48 Weeks
2 and 3	>2 × 10⁶ copies/mL	64	60	33
2 and 3	<2 × 10⁶ copies/mL	64	67	34
1	>2 × 10⁶ copies/mL	28	8	4
1	<2 × 10⁶ copies/mL	36	35	29

veloping cirrhosis or reduce the progression of disease if cirrhosis is already present. But in other patients in whom cirrhosis is already established before treatment (e.g., hemochromatosis, alcohol induced cirrhosis) it is well recognized that despite successful phlebotomy or alcohol abstinence, subsequent HCC is not prevented. In one study, application of multiple regression analysis for risk factors for disease severity indicated that the "apparent" beneficial effect of IFN alfa therapy in reducing the rate of HCC disappeared.[21] Nevertheless, the recent results of a much larger analysis of IFN treated subjects (>2000) from Japan lends support to the inference that treatment of hepatitis C may reduce the risk of HCC, at least in Japanese patients.[22]

A recent study has suggested that liver histology may improve even in the absence of a viral response to standard treatments.[23] It remains to be established whether this improvement can be maintained after cessation of therapy or whether subsequent "catch up" takes place. Trials of prolonged therapy are currently being initiated in patients who have severe disease and who have not had a sustained virologic response to standard therapies.

Patients with Mild Histologic Disease— Should They Be Treated Now?

The data on the natural history of the histologic progression of hepatitis C are fairly sparse. However, it is known that the overall mortality after hepatitis C acquired after a blood transfusion is no different from patients transfused at the same time but who did not acquire hepatitis C, at least for the first 20 years[24] (Fig. 1). Data from liver biopsies performed on persons infected for a known period of time either via blood transfusion[25] or contaminated γ-globulin fractions[26] indicate that up to 20 yrs after the acute infection, cirrhosis is found in only 1% and 2%, respectively, when infection occurrs in

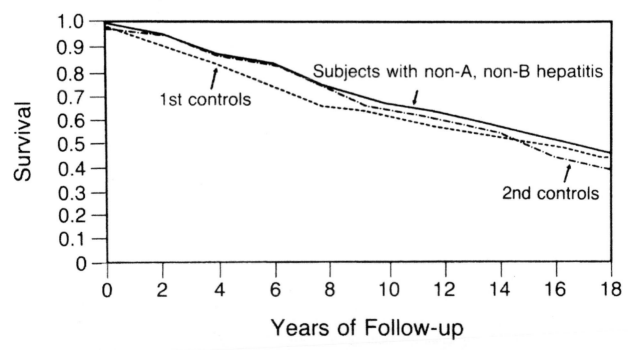

FIG. 1. Mortality from all causes among subjects with non-A, non-B hepatitis, first controls, and second controls. (From Ref. 24.)

childhood or in young female adults. A recent 45-year follow-up study of 8568 young male army recruits (of whom 0.1% of white and 1.8% of African-Americans were confirmed anti-HCV positive) showed that mortality from liver disease was negligible. Only one of the six deaths (16.8%) in those with HCV infection was due to liver disease; the death rate from liver disease in the uninfected recruits was 6.8%.[27] Two Japanese studies (one with 1500 cases of chronic hepatitis C[28] and the other with 70[29]) of serial liver biopsies in untreated patients with varying severities of liver disease due to hepatitis C, present for an unknown duration, indicated that the rate of progression to cirrhosis can be predicted from the pattern seen on baseline histology; that is, if minimal or no fibrosis and/or inflammation is present the likelihood of cirrhosis developing over the next 15 years was 10 to 30%, whereas a score of 3 out of 4 for fibrosis and/or inflammation virtually guarantees cirrhosis within 15 years.

The rate of progression of fibrosis is greatly influenced by the degree of alcohol consumption; in addition, male gender, age at acquisition, and background immune suppression appear to be additional risk factors for disease progression.[30] This and other studies report that the average rate of progression to cirrhosis in subjects with untreated hepatitis C ranges from 0.133 to 0.15 fibrosis units per year.[30,31] Hence, in most, hepatitis C is a very slowly progressive disease, certainly within the first 20 years of infection. Although more rapid progression is observed in those who acquire their infection over the age of 50 years this has little effect on overall mortality because of their age.[32]

Calculation of standardized mortality ratios in 838 German patients referred at different stages of their hepatitis C to a tertiary center indicated that those who were infected when they were less than 50 years of age and particularly those who had been infected for more than 15 years and who had cirrhosis at presentation were more likely to die of a hepatitis C related illness (SMR 30 [ratio of the overall mortality from hepatitis C relative to the general population]) than those who presented when they were greater than 50 years and had likely been infected for more than 15 years, with cirrhosis (SMR 3.9). Both the patient selection due to referral bias and the fact that the exact duration of infection and presence or absence of risk factors for progression were rarely known may have influenced these results. Such a study needs to be contrasted with the previously described long-term follow-up studies of persons infected at a known point in time. It is clear that once a diagnosis of hepatitis C has been made, a patient should be advised that regular consumption of alcohol will enhance the rate of progression of their chronic hepatitis C. If advice to abstain or consume only minimal amounts of alcohol is heeded, this will likely have a marked benefit on the natural history of their hepatitis C infection.

The Role of Liver Biopsy

A pretreatment liver biopsy is helpful in determining the urgency with which therapy should be instituted. If noninvasive investigations such as ultrasonography or computer tomography scan suggest that cirrhosis is clearly present, then a liver biopsy is not required. But in the absence of such findings, there is currently no other reliable test to assess the degree of hepatic fibrosis. Studies indicate that percutaneous liver biopsies can be performed safely in the outpatient setting, with a relatively low complication rate,[33,34] thus minimizing cost. If and when the therapeutic options become highly effective and less toxic, one might advocate treatment for all those infected with hepatitis C and thus perhaps forgo the biopsy. Until that time, a liver biopsy that indicates little or no fibrosis can reassure a patient who feels the cost-to-benefit ratio of treatment is high and that it is likely quite safe to wait a few years (in the absence of daily alcohol consumption) for more effective therapies. On the other hand, it could be argued that as the efficacy of current therapies may be greater in young persons with mild disease,[8] it might be best to treat sooner rather than later. The decision to treat should be determined by the patient's own level of comfort with untreated disease. Although a liver biopsy adds to both the risk and the cost of investigation, these costs have to be weighed against both the risk and cost of treatment, which may not be necessary at a time when only mild disease is present. Such patients who opt for no treatment because their disease is mild should be followed and advised to undergo repeat liver biopsy in 3 years or so, as a third (so called "rapid fibrosis") may develop progressive disease over this period of time.[35]

Will Treatment Improve the Quality of Life in Symptomatic CHC?

Subjects with hepatitis C recruited to randomized controlled trials (RCTs) conducted at tertiary referral centres are not representative of the population at large who have chronic hepatitis C. For one reason or another (often because of symptoms), patients recruited to trials have sought medical attention and are willing to subject themselves to the rigors of a clinical trial. Two reports from large studies, one on the effect of IFN monotherapies (either alfa 2b or alfa-con-1)[36] and the other comparing IFN-alfa-2b monotherapy with IFN-alfa-2b combined with ribavirin in the retreatment of patients who had relapsed after treatment with IFN monotherapy,[37] have rigorously assessed the quality of life (QOL) before and after treatment using the SF-36 survey. The SF-36 survey has been well validated in several chronic disease states. The questionnaire covers a broad range of items that may affect a persons quality of life, in a nondisease specific way, but it does not specifically ask questions regarding fatigue—a complaint of many patients with CHC. The SF-36 survey only takes 15 minutes or less to complete and has been shown to be reliable. Both studies reported that some but not all aspects of patient QOL were improved if a sustained response (biochemical with or without a virological response) is achieved. Unavoidable bias is present due to the natural desire of patients to know at the time their blood samples are taken of the effect of treatment on these blood tests performed during and after therapy. This knowledge likely influences the replies to any such questionnaire, hence improvement in aspects of QOL were seen both in those with only a biochemical response (return of serum aminotransferase levels to normal) and in those with a sustained biochemical and virologic response.[36] Unfortunately, "labeling" someone as being infected with hepatitis C appears to have a profound psychological effect, as demonstrated in one large study of women infected with "tainted" globulin factors.[38] To treat chronic hepatitis C only to improve the QOL alone is probably inappropriate as there is no guarantee that a patient's most troublesome pretreatment symptoms will disappear even if a sustained virological response is achieved.

Situations Where There is Currently No Documented Proof that Treatment for Hepatitis C Infection Will Be Beneficial

Patients with Normal Serum Aminotransferase Values

There have been no RCTs of sufficient size to indicate that current antiviral therapy is efficacious in patients who have consistently *normal ALT levels* in the presence of HCV RNA in serum, despite ongoing hepatitis on liver histology. Such patients tend to have milder disease than those with persistently elevated ALT values.[39] However, the biochemical pattern may fluctuate, and hence such patients should be observed regularly.

Coinfection with HIV and/or Hepatitis B

The long-term efficacy of IFN alfa monotherapy in patients with chronic hepatitis C coinfected with HIV may be less than in HIV negative subjects although the response rate in HIV coinfected individuals likely varies according to the degree of immune competence.[40,41] Another study[42] indicated that a sustained virologic response of 22.5% using IFN monotherapy was

obtained in HIV-positive patients that was not significantly different from that observed in HIV-negative patients recruited to the same trial (SR 25%). Relapse rates were no different in HIV-positive and HIV-negative patients. The institution of highly active antiretroviral therapy has markedly improved the survival of HIV-infected subjects. Studies of the natural history of HCV and coinfection with HIV have indicated a more rapidly progressive HCV-associated liver disease occurs, but these studies mostly eminate before the introduction of highly active antiretroviral therapy.[43] The need to more effectively treat these HCV/HIV coinfected patients is urgent. There are several ongoing trials of different antiviral regimens in subjects coinfected with HCV and HIV. It is of concern that in vitro ribavirin inhibits the action of zidovudine, and hence this drug should probably be withdrawn and appropriately replaced before instituting any treatment for HCV.[44] As we do not know if ribavirin may affect the efficacy of other new drugs used to treat HIV, careful monitoring of HIV RNA levels and possibly CD4 numbers needs to be maintained during these trials. HCV/HIV coinfected patient should not be treated outside the context of a formal carefully monitored trial.

As the long-term outcome of individuals coinfected with hepatitis C and B suggests a higher rate of progressive liver disease and HCC, effective treatment for such individuals is of particular importance. One viral infection generally inhibits the other, so it is essential to measure both HBV DNA and HCV RNA to determine which infection is active and treat accordingly. The optimum therapy for active hepatitis B is not the topic of this chapter.

Patients with Chronic Hepatitis C and Other Concurrent Diseases

Persons who require repeated treatments with blood or blood products (i.e., subjects with thalassemia and other hemolytic anemias and those with congenital coagulation abnormalities) have a very high rate of liver disease due to infection with hepatitis C with or without coinfection with HIV.[45] There have been few reported therapeutic trials for hepatitis C in persons with thalassemia. Such patients tend to have marked iron overload. It has been suggested that this may reduce the effectiveness of antiviral therapy, although the data supporting this are weak. A pilot study of IFN alfa 2b and ribavirin in subjects with thalassemia indicating that as long as the hemoglobin could be maintained with transfusion, the treatment was safe, but the trial was too small to have the power to assess efficacy.[46] There have been a number of trials of IFN alfa therapy in subjects with hemophilia and hepatitis C. Some suggest response to treatment in this setting is poor; more recent reports of trials using combination therapy have indicated similar antiviral efficacy to subjects with HCV infection without hemophilia.[47] In this study, liver biopsies performed with appropriate factor coverage were reported to be safe and most patients were found to have mild disease (these patients were not coinfected with HIV).

As previously mentioned, ribavirin cannot be given to patients with renal failure. IFN alfa is poorly tolerated in patients with end-stage renal disease, and thus no good data support its use in this clinical setting.[48] The outcome of renal transplantation in patients with renal failure and chronic hepatitis C shows that both the graft and patient survival at 10 but not at 5 years posttransplant is significantly less than in uninfected patients with a renal transplant.[49] Treatment cannot be given to patients with hepatitis C who already have a kidney transplant because IFN causes an unacceptable rate of rejection.[50]

Nonhepatic Disease Caused by HCV

Symptomatic cryoglobulinenemia caused by HCV infection is associated with significant morbidity and mortality, independent of any liver disease. Death may result from renal failure or systemic vasculitis. There may also be an association with nonHodgkin's lymphoma, generally but not always confined to the bone marrow, in patients with cryoglobulinenemia. One randomized controlled trial of IFN alfa-2a monotherapy[51] and several case series[52–59] indicated that treatment with alfa-IFN is effective in eradicating the cryoglobulinenemia, improving renal function, and eliminating the symptoms of vasculitis although no beneficial effect on neuropathy is said to occur. However, the general experience is that posttreatment relapse is common, this may not be the case when IFN-alfa-2b plus ribavirin is used. Studies have indicated that IFN-alfa therapy causes regression of low-grade lymphoma whether systemic or confined to the bone marrow.[54,56] As in other situations where a disease is rare, it is unlikely that there will ever be studies of sufficient size to indicate the true effectiveness of therapy in hepatitis C associated cryoglobulinenemia. Hence, the difficulty in persuading insurance companies to fund treatment for such patients, which often requires long term therapy to maintain symptomatic improvement.

Reinfection of Liver Allograft

The immunosuppressive therapy required to prevent rejection enhances viral replication so that very high viral titers develop postliver transplant and thus an antiviral effect from therapy with IFN alfa, although it may occur, is rare and transient.[60,61] In one study which employed IFNα2b plus ribavirin for the first 6 months post liver transplant, followed by a further 6 months of ribavirin monotherapy, loss of detectable HCV RNA in serum, and

normalization of ALT was observed in 50%.[62] Long term follow-up data are not currently available. Azathioprine was avoided in these patients because of its potential interaction with ribavirin. Antiviral therapy, either IFN monotherapy or in combination with ribavirin, is very poorly tolerated in subjects with a liver transplant. Data indicate that a high viral load pretransplant may predict more rapidly progressive liver disease after liver transplantation due to recurrent hepatitis C.[63] Pretransplant IFN treatment to lower the viral load is very risky, as reduction in the absolute neutrophil count may precipitate septicemia in a patient with decompensated cirrhosis. Induction of "rejection" is not a problem when IFN alfa is given to patients with a reinfected liver allograft.

HOST AND VIRAL FACTORS WHICH MAY INFLUENCE DECISIONS REGARDING TREATMENT

Host Factors

Age, Gender, and Racial Influences

A number of host factors appear to affect response to antiviral therapy in hepatitis C. Again, these issues need to be discussed with patients so they can weigh the risks and benefits of therapy. Younger patients respond better than older, and females respond better than males.[8] It has been noted that Afro-Americans have a significantly poorer response to IFN-alfa monotherapy[64] but not to treatment with IFN alfa-2b and ribavirin.[65] Whereas "ageism" may be appropriate, "sexism" and "racism" is not!

Cirrhosis

Recently published reports on the efficacy of IFN-alfa monotherapy in purely cirrhotic populations with hepatitis C suggest that a sustained virologic response similar to that observed in the non-cirrhotic can be achieved.[66–68] One large study also restricted to subjects with chronic hepatitis C and cirrhosis or "transition" to cirrhosis (reported in abstract form only) indicated that the long-acting PEG40kd IFN-alfa-2a (given once a week) is both safe and more effective than standard IFN-alfa-2a.[69] The effectiveness of combination therapy in cirrhotics cannot be accurately evaluated in the population studied so far, because there were too few patients with fibrosis and/or cirrhosis in the two large trials.[6,7] Even when the data from these two studies were combined, the number of subjects with severe fibrosis/cirrhosis was still too small to make any meaningful comparisons of efficacy with the very large number of patients with only grades 1 and 2 fibrosis.[8]

Immunologic Factors

Interferons are immunostimulants and so IFN-alfa therapy should not be given to patients with autoimmune disease. An "autoimmune hepatitis" induced by INF has been described,[70] but pretreatment screening for autoantibodies was not helpful in predicting this response, and hence testing serum for antinuclear antibody (ANA) and smooth muscle antibody (SMA) is probably unnecessary before starting therapy. Specific class II human leukocyte antigen (HLA) types have been linked with the likelihood of response to therapy, but these are only small factors in determining response to therapy and tissue typing does not need to be performed.[71]

Viral Factors

All therapeutic trials of antiviral therapy in chronic hepatitis C have consistently shown that *viral genotype* and pre-treatment *viral titre* are major factors which determine response to current antiviral therapies. This is the case whether alfa IFNs are given as monotherapy[72–74] or combined with Ribavirin.[75]

Viral Genotype

Testing for viral genotype using current techniques is reliable and dual infections are uncommon. Genotypes 1a and 1b, which predominate in North America are the most resistant to currently available antiviral therapies, and the reasons have not been clarified. The less common genotypes in North America namely genotypes 2 and 3 (more common in Europe and Australia) respond much better to antiviral therapy. Genotypes 4, 5, and 6 appear to respond to combination therapy less well than genotypes 2 and 3 but better than 1a and 1b; however, the number of patients with genotypes 4, 5 and 6 was very small in the large U.S. trial.[6]

Viral Load

The measurement of viral load (actually, serum viral particle concentration) is unreliable in that it is very technique dependent. There is currently no gold standard for the measurement of HCV RNA. The qualitative tests are more sensitive than the quantitative tests, but it is the latter that are most helpful in deciding treatment plans for the patient. A factor that has not been examined extensively but may be very important is whether measurement in whole blood is more accurate than in plasma.[16] What is considered a low or a high viral titer is to a considerable degree arbitrary. A value of 2 million copies/mL was used as the boundary separating low (<2 million) from high (>2 million) titers in the initial reports from large studies comparing IFN-alfa-2b monotherapy with IFN-alfa-con-1 and again when comparing the former with the same IFN combined with ribavirin.[6,7] But there is likely quite a range around this figure that predicts the likelihood of response to therapy. In the reanalysis of these two large trials of combination therapy, the cutoff was changed to 3.5 million copies/mL this being considered by the authors to be the more appropriate dividing line.[8] If treatment with IFN-alfa monotherapy is given then it appears that both IFN-alfa-con-1[72] and IFN-alfa-n-1[73] (not licensed in the United States) are more likely to give rise to a sustained virologic response than IFN alfa 2b, when the baseline viral load is high (Fig. 2).

The first studies using IFN alfa 2b combined with ribavirin indicated that the sustained antiviral effect was significantly greater than with IFN-alfa 2b monotherapy in all patients, including those with high viral loads.[75] In the European trial[7] when combination therapy was used to treat genotype 2 and 3 infections, the treatment response appeared to be independent of viral load or duration of therapy, (i.e., 6 or 12[7] months) (Tables 3 and 4). In addition, the data presented showed that genotype 1 infections in patients with a viral load of <2 million copies/mL could attain a similar response rate following treatment with 6 or 12 months, whereas patients with genotype 1 infection and a viral load of >2 million copies/ml had a greater sustained virologic response after 12 months than they did after only 6 months of treatment. Now that the results from this study have been combined with a similar study from the United States, and the cutoff values for high and low viral load changed to >3.5 or <3.5 million copies/mL, the response rates according to duration of therapy and geno-

TABLE 4. Percent of Sustained Virologic Response: IFN-a-2b + Ribavirin vs. IFN-a-2b Monotherapy—European[7] vs. U.S.[6] Studies

	Combination Therapy for 48 Weeks		Combination Therapy for 24 Weeks		IFN for 48 Weeks	
	European	United States	European	United States	European	United States
Overall efficacy	42	38	17	31	19	12
Genotype						
1	31	28	18	16	16	7
2, 3, other	64	66	65	69	33	29

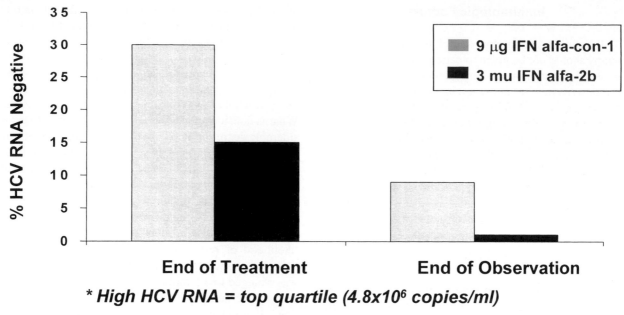

FIG. 2.   HCV RNA response in patients with high HCV RNA titers.* (From Ref. 73.)

type are different. The sustained virologic response rates for genotypes 1, 4, 5 or 6 infections when the "low" cutoff has been reset at the higher level of 3.5×10^6 c/mL is now 33% after 48 weeks versus 26% after 24 weeks of combination therapy.[8] In those with genotype 2 or 3 who had fibrosis, the sustained virologic response was in 17 of 26 patients (65%) treated for 24 weeks versus 20 of 25 patients (80%) in those treated for 48 weeks ($p = 0.30$). However, the authors conclude that 48 weeks of therapy should be given to almost all patients.

Quasispecies

More recently, the number and diversity of quasispecies (see review by Farci and Purcell in *Seminars in Liver Disease,* Volume 21, number 1, 2000) have been identified as another possible determinant of response to therapy in both naive and treated patients. However, identification of quasispecies demands time consuming and expensive sequence analyses, and hence, for the present, will remain within the confines of the research laboratory.

Overall Risk Assessment

The data collected in the European trial of IFNα2b versus IFNα2b + Ribavirin[7] and now the data from the combination of the data from this trial with that from the US trial[8] indicate that aside from genotype and viral load there are a number of risk factors which play a role

(said to be responsible for only 20% of the variability in response rates) in predicting the likelihood of a sustained response to therapy in an individual patient. These factors being: gender, age of patient, stage of fibrosis. However, when therapeutic studies have been confined to cirrhotic populations,[66–68] it is not so obvious that patients with cirrhosis have a lower response rate to antiviral therapy, and unless their liver disease is decompensated, the presence of cirrhosis should not exclude patients from antiviral therapy. The cost effectiveness ratio of treating older patients becomes prohibitive, and when ribavirin is employed, a marked increase in toxicity is likely because of the higher prevalence of vascular disease in the elderly.

TREATMENT/MONITORING SCHEDULES FOR PATIENTS WITH CHRONIC HEPATITIS C

Treatment of Naive Patients

Once it is decided that antiviral therapy is appropriate in a given patient the consensus, at least in Canada and Europe,[4,5] based on results of peer reviewed literature, has been to opt for treatment with standard IFN-alfa-2b given subcutaneously three times a week combined with ribavirin 1000 to 1200 mg/day po (in the absence of absolute contraindications to either drug). No dose ranging data indicate that this is the optimal dose of combination therapy—it could well be that smaller doses of ribavirin may be just as effective with fewer side effects. However, studies are needed to assess this. In addition results of oral ribavirin given in combination with INF other than IFN-alfa-2b are eagerly awaited, especially when given in combination with long acting (pegylated) IFNs. An abstract of a pilot study suggests an advantage to this combination.[76] The long-acting pegylated IFNs, given once weekly, are much more efficacious than standard short-acting IFN-alfas given on an intermittent, usually three times a week, basis,[69] likely because serum IFN levels do not fluctuate with the former. Hence pegylated interferons once licensed are likely to become the "standard" of care, likely in combination with ribavirin.

The published data indicate that it is essential to establish both the viral genotype and viral titer pretreatment to determine the appropriate duration of therapy. The data from trials using IFN-alfa monotherapy showed that if serum HCV RNA (using the more sensitive qualitative analysis) remains detectable at 12 weeks into therapy, the patient can be considered a "nonresponder"[77–79] and consideration should be given to abandoning further treatment at this time. In those whose HCV RNA becomes undetectable at any time up to 12 weeks, therapy should be continued for the full duration. When testing for HCV RNA is measured in serum, there is currently no way to predict who will have a sustained viral loss after cessation of an adequate course of treatment or who will relapse of those whose HCV RNA became undetectable during treatment. If the qualitative test for HCV RNA (lower limit of detectability, 100 copies/mL) is still positive at 12 weeks, data published in abstract form only suggests that there is up to a 9% chance that if treatment with IFN-α2b plus ribavirin is continued the patient will eventually become a sustained responder.[80]

It is likely that once quantitative HCV RNA testing is better established, the log decline of serum HCV RNA over the first few weeks or months of therapy may be sufficient to predict at least those patients who will definitely be a nonresponder, thus permitting savings both financially (from continued monitoring and treatment) and personally (from drug side effects) by stopping treatment at this point. The reanalysis of the combined data from the two large trials of combination therapy stated that in patients with more than 400,000 copies/mL 4 weeks into treatment have no chance of responding when 24 weeks of therapy is given. For those patients given 48 weeks of treatment, the negative predictive value of greater than 400,000 copies/mL at week 4 and week 12 was 96.7% and 100%, respectively; however, the authors did not suggest that treatment should be stopped at 12 weeks if the viral load fails to fall below 400,000 copies/mL. This study indicates that it would seem more appropriate to perform quantitative HCV RNA at 12 weeks using a test that has a cut off of <400,000 copies/mL. Two small studies,[81,82] the latter published in abstract form only, both indicate that non-responders to treatment with either IFN-alfa-2b monotherapy or with IFN-alfa-2b and ribavirin can be predicted by the degree decline of serum HCV RNA (quantitative testing necessary), within the first few weeks, using either therapy.

Monitoring of Toxicity and Response

Initially, weekly checks of the hemoglobin, absolute neutrophil count, and platelet count are required to detect toxicity. Instructions regarding dose reduction and the need for cessation of treatment are well documented in consensus reports. Because the effects of combination therapy on the complete blood count are maximal during the first months of treatment, it is essential that the patient and treating medical personnel are readily available to discuss the potential need to change drug doses. It is equally important that the tolerability of therapy is discussed with the patient and perhaps even with their household members. Some patients may find that the treatment interferes with their work performance. In some instances, a change in work schedule, (e.g., shift change) may alleviate this problem. Outside the context of clinical trials, the withdrawal rate during treatment is unknown. Data from published trials with an unusually high level of commitment have indicated that both increasing the duration of therapy and the use of combination therapy increase the withdrawal rate. The withdrawal rate in those randomized to 48 weeks of IFN monotherapy was 13 to 14%. In those randomized to combination therapy, 8% withdrew before 24 weeks and those randomized to 48 weeks of combination therapy 19 to 21% withdrew. Clearly, the tolerability to combination therapy wanes after 24 weeks, so that the new proposal that most patients should be treated for this period of time[8] may in practice be unrealistic (hence the urgent need for better and less toxic therapies).

After the cessation of treatment, it is necessary to assess whether the end of treatment response (normalization of ALT, undetectability of HCV RNA) is maintained so as to determine whether a sustained response has been achieved. The measurement of HCV RNA (using the more sensitive qualitative technique) at 6 months after the cessation of treatment is a reliable indicator of whether the response to either IFN alfa monotherapy or to combination therapy will be durable in the long term.[9,11,13–15] Because the lower limit of detection of HCV RNA varies between methods, it is essential that the most sensitive technique is used to be confident of the results. It is unusual (<5%) that once serum HCV RNA is undetectable by qualitative polymerase chain reaction at 6 months after treatment cessation, relapse will occur. However, it is probably wise to check the serum HCV RNA in "responders" annually for at least 2 years after cessation of therapy, as just occasionally HCV RNA detection is intermittent. Repeat liver biopsy at the end of successful treatment is unnecessary because published studies have shown liver histology remains stable or improves in patients with a sustained virologic response to current antiviral therapies.[9,11] Reinfection may occur, hence the reason not to start treatment in those actively using intravenous drugs and/or cocaine.

Relapsers to IFN Alfa Monotherapy

When alfa IFNs were the only therapeutic options for hepatitis C and particularly when treatment was given for only 6 months, relapse after successful treatment (defined as normalization of ALT $\pm$ loss of detectable HCV RNA) was common. The introduction of combination therapy for naive patients has reduced the end of treatment relapse rate considerably. For those patients who did respond to IFN-alfa monotherapy but who subsequently relapsed, retreatment either with combination therapy for 6 months or high dose IFN-alfa-con-1 (15 μg, tiw) for 12 months has been shown to induce a sustained response rate of 49% and 58% respectively.[(83,84)] One study that randomized previous IFN monotherapy relapsers or nonresponders to either retreatment with IFN-alfa-2a 4.5 Mu three times a week or IFN-alfa-2a (4.5 mu ttw) plus Ribavirin 1000–1200 mg/d for the same duration (6 months) found no difference in the sustained virologic response between these two groups, but the responses were very much genotype dependant.[85] Two recent reports, one from the combined data of six trials of combination therapy for relapsers from previous IFN monotherapy[86] and the other a single study,[87] showed lower sustained response rates, 13% for genotype 1 and 36% for genotypes 2 and 3 in one[86] and an overall sustained response of 30% to retreatment after 24 months of combination therapy in the other.[87] Now that the role of viral genotype and viral load as predictors of response have been clarified, it is likely that the duration of combination therapy for IFN monotherapy relapsers should be as for naive patients. Approximately 25% of those who previously responded and subsequently relapsed after IFN-alfa monotherapy fail to respond to retreatment. It has been speculated that this reflects the development of resistant quasispecies.[88]

Non-responders to IFN Alfa Therapy

High dose IFN-alfa-2b monotherapy does not appear to enhance the sustained virologic response rate in chronic hepatitis C.[89] Whereas the success of retreatment of primary nonresponders to IFN-alfa monother-

apy with combination therapy depends on genotype, it appears to be independent of background histology. A sustained response in genotype 2 or 3 infections may be observed in up to 29% of cirrhotic prior nonresponders to IFN monotherapy, but in genotype 1 infections the sustained virological response rate in cirrhotics is only 8%.[86] Thus the decision to retreat a nonresponder to IFN-alfa monotherapy with combination therapy may not be warranted except for those infected with genotype 2 or 3. Some so called nonresponders are in fact "breakthroughs,"[90] that is, patients in whom sometime during antiviral therapy HCV RNA becomes undetectable but, despite continued treatment, reappears by the end of treatment. Patients who breakthrough can only be detected if repeated HCV RNA testing is conducted during treatment. However, this is not cost effective and is only performed in the context of a clinical trial. It has been shown that breakthrough patients are more likely to respond to subsequent re-treatment than true nonresponders.[91]

Recent reports suggest that continued treatment with antiviral therapy despite the absence of a sustained virologic response may induce a histological response at least in those who showed a histologic improvement after their initial course of treatment was completed and a fall in viral load by greater than a log.[23,92] This has prompted long term trials of therapy be conducted in such patients. At present, retreatment in this situation should be restricted to clinical trials.

Nonresponders to Combination Therapy, Such as IFN-alfa-2b Plus Ribavirin

No satisfactory antiviral therapy for such patients has been reported. "Induction" IFN alfa therapy (i.e., high dose) daily treatment for the first few months followed by standard intermittent IFN-alfa therapy may increase the end of treatment response, but fails to enhance the sustained response rate.[93] The addition of other agents eg: nonsteroidal anti-inflammatory agents,[94] ursodeoxycholic acid[95] do not enhance the antiviral response. Adjunctive therapy with the immunomodulary agent thymosinα may enhance the end of treatment viral response, but there is insufficient data indicate its long-term effectiveness.[96]

SUMMARY

Patients chronically infected with hepatitis C who have an ongoing hepatitis as judged by persistent elevation in serum ALT levels and histologic evidence of progressive liver disease (i.e., marked inflammation and/or fibrosis or cirrhosis who have no absolute contraindications to currently licensed treatments) should be offered therapy. However, it is essential that before the initiation of treatment, the patient be fully cognizant of the likelihood of their achieving a sustained response, the potential duration of therapy, the full array of treatment side effects, and the need to practice "safer sex" and to comply with regular monitoring of blood tests and QOL issues throughout treatment. The timing of the treatment should be tailored to the patients other activities, because once treatment is started it requires considerable commitment both on the part of the patient, their family, and the attending health care personnel. In addition, patients with serious extrahepatic manifestations of hepatitis C (e.g., cryoglobulinemia and all its complications) may also benefit, at least symptomatically, from treatment of their hepatitis C regardless of their liver status.

Whether subjects who have mild inflammation and little to no fibrosis should be treated immediately or await more effective less toxic therapies is debatable. Their 10-year prognosis is excellent, although some, about a third, will develop progressive fibrosis and hence repeat biopsy is necessary within 3 years if a delay in therapy is chosen. The ultimate decision to treat or not to treat in these circumstances lies with the patient.

No data from randomized controlled clinical trials prove that antiviral therapy enhances patient survival either from liver disease and its complications or the nonhepatic manifestations of chronic hepatitis C infection. This is because long term follow-up studies of randomized controlled trials have not been done, because treatment became licensed shortly after the defining therapeutic trials had been completed. However, it is logical to presume that a sustained virologic response that halts liver disease progression will enhance patient survival (at least from their liver disease and perhaps even from the complications thereof, e.g., HCC). At the same time, it is important to bear in mind that most persons infected with hepatitis C are not only currently unaware of their infection, but for many, their untreated infection with hepatitis C will not alter their overall survival.

ABBREVIATIONS

CHC   chronic hepatitis C
HCC   hepatocellular carcinoma
HCV   hepatitis C virus
IFN   interferon
QOL   quality of life

REFERENCES

1. Maddrey W. Safety of combination interferon alfa-2b/ribavirin therapy in chronic hepatitis C-relapsed and treatment-naïve patients. Seminars Liver Dis 1999;19:67–75

2. Renault P and Hoofnaagle J. Side effects of alpha interferon. Semin in Liver Dis 1989;9:273–277

3. Glue P. The clinical pharmacology of ribavirin. Sem Liver Dis 1999;19:17–24

4. Please see www.lhsc.on.ca/casl/

5. Consensus statement. EASL international consensus conference on hepatitis C. Paris, 26–28 February 1999. J Hepatol 1999; 30:956–961

6. McHutchison J, Gordon S, Schiff E, et al. Interferon alfa 2b alone or in combination with ribavirin as initial treatment for chronic hepatitis C. N Eng J Med 1198;339:1485–1492

7. Poynard T, Marcellin P, Lee S, et al. Randomised trial of interferon alpha 2b plus ribavirin for 48 weeks or for 24 weeks versus interferon alpha 2b plus placebo for 48 weeks for treatment of chronic infection with hepatitis C virus. Lancet 1998;352: 1426–1432

8. Poynard T, McHutchison J, Goodman Z, Ling M, and Albrecht J. Is an "a la carte" combination interferon alfa-2b plus ribavirin regimen possible for the first line treatment in patients with chronic hepatitis C? Hepatology 2000;31:211–218

9. Marcellin P, Boyer N, Gervais A, et al. Long-term histologic improvement and loss of detectable intrahepatic HCV RNA in patients with chronic hepatitis C and sustained response to interferon-α therapy. Ann Intern Med 1997;127:875–881

10. Camma C, Di Marco V, Lo Iacono O, et al. Long-term course of interferon-treated chronic hepatitis C. J Hepatol 1998;28: 531–537

11. Lau D, Kleiner DE, Ghany MG, Park Y, Schmid P, Hoofnagle J. 10-Year follow-up after Interferon-α therapy for chronic hepatitis C. Hepatology 1998;28:1121–1127

12. Niederau C, Lange S, Heintges T, et al. Prognosis of chronic hepatitis C: Results of a large, prospective cohort study. Hepatology 1998;28:1687–1695

13. Sim H, Yim C, Krajden M, Heathcote J. Durability of serological remission in chronic hepatitis C treated with Interferon alpha-2b. Am J Gastroenteral 1998;93:39–43

14. Reichard O, Glaumann H, Fryden A, Norkans G, Wejstal R, Weiland O. Long-term follow-up of chronic hepatitis C patients with sustained virological response to alpha-interferon. J Hepatol 1999;30:783–787

15. Davis G, McHutchison J, Poynard T, et al. Durability of viral response to interferon alone or in combination with oral ribavirin in patients with chronic hepatitis C [Abstract # 570]. Hepatology 1999;30:303A

16. Schmidt WS, Wu P, Brashear D, et al. Effect of Interferon therapy on hepatitis C virus RNA in whole blood, plasma and peripheral mononuclear cells. Hepatology 1998;28: 1110–1116

17. Nishiguchi S, Kuroki T, Nakatani S, et al. Randomized trial of effects of interferon-α on incidence of hepatocellular carcinoma in chronic active hepatitis C with cirrhosis. Lancet 1995;346: 1051–1055

18. Mazzella G, Accogli E, Sottili S, et al. Alpha interferon treatment may prevent hepatocellular carcinoma in HCV-related liver cirrhosis. J Hepatol 1996;24:141–147

19. Imai Y, Kawata S, Tamura S, et al. Relation of interferon therapy and hepatocellular carcinoma in patients with chronic hepatitis C. Ann Intern Med 1998;129:94–99

20. Kasahara A, Hayashi N, Mochizuki K, et al. Risk factors for hepatocellular carcinoma and its incidence after interferon treatment in patients with chronic hepatitis C. Hepatology 1998;27: 1394–1402

21. Fattovich G, Giustina G, Degos F, et al. Effectiveness of interferon alfa on incidence of hepatocellular carcinoma and decompensation in cirrhosis type C. J Hepatol 1997;27:201–205

22. Yoshida H, Shiratori Y, Moriyama M, et al. Interferon therapy reduces the risk for hepatocellular carcinoma: National surveil-

lance program of cirrhotic and noncirrhotic patients with chronic hepatitis C in Japan. Ann Intern Med 1999;131:174–181

23. Shiffman M, Hofmann C, Contos M, et al. A randomized controlled trial of maintenance Interferon therapy for patients with chronic hepatitis C virus and persistent viremia. Gastroenterology 1999;117:1164–1172

24. Seeff L, Buskell-Bales Z, Wright E, et al. Long-term mortality after transfusion-associated non-a, non-b hepatitis. N Eng J Med 1992;327:1906–1911

25. Vogt M, Lang T, Frosner G, et al. Pevalence and clinical outcome of hepatitis C infection in children who underwent cardiac surgery before the implementation of blood-donor screening. N Eng J Med 1999;341:866–870

26. Kenny-Walsh E. Clinical outcomes after hepatitis C infection from contaminated anti-D immune globulin. N Eng J Med 1999;340:1228–1233

27. Seeff LB, Miller RN, Rabkin CS, et al. 45 year follow-up of hepatitis C virus infection in healthy young adults. Ann Intern Med 2000;132:105–111

28. Ikeda K, Saitoh S, Suzuki Y, et al. Disease progression and hepatocellular carcinogenesis in patients with chronic viral hepatitis: A prospective observation of 2215 patients. J Hepatol 1998; 28:930–938

29. Yano M, Kumada H, Kage M, et al. The long-term pathological evolution of chronic hepatitis C. Hepatology 1996;23: 1334–1340

30. Poynard T, Bedossa P, Opolon P. Natural history of liver fibrosis progression in patients with chronic hepatitis C. Lancet 1997;349:825–832

31. Wali M, Lewis S, Hubscher S, et al. Histological progression during short-term follow-up of patients with chronic hepatitis C virus infection. J Viral Hepat 1999;6:445–452

32. Niederau C, Lange S, Heintges T, et al. Prognosis of chronic hepatitis C: Results of a large, prospective cohort study. Hepatology 1998;28:1687–1695

33. Garcia-Tsao G, Boyer J. Outpatient liver biopsy: How safe is it? Ann Intern Med 1993;118:150–153

34. Piccinino F, Sagnelli E, Pasquale G, et al. Complications following percutaneous liver biopsy: A multicentre retrospective study on 68,276 biopsies. J Hepatol 1986;2:165–173

35. Sobelsky R, Mathurin P, Charlotte F, et al. Modeling the impact of interferon alfa treatment on liver fibrosis progression in chronic hepatitis C: A dynamic view. Gastroenterology 1999; 116:378–386

36. Bonkovsky H, Woolley M, the Consensus Interferon Study Group. Reduction of health-related quality of life in chronic hepatitis C and improvement with Interferon therapy. Hepatology 1999;29:264–270

37. Ware JE, Bayliss M, Mannocchia M, Davis G, the International Hepatitis Interventional Therapy Group. Health-related quality of life in chronic hepatitis C: Impact of disease and treatment response. Hepatology 1999;30:550–555

38. Goh J, Coughlan B, Quinn J, O'Keane JC, Crowe J. Fatigue does not correlate with the degree of hepatitis or the presence of autoimmune disorders in chronic hepatitis C infection. Eur J Gastroenterol Hepatol 1999;11:833–838

39. Mathurin P, Moussalli J, Cadranel J, et al. Slow progression rate of fibrosis in hepatitis C virus patients with persistently normal alanine transaminase activity. Hepatology 1998;27:868–872

40. Boyer N, Marcellin P, Degott C, et al. Recombinant Interferon-α for chronic hepatitis C in patients positive for antibody to human immunodeficiency virus. J Infect Dis 1992;165:723–726

41. Marriott E, Navas S, del Romero J, Garcia S, Castillo I, Quiroga JA, Carreno V. Treatment with recombinant α-interferon of chronic hepatitis C in anti-HIV positive patients. J Med Virol 1993;40;107–111

42. Soriano V, Garcia-Samaniego J, Bravo R, et al. Interferon alpha for the treatment of chronic hepatitis C in patients infected with human immunodeficiency virus. Clin Infect Dis 1996;23: 585–591

43. Collier J, Heathcote J. Hepatitis C viral infection in the immunosuppressed patient. Hepatology 1998;27:2–6

44. Vogt MW, Hartshorn KL, Furman PA, et al. Ribavirin antagonizes the effect of azidothymidine on HIV replication. Science 1987;27:1376–1379

45. Darby S, Ewart D, Giangrande P, et al. Mortality from liver cancer and liver disease in haemophilic men and boys in UK given blood products contaminated with hepatitis C. Lancet 1997;350: 1425–1431

46. Telfer P, Garson J, Whitby K, et al. Combination therapy with interferon alpha and ribavirin for chronic hepatitis C virus infection in thalassaemic patients. Br J Haematol 1997;98:850–855

47. Lethagen S, Widell A, Berntorp E, Verbaan H, Lindgren S. Interferon and ribavirin treatment in patients with hemophilia or von Willebrand disease infected with hepatitis C: An update [Abstract # 430]. Haemophilia 1998;4:263

48. Fernandez JL, Rendo P, del Pino N. A double-blind controlled trial of recombinant interferon-α2b in hemodialysis patients with chronic hepatitis C virus infection and abnormal aminotransferase levels. J Viral Hepat 1997;4:113–119

49. Mathurin P, Mouquet C, Poynard T, et al. Impact of hepatitis B and C on kidney transplantation outcome. Hepatology 1999;29: 257–263

50. Rostaing L, Izopet J, Baron E, Duffaut M, Puel J, Durant D. Treatment of chronic hepatitis C with recombinant interferon alpha in kidney transplant recipients. Transplantation 1995;59: 1426–1431

51. Misiani R, Bellavita P, Fenilli D, et al. Interferon alfa-2a therapy in cryoglobulinemia associated with hepatitis C virus. N Eng J Med 1994;330:751–756

52. Disdier P, Harle JR, Weiller PJ. Interferon for mixed cryoglobulinemia associated with hepatitis C. Am J Med 1992;93:115–116

53. Taillan B, Ferrari E, Garnier G, et al. Low-dose Interferon-α for mixed cryoglobulinemia associated with hepatitis c virus. Am J Med 1992;93:476

54. Mazzaro C, Franzin F, Tulissi P, et al. Regression of monoclonal B-cell expansion in patients affected by mixed cryoglobulinemia responsive to α-Interferon therapy. Cancer 1996;77:2604–2613

55. Ferri C, Zignego G, Longombardo M, et al. Effect of alpha-Interferon on hepatitis C virus chronic infection in mixed cryoglobulinemia patients. Infection 1993;2:93–97

56. Hermine O, Lefrere J, Bronowicki X, et al. Patients with splenic lymphoma with villous lymphocytes associated with hepatitis C infection may enter in complete clinical response after reduction of viral load. American Society of Hematology 41st Annual Meeting, December 6, 1999

57. Polzien F, Schott P, Mihm S, Ramadori G, Hartmann H. Interferon-α treatment of hepatitis C virus-associated mixed cryoglobulinemia. J Hepatol 1997;27:63–71

58. Sarac E, Bastacky S, Johnson J. Response to high-dose Interferon-α after failure of standard therapy in MPGN associated with hepatitis c virus infection. Am J Kidney Dis 1997;30: 113–115

59. Cresta P, Musset L, Cacoub P, et al. Response to interferon α treatment and disappearance of cryoglobulinaemia in patients infected by hepatitis C virus. Gut 1999;45:122–128

60. Wright T, Combs C, Kim M, et al. Interferon-α therapy for hepatitis C virus infection after liver transplantation. Hepatology 1994;20:773–779

61. Sheiner P, Boros P, Klion M, et al. The efficacy of prophylactic interferon alfa-2b in preventing recurrent hepatitis C after liver transplantation. Hepatology 1998;28:831–838

62. Bizollon T, Palazzo U, Ducerf C, et al. Pilot study of the combination of interferon alfa and ribavirin as therapy of recurrent hepatitis C after liver transplantation. Hepatology 1997;26: 500–504

63. Charlton M, Seaberg E, Wiesner R, Everhart J, et al. Predictors of patient and graft survival following liver transplantation for hepatitis C. Hepatology 1998;28:823–830

64. Reddy K, Hoofnagle J, Tong M, et al. Racial differences in responses to therapy with interferon in chronic hepatitis C. Hepatology 1999;30:787–793

65. McHutchison J, Poynard T, Gordon S, et al. The impact of race on response to anti-viral therapy in patients with chronic hepatitis C [Abstract # 568]. Hepatology 1999;30:302A

66. Everson G, Jensen DM, Craig JR, et al. Efficacy of Interferon treatment for patients with chronic hepatitis C: Comparison of response in cirrhotics, fibrotics or nonfibrotics. Hepatology 1999;30:271–276

67. Valla DC, Chevallier M, Marcellin P, et al. Treatment of hepatitis C virus-related cirrhosis: A randomized controlled trial of Interferon alfa-2b versus no treatment. Hepatology 1999;29: 1870–1875

68. Shiratori Y, Yokosuka O, Nakata R, et al. Prospective study of Interferon therapy for compensated cirrhotic patients with chronic hepatitis C by monitoring serum hepatitis C RNA. Hepatology 1999;29:1573–1580

69. Heathcote E, Shiffman M, Cooksley G, et al. Multinational evaluation of the efficacy and safety of once-weekly peginterferon alfa 2a (PEG-IFN) in patients with chronic hepatitis C (CHC) with compensated cirrhosis [Abstract # 621]. Hepatology 1999;30:316A

70. Garcia Buey L, Garcia-Monzon C, Rodriguez S, et al. Latent autoimmune hepatitis triggered during interferon therapy in patients with chronic hepatitis C. Gastroenterology 1995;108: 1770–1777

71. Sim KH, Wojcik JP, Margulies M, Wade J, Heathcote J. Human leukocyte antigen class II alleles may affect response of chronic hepatitis C to interferon therapy. J Viral Hepat 1998;5:249–253

72. Bell H, Hellum K, Harthug S, et al. Genotype, viral load and age as independent predictors of treatment outcome of interferon-α2a treatment in patients with chronic hepatitis C. Scand J Infect Dis 1997;29:17–22

73. Tong M, Reddy R, Lee W, et al. Treatment of chronic hepatitis C with consensus interferon: A multicenter, randomized, controlled trial. Hepatology 1997;26:747–754

74. Farrell G, Bacon B, Goldin R, the Clinical Advisory Group for the Hepatitis C Comparative Study. Lymphoblastoid interferon alfa-n1 improves the long-term response to a 6-month course of treatment in chronic hepatitis C compared with recombinant interferon alfa-2b: Results of an international randomized controlled trial. Hepatology 1998;27:1121–1127

75. Reichard O, Norkrans G, Fryden A, et al. Randomised, double-blind, placebo-controlled trial of interferon alfa 2b with and without ribavirin for chronic hepatitis C. Lancet 1998;351: 83–87

76. Sulkowski M, Reindollar R, Clin C, Yu J. Combination therapy with peginterferon alfa-2a (PEG-IFN) and ribavirin in the treatment of patients with chronic hepatitis C (CHC): A phase II open-label study [Abstract # 145]. Hepatology 1999;30:197A

77. Gavier B, Martinez-Gonzalez M, Riezu-Boj J, et al. Viremia after one month of interferon therapy predicts treatment outcome in patients with chronic hepatitis C. Gastroenterology 1997: 113:1647–1653

78. Neumann A, Lam N, Dahari H, et al. Hepatitis C viral dynamics in vivo and the antiviral efficacy of interferon alfa therapy. Science 1998;282:103–107

79. Zeuzem S, Lee J, Franke A, et al. Quantification of the initial decline of serum hepatitis C virus RNA and response to interferon alfa. Hepatology 1998;27:1149–1156

80. McHutchison JG, Gordon SC, Morgan T, et al. Predicting response to initial therapy with interferon alpha and ribavirin in chronic hepatitis C using serum HCV RNA during therapy [Abstract # 818]. Hepatology 1999;30:365A

81. Brouwer J, Hansen B, Niesters H, Schalm S. Early prediction of response in interferon monotherapy and in interferon-ribavirin combination therapy for chronic hepatitis C: HCV RNA at 4 weeks versus ALT. J Hepatol 1999;30:192–198

82. Neumann A, Dahari H, Univ B, et al. Early prediction and mechanism of the ribavirin/IFN alpha dual therapy effect on chronic hepatitis C virus (HCV) infection [Abstract # 595]. Hepatology 1999;30:309A

83. Davis GL, Esteban-Mur R, Rustigi V, et al. Interferon alfa 2b alone or in combination with ribavirin for the treatment of relapse of chronic hepatitis C. N Eng J Med 1998;339:1493–1499

84. Heathcote J, Keefe E, Lee S, et al. Re-treatment of chronic hepatitis C with consensus Interferon. Hepatology 1998;27: 1136–1143

85. Bell H, Hellum K, Harthug S, et al. Treatment with interferon-alpha2a alone or interferon-alpha2a plus ribavirin in patients with chronic hepatitis C previously treated with inteferon-alpha2a. Scand J Gastroenterol 1999;34:194–198

86. Schalm S, Weiland O, Hansen B. et al. Interferon-ribavirin for chronic hepatitis C with and without cirrhosis: Analysis of individual patient data of six controlled trials. Gastroenterology 1999;117:408–413

87. Barbaro G, Di Lorenzo G, Belloni G, et al. Interferon alpha-2b and ribavirin in combination for patients with chronic hepatitis C who failed to respond to, or relapsed after, interferon alpha therapy: A randomized trial. Am J Med 1999;107:112–118

88. Hassoba HM, Bzowej N, Berengner M, et al. Evolution of viral quasispecies in interferon treated patients with chronic hepatitis C infection. J Hepatol 1999;31:618–627

89. Lindsay K, Davis G, Schiff E, et al. Response to higher doses of Interferon alfa-2b in patients with chronic hepatitis C: A randomized multicenter trial. Hepatology 1996;24:1034–1040

90. Roffi L, Colloredo M, Antonelli G, et al. Breakthrough during recombinant Interferon alfa therapy in patients with chronic hepatitis C virus infection: Prevalence, etiology and management. Hepatology 1995;3:645–649

91. Heathcote E, James S, Mullen K, Hauser SC, Rosenblate H, Albert D, the Consensus Interferon Study Group. Chronic hepatitis C virus patients with breakthroughs during Interferon treatment can successfully be retreated with Consensus Interferon. Hepatology 1999;30:562–566

92. Shiffman M, Hofmann C, Thompson E, et al. Relationship between biochemical, virological, and histological response during Interferon treatment of chronic hepatitis C. Hepatology 1997;26:780–785

93. Shiffman ML. Use of high-dose interferon in the treatment of chronic hepatitis C. Semin Liver Dis 1999;19(s1):25–34

94. Zarski JP, Maynard-Muet M, Chousterman S, et al. Tenoxicam, a non-steroid anti-inflammatory drug, is unable to increase the response rate in patients with chronic hepatitis C treated by alpha Interferon. Hepatology 1998;27:862–867

95. Boucher E, Jouanolle H, Andre P, et al. Interferon and Ursodeoxycholic Acid combined therapy in the treatment of chronic viral C hepatitis: Results from controlled randomized trial in 80 patients. Hepatology 1995;21:322–327

96. Sherman K, Sherman SN. Interferon plus thymosin α-1 treatment of chronic hepatitis C infection: A meta analysis. Therap Viral Hepat 1998;48:379–383

Hepatitis C After Liver Transplantation

PATRICIA A. SHEINER, M.D.

ABSTRACT: *Hepatitis C is the most common cause of end-stage liver disease leading to liver transplant. The disease can recur after transplant, resulting in clinical hepatitis in up to 75% of patients and severe disease in approximately 7%. Treatment of rejection with steroid boluses and treatment of steroid-resistant rejection with OKT3 have both been shown to increase the incidence of recurrent hepatitis C. The use of OKT3 for steroid-resistant rejection is reportedly associated with more severe recurrence. The calcineurin inhibitors tacrolimus and cyclosporine have not been conclusively associated with different rates or severity of recurrence. Viral levels rise 10- to 15-fold after transplant and appear to be associated with the use of immunosuppression. Studies suggest that high viral levels, either pretransplant or early after transplant, may be associated with severe recurrent disease. Although the role of genotype is still unclear, genotype 1b is known to be associated with a poorer prognosis in nontransplanted patients and a lesser response to treatment than other genotypes. Furthermore, some reports suggest that after transplant, recurrent disease may progress more rapidly in patients with genotype 1. Treatment options after recurrence remain poor. Neither interferon nor ribavirin alone provides any true benefit. Combination therapy appears to have a better short-term outcome but may be poorly tolerated, and long-term benefits are unknown. Prophylaxis with combination therapy may be a better option but requires further study. Finally, retransplantation for recurrent hepatitis C is complicated not by rapid recurrence of disease in the new allograft but by high perioperative mortality that may be predicted by the presence of renal failure or sepsis pretransplant.*

KEY WORDS: hepatitis C, liver transplantation, recurrence, immunosuppression

Objectives

Upon completion of this article, the reader should be able to 1) understand the natural history of hepatitis C posttransplant and summarize risk factors for severe recurrence, 2) know results of treatment with the present available medications, and 3) be aware of factors that predict a high mortality rate with retransplantation.

Accreditation

The Indiana University School of Medicine is accredited by the Accreditation Council for Continuing Medical Education to provide continuing medical education for physicians.

Credit

The Indiana University School of Medicine designates this educational activity for a maximum of 1.0 hours credit toward the AMA Physicians Recognition Award in category one. Each physician should claim only those hours of credit that he/she actually spent in the educational activity.

Disclosure

Statements have been obtained regarding the author's relationships with financial supporters of this activity. There is no apparent conflict of interest related to the context of participation of the author of this article.

Department of Surgery, The Mount Sinai School of Medicine, Chief, Adult Liver Transplantation Surgery, The Recanati/Miller Transplantation Institute, New York, New York.

Reprint requests: Patricia A. Sheiner, M.D., Mount Sinai Hospital, Box 1104, One Gustave L. Levy Place, New York, NY 10029. E-mail: patricia.sheiner@mountsinai.org

Copyright © 2000 by Thieme Medical Publishers, Inc., 333 Seventh Avenue, New York, NY 10001, USA. Tel.: +1(212) 584-4662.
0272-8087,p;2000,20,02,201,210,ftx,en;sld00057x

Hepatitis C virus (HCV) is now the major cause of end-stage liver disease leading to transplantation. According to United Network for Organ Sharing (UNOS) data, between 1987 and 1993, 2,378 transplants were performed for HCV or for HCV in combination with alcoholic liver disease; between 1994 and 1998, 3,883 transplants were performed for the same indication.[1]

It is now well known that hepatitis C recurs in the new liver.[2] Although most studies have yet to show a difference in survival between patients transplanted for hepatitis C and those transplanted for other diseases,[1,3] recurrent disease is a major source of morbidity and mortality after transplant.[4,5]

RECURRENCE RATE OF HEPATITIS C

In 1991, Martin et al.[6] were the first to describe recurrence in six patients who had undergone transplantation for hepatitis C. Five remained HCV antibody positive, three had biopsy-proven hepatitis, and one died a year posttransplant of recurrence, after receiving a second transplant for recurrent disease. Since then, sensitive tests such as polymerase chain reaction have revealed that HCV is present after transplant in virtually all patients transplanted for hepatitis C. In one of the earliest studies using these tests, Wright et al.[7] at UCSF followed 41 patients who were either HCV RNA (+) or anti-HCV(+) before liver transplant. Posttransplant, 39 (95%) were viremic and 41% had hepatitis. Quantitative studies such as the Chiron branched-chain DNA assay show that viral levels tend to run 10- to 20-fold higher posttransplant compared with pretransplant.[8]

Clinical hepatitis, defined as the presence of lobular inflammation and necroinflammatory lesions, develops in up to 75% of patients posttransplant.[9] A more severe form of hepatitis—fibrosing cholestatic hepatitis—occurs in approximately 7% of patients after orthotopic liver transplantation (OLT).[10]

NATURAL HISTORY AND SEVERITY OF RECURRENCE

Initially, early reports suggested that recurrent hepatitis C was mild[11] and would follow the indolent course of disease seen in patients with chronic hepatitis C pretransplant.[12] It is becoming increasingly clear, however, that in contrast to the slow course of hepatitis C pretransplant, recurrent disease can progress rapidly over the course of just a year. Greenson et al.,[9] for example, analyzed 81 liver biopsies from 19 patients, 14 of whom developed hepatitis. When the biopsies were separated into three groups—no hepatitis, acute lobular hepatitis, and

chronic hepatitis—there was a definite correlation between biopsy findings and interval since transplant. Biopsies without hepatitis were seen early posttransplant (usually in the first 30 days), whereas biopsies showing acute lobular hepatitis and chronic hepatitis were noted at averages of 135 and 356 days, respectively.

Not only is recurrence common, but it can be severe as well. There appear to be two types of severe recurrent hepatitis C: end-stage liver disease from cirrhosis and fibrosing cholestatic hepatitis, with fibrosis and cirrhosis developing within a short time after transplant. Johnson et al.[4] reported on 67 patients who had undergone transplant for hepatitis C. At a mean follow-up of only 22 months, 56% had developed clinical hepatitis, 29% had developed fibrosis or cirrhosis, and 4 had required retransplantation for hepatitis C. Gane et al.[5] noted cirrhosis in 10 of 130 (5.4%) patients at a median of 51 months posttransplant. Five developed liver failure and either underwent retransplantation or died. In a study of 96 patients transplanted for hepatitis C at the Mount Sinai Medical Center, we found clinical recurrence in 43; 7 of the 43 required retransplant and 1 patient died of recurrent hepatitis C.[13] In a later report, we described fibrosing cholestatic hepatitis, which had previously been reported in association with recurrent hepatitis B,[14,15] in 10 of 135 patients (7.4%) transplanted for hepatitis C.[10] In all cases, fibrosing cholestatic hepatitis led to retransplant or death. Others have reported similar poor outcomes in patients with recurrent hepatitis C and fibrosing cholestatic hepatitis.[16]

RISK FACTORS FOR RECURRENCE

Immunosuppression

It is becoming increasingly clear that immunosuppression, especially steroids, plays a role in the recurrence of hepatitis C. In a controlled trial in patients with non-A, non-B hepatitis who had not undergone transplant, progression of liver disease was significantly greater in patients treated with steroids compared with untreated patients.[17] In nontransplanted patients with chronic hepatitis C, steroid administration has been shown to result in a 5- to 10-fold increase in HCV RNA levels during treatment.[18,19] In another study, HCV RNA levels in patients with both HCV and HIV were higher than in HCV(+) patients who were HIV(−).[20]

Augmented immunosuppression for treatment of rejection has been shown to be a particular risk factor for recurrence. In 96 patients who underwent transplant for hepatitis C, we noted recurrence in 43.[13] Recurrence and number of rejection episodes were clearly associated: 6 of 33 (18.2%) with no rejection had recurrence, versus 11 of 26 (42.3%) with one rejection episode and 26 of 37

(70.2%) with more than one episode. Fifteen of 21 patients (71.4%) who required OKT3 for steroid-resistant rejection (SRR) had recurrence, versus 28 of 75 (37.3%) who either had no SRR or developed it after recurrence was diagnosed. Furthermore, patients who had SRR recurred earlier (127 ± 31 days) than those who recurred but did not have SRR (246 ± 42 days). Others have reported similar findings. Rosen et al.[21] compared 19 patients who received OKT3 for SRR to 33 matched controls who received steroids alone for rejection. Patients receiving OKT3 had a higher recurrence rate (84.2% versus 51.5%) and a shorter interval to diagnosis of recurrence. Additionally, on long-term follow-up, 26.3% of patients who received OKT3 for SRR developed cirrhosis versus 6% of patients who received steroids alone.

Rejection episodes have also been associated with severe recurrence leading to cirrhosis. Prieto et al.[22] reported on 81 HCV(+) liver recipients followed for an average of 32 months. All underwent yearly biopsies. At time of last biopsy, 97% of patients had hepatitis; 12 had developed cirrhosis at a median of 24 months (range, 12–48) and 7 had evidence of liver failure. The actuarial rate of cirrhosis was 28% at 4 years. Rejection was significantly more common among patients with cirrhosis than among those without (83% versus 48%). Rates of cirrhosis were 5% in patients with no rejection, 15% in patients with one rejection episode, and 50% in those with two episodes. Similarly, on 2-year protocol biopsies performed in 63 transplant recipients with HCV genotype 1b, Berenguer et al.[23] noted that rejection, treatment for rejection, and a trend toward higher cumulative steroid and azathioprine doses were correlated with the presence of chronic active hepatitis. In the report from the NIDDK liver transplantation database, acute rejection and SRR each increased the risk for mortality after transplantation for hepatitis C. Similar effects were not seen in patients transplanted for other diseases, such as primary sclerosing cholangitis (PSC) or primary biliary cirrhosis (PBC).[24]

An alternative view—that hepatitis C infection promotes rejection rather than vice versa—must also be considered. Viral infection, such as with cytomegalovirus, may upregulate the immune system, and there are reported associations between cytomegalovirus infection and acute and chronic rejection.[25,26] Farges et al.[27] studied the incidence of rejection among patients transplanted for different etiologies and noted a lower rejection rate in patients transplanted for alcoholic liver disease but no difference in rejection rates between patients transplanted for hepatitis C and other nonalcoholic diseases. We[13] reported, as did Singh et al.,[28] that overall incidences of rejection and SRR did not differ between patients transplanted for hepatitis C and those transplanted for primary biliary cirrhosis or primary sclerosing cholangitis. There have, however, been reports of chronic rejection associated with hepatitis C

(unrelated to interferon use). Loinaz et al.[29] reported a 24% incidence of chronic rejection in patients transplanted for hepatitis C versus 10.3% in patients transplanted for other diseases. Similarly, Hoffmann et al.[30] reported a 23% (4/17) incidence of ductopenic rejection in patients transplanted for hepatitis C compared with patients transplanted for other diseases (6/103, 5.3%).

IMMUNOSUPPRESSIVE AGENTS

Although it is clear that steroids play an important role in recurrence of hepatitis C, little is known about the impact of other immunosuppressive agents, such as tacrolimus and cyclosporine. When cyclosporine was used to treat chronic hepatitis C in nontransplanted patients, there was a decrease in alanine transferase (ALT), but more importantly, however, viral levels did not change during treatment, which suggests that the role of cyclosporine in recurrence is not as important as that of steroids.[31] Nevertheless, whether one interleukin-2 blocker is better than the other in patients with hepatitis C is still largely unknown. It is also unclear whether primary induction immunosuppression plays a role in recurrent hepatitis C. Early studies suggested some advantage of one agent over the other, but none were randomized and all were small series. In our series of 96 patients, recurrence was more rapid in the small group of nine patients who received tacrolimus for primary immunosuppression. We also noted that OKT3 induction delayed the diagnosis of recurrent disease, presumably via a decrease in the incidence of early or severe rejection.[13] In a more recent study,[32] no advantage was seen with OKT3 induction. Johnson et al.[4] followed 74 patients transplanted for HCV, 67 of whom survived more than 2 months. Of these, 56% developed clinical hepatitis, 29% developed fibrosis or cirrhosis, and 5.9% were retransplanted for recurrent hepatitis C. There was no difference in recurrence rates among patients treated with cyclosporine, tacrolimus, or OKT3, but disease was more severe in tacrolimus-treated patients. These patients, however, had been given tacrolimus for rescue from rejection; they had received high levels of immunosuppression and previous treatment for rejection. Flamm et al.[33], in a small retrospective study, analyzed data on 32 patients transplanted for hepatitis C, 22 of whom received cyclosporine and 10 of whom received tacrolimus. Survival was significantly lower among patients treated with tacrolimus. Casavilla et al.[34] also reported a significant decrease in 2- and 3-year survival in patients transplanted for hepatitis C under a tacrolimus regimen. More recently, this same group noted that with reduction of standard tacrolimus dosing, survival after transplantation for hepatitis C is similar to that after transplantation for other diseases.[35] Lake et al.[36] presented 5-year survival data on 113 patients transplanted for hepatitis C within the U.S. FK506 multicenter trial. Survival was significantly worse among patients randomized to receive cyclosporine.

Others, however, have found no effect of cyclosporine or tacrolimus on either the risk of recurrence or on survival. In one of the few randomized trials to compare tacrolimus with microemulsion cyclosporine (Neoral) for primary immunosuppression after transplantation for hepatitis C, Zervos et al.[37] found more rejection episodes in the Neoral group but no difference in recurrence rate between the groups. In an analysis of data from the NIDDK liver transplant database, Charlton et al.[24] reported no difference in outcome in patients transplanted for hepatitis C according to primary immunosuppression regimen. In another large series, Ghobrial et al.[38] also found no difference in patient or graft survival between patients treated primarily with either tacrolimus or cyclosporine.

The effects of the newer immunosuppressive agents, such as mycophenolate mofetil (MMF) or rapamycin, on hepatitis C are still unknown. In vitro, MMF has been reported to have antiviral effects.[39] Few clinical studies have looked at the effect of MMF on hepatitis C posttransplant. In a small series of six patients placed on MMF after the diagnosis of recurrent disease, Platz et al.[40] noted a reduction in HCV RNA levels on therapy. Paterson et al.[41] reported no difference in the incidence of infection, including infection with HCV, in patients placed on MMF versus patients receiving non-MMF immunosuppression. There is little clinical information on the effects of new agents such as rapamycin, daclizumab, and Simulect on the recurrence of hepatitis C. Whether prevention of acute rejection (perhaps allowing for early steroid withdrawal) will be of benefit will only be determined with longer follow-up.

Viral Levels

Viral levels rise dramatically posttransplant, but the role of pre- and posttransplant viral levels in predicting recurrence or severity of recurrence remains to be clarified. Chazouilleres et al.[42] analyzed viral levels before and after transplant and found that post-OLT levels were 16-fold higher than pretransplant and that patients with higher levels pretransplant tended to have higher levels posttransplant. Interestingly, there was no correlation between recurrence or severity of recurrence and viral levels. In another study, Freeman et al.[43] followed 28 patients for a mean of 22 months after transplant and found that in 75%, viral levels rose post-OLT—but again, there was no clear correlation between recurrence and viral levels.

More recent data, however, suggest that viral levels, especially pre- or early posttransplant, may be an important prognostic factor. In the report by Charlton et al.[44] on data from the NIDDK liver transplant database, patients transplanted for hepatitis C with higher pretransplant viral levels had much lower 5-year survival (57%) than those with low pretransplant levels (85%). Similarly, Doughty et al.[45] found that patients who developed fibrosing cholestatic hepatitis were more likely to have had high pretransplant viral levels.

Others, including ourselves, have found that pretransplant levels do not predict severe recurrence but that high viral levels early after transplant may have prognostic significance. In 19 patients, we found that only 1 had a negative viral level at 1-year posttransplant.[32] Pretransplant viral level did not predict recurrence in this study, but viral level at 1 month after transplant was an independent predictor of recurrence. Gane et al.[46] reported that viral levels rose 4- to 100-fold after steroid treatment of rejection; furthermore, they observed higher RNA levels in patients with acute hepatitis, with the highest levels in patients with more severe hepatitis. In a study by Berg et al.[47] of 79 patients, 40 (51%) developed recurrent hepatitis and 7 (9%) developed cirrhosis—but neither pre- nor posttransplant HCV RNA level was significantly associated with graft hepatitis. Among patients infected with subtype 1b, however, Berg's group noted a trend toward more severe recurrence in those with high viral levels early after transplant. Moll et al.[48] reported that patients with higher viral levels in the first 60 days post-OLT were more likely to develop complications of recurrent hepatitis C than those with low viral levels during that period.

Viral Genotype

In patients with chronic hepatitis C, pretransplant genotype 1b is associated with a poorer prognosis and a lesser response to treatment.[49-51] The impact of genotype on posttransplant outcome is less clear. Studies differ in terms of diagnostic criteria for severe recurrence, length of follow-up, and end points.

Initially, many studies found a relationship between genotype 1b and severity of liver disease posttransplant. Feray et al.[52] followed 60 hepatitis C(+) liver recipients, among whom the predominant genotype was 1b. Actuarial rates of acute and chronic hepatitis at 3 years were significantly higher in transplant recipients with genotype 1b (77% and 59%, respectively, versus 40% and 22%, respectively, in recipients with other genotypes). Similarly, Gordon et al.[53] noted that although recurrence rates did not differ between genotype 1b patients and non-1b patients, hepatic activity index (HAI) scores and histologic stage were higher in genotype 1b patients. Furthermore, 35% of genotype 1b patients developed cirrhosis, compared to only 8% of patients with other genotypes.

Genotype 1a has also been reported to be associated with more severe disease. Pageaux et al.[54] reported higher HCV RNA levels and more severe recurrence in patients with genotype 1 (1a and 1b). In our report on 14 patients who underwent retransplant for severe recurrent disease, all seven patients on whom genotyping was performed were genotype 1a.[55]

There are, however, a number of reports to suggest that genotype has no effect on either rate or severity of recurrence. Zhou et al.[56] followed 112 patients who were genotyped after transplant; the most predominant genotypes were 1b (32.2%) and 1a (27.3%). After a mean follow-up of 25 months (range, 1–75), there was no difference in level of viremia, ALT, aspartate aminotransferase (AST), bilirubin, or total histologic score between patients with genotype 1b versus others or genotype 1 versus all nongenotype 1 recipients. Furthermore, there was no difference in graft or patient survival at 3 years between genotypes.

Newer studies have questioned the role of genotype. Vargas et al.[57] examined the influence of genotype on recurrence of hepatitis and progression to cirrhosis after transplant in 150 patients with known genotype. After a mean of 874 days (range, 40–1,800), there was no difference in recurrence rates, survival, HAI index, or progression to cirrhosis. Similarly, in the report by Charlton et al.[44] on data from the NIDDK liver transplant database, genotype was not found to be a predictor of patient or graft survival. Longer follow-up and more multicenter studies may help elucidate the role of genotype in determining outcome after liver transplant.

TREATMENT OF RECURRENT HEPATITIS

When hepatitis C was found to recur after transplant, there were many initial reports of treatment with interferon—most with poor results. Wright et al.[58] administered interferon to 11 patients with recurrent hepatitis C, but only 1 patient responded with normalization of liver function tests (LFTs). Wright et al.[59] reported on 18 patients treated with 3 million units interferon-α subcutaneously tiw for at least 4 months. Five responded with normalizing LFTs. Similar to experience with nontransplant patients,[60,61] responders had lower pretreatment viral and bilirubin levels than nonresponders.

Unfortunately, given the varying natural history of patients with hepatitis C and in the absence of a large randomized trial, it is difficult to ascribe any long-term benefit to treatment with interferon. Furthermore, an important potential side effect of interferon is an increase in the risk of rejection (secondary to upregulation of the immune system). Feray et al.[62] reported on 14 patients treated for recurrent disease with interferon-α at 3 million units tiw. Patients were started on therapy late after transplant, at a mean of 31 months. Five patients developed chronic rejection, compared with 1 of 32 patients who were not treated with interferon. Although the concern about chronic rejection is important, others—including Jain et al.,[63] who compared 105 patients who received interferon therapy to 132 patients who did not—have noted no difference in rejection rate or rate of chronic rejection with interferon treatment.

Ribavirin, a synthetic nucleotide with antiviral activity, has also been used against recurrent hepatitis C. Cattral et al.[64] treated 18 patients with ribavirin monotherapy. Initially, all responded with improvement in ALT; in five patients, ALT normalized. HCV RNA levels did not change during treatment, and repeat biopsy showed worsening of fibrosis in 12 patients and cirrhosis in 5. Gane et al.[65] randomized 30 patients to monotherapy for 24 months with either interferon or ribavirin. Groups were similar in age, gender, time from transplant to diagnosis of hepatitis C recurrence, or initiation of treatment. Sixteen patients received ribavirin (either 500 or 600 mg po bid, depending on body size; patients less than 70 kg received the lower dose). Ribavirin-treated patients were more likely to normalize ALT than interferon-treated patients (13/16 versus 6/14) but were less likely to have undetectable serum levels of HCV RNA (0/16 versus 5/14). Both groups, however, had either no change on liver biopsy or an increase in fibrosis, suggesting that therapy was ineffective. Both groups experienced side effects. Eight of 16 patients on ribavirin required dose reduction for hemolysis and 4 required drug discontinuation. Three patients on interferon required dose reduction for leukopenia.

Given that neither drug alone is effective against recurrent hepatitis C, combination therapy has been attempted. Bizollan et al.[66] treated 21 patients with a combination of interferon-α, 3 million units tiw, and oral ribavirin (dosage depending on body weight) for 6 months followed by ribavirin monotherapy for 6 months. The interval from transplant to initiation of antiviral treatment ranged from 3 to 24 months (mean, 9 months). Mean ALT at initiation of therapy was 233 ± 199; the mean bilirubin level was normal (1.2 ± 0.3). Twenty of the 21 patients were genotype 1b. After the first 6 months of therapy, ALT levels had normalized in all 21. Furthermore, 10 patients had undetectable HCV RNA levels, and the others had levels less than 50% of baseline. During monotherapy, one relapsed biochemically on treatment. Three patients did not tolerate ribavirin due to anemia (all had biochemical relapse). Of the 10 patients with negative RNA levels, 5 became HCV RNA positive on monotherapy with no increase in ALT. Before treatment, patients' mean HAI score was 6.3 ± 2; at 12 months after treatment, the mean score was 3 ± 1. Although this is an early treatment study with short follow-up, the results suggest that combination therapy with interferon/ribavirin is more effective than monotherapy. The finding that half the people who lost their RNA while on combination treatment became positive again on monotherapy raises the question of whether combination therapy for longer periods would be a more optimal treatment.

Most patients in Bizollon's study, however, had normal bilirubin levels when treatment began. Interferon alone has been shown to be less effective when pretreatment bilirubin is high. Whether treatment would be effective in patients with abnormal bilirubin is unclear. At Mount Sinai, we placed 15 patients with recurrent HCV (mean age, 51.4 years; r, 20–73; 4 females, 11 males) on a 12-month course of interferon/ribavirin. The mean time from OLT to start of interferon/ribavirin was 403 days (range, 30–1,055). In eight patients, interferon/ribavirin was discontinued at a mean of 46 days (range, 23–96) for adverse effects: anemia ($n = 2$), leukopenia ($n = 3$), and fatigue with weakness and nausea ($n = 3$). One of these eight required re-OLT for recurrent disease. Of the seven patients who tolerated treatment, one required re-OLT for disease progression. Three patients completed a year of treatment. Of the three who are still receiving interferon/ribavirin, one has been treated for less than 30 days and the other two have been treated for 98 and 265 days. Overall, the mean length of treatment for the three who completed the course and the two who remain in the protocol and have been treated for at least 30 days is 311 days. In these five patients, LFTs did not significantly differ from baseline at 3 months but were significantly different for ALT (291 ± 215 versus 54 ± 34; $p = 0.05$) and AST (275 ± 170 versus 57 ± 20; $p = 0.05$) at last follow-up. All five treated patients had reductions in transaminases and bilirubin. Two patients with baseline bilirubin levels above 5.0 remained in therapy for more than 1 year, with decreases in bilirubin level from 7.5 to 2.4 and 17.2 to 3.9. Patients who withdrew from therapy early had no statistically significant difference in AST or ALT from baseline, at a mean of 193 days after withdrawal. Only two patients became HCV RNA negative while on therapy. Overall, interferon/ribavirin was poorly tolerated, with fewer than half the patients able to stay on therapy. However, despite disease progression in one patient while on therapy, there appeared to be a biochemical response in those who tolerated treatment. Once again, the long-term outcome is still unknown in this small group of patients.

PROPHYLAXIS

Given that the long-term effectiveness of treatment, even with combinations of drugs, is still unproved, prophylaxis of posttransplant recurrence is a particularly important focus of research. At Mount Sinai, we con-

ducted a randomized trial to determine whether administration of interferon-α2b after liver transplant would prevent or delay recurrence of hepatitis C and whether viral load affected response to therapy.[32] Because interferon/ribavirin appears to work best when pretreatment viral levels are low[59] and because in most liver recipients viral levels are lowest early after transplant, we initiated the drug within the first 2 weeks after transplant. Treatment was continued for a year in the absence of indications to discontinue. Thirty patients were randomized to interferon, 3 million units tiw; 41 patients received no treatment. Clinical features at study entry were similar between groups. Mean follow-up was 628 ± 264 days (range, 168–1,040) in interferon/ribavirin patients and 594 ± 266 days (range, 204–1,064) in no-interferon/ribavirin patients. All patients received protocol immunosuppression, including OKT3 induction immunotherapy followed by triple immunosuppression with cyclosporine, azathioprine, and steroids. Patients were converted to tacrolimus for recurrent or severe rejection or for side effects of cyclosporine. We found that patients treated with interferon were less likely to develop recurrent hepatitis than patients who were not treated. Eight interferon/ribavirin patients recurred at 194 ± 168 days (range, 69 – 496) versus 22 no-interferon/ribavirin patients at 220 ± 144 days (range, 45–830) ($p = 0.02$, log-rank test).

Viral level at 1 month was important in predicting both recurrence and response to interferon. One-month viral level was an independent predictor of recurrence. An HCV RNA level $>100 \times 10^5$ Eq/mL at 1 month increased the risk by a factor of 3.1 ($p = 0.01$). Although the use of interferon/ribavirin overall reduced the risk of recurrence by a factor of 0.4 ($p = 0.04$, Cox proportional hazards model), recurrence rates differed significantly depending on 1- and 3-month viral levels. Low, moderate, and high viral levels at 1 and 3 months were associated with significantly different recurrence rates in interferon/ribavirin patients, with significantly less recurrence in patients on interferon/ribavirin with low viral levels. In the untreated patients, high viral levels at 1 month were associated with high recurrence rates compared with patients with lower viral levels, but the difference did not achieve statistical significance.

Unfortunately, despite the decreased incidence of recurrent hepatitis in patients treated with interferon, we were unable to prevent fibrosing cholestatic hepatitis. Two patients in the treated group underwent retransplant for fibrosing cholestatic hepatitis, compared with two in the untreated group. This outcome suggests that interferon alone, even given as prophylaxis, will not solve the issue of severe recurrent hepatitis C. In a smaller study, Singh et al.[67] compared the incidence of recurrent hepatitis and severity of recurrence in 12 patients treated with prophylactic interferon and 12 patients not treated; they found no difference between the two groups in incidence or severity but found that time to recurrence was delayed.

Combination therapy with interferon and ribavirin has also been studied for prophylaxis. In a nonrandomized trial, Mazzaferro et al.[68] placed 21 patients on interferon and ribavirin within 2 weeks after transplant. Twenty patients were available for follow-up at a median of 12 months. Four had developed biopsy-proven hepatitis, and one had developed chronic active hepatitis. No patient developed cirrhosis—although median follow-up was too short to be able to draw conclusions. More importantly, HCV RNA was negative in nine patients (41%). Side effects were seen in nine patients, usually hemolysis or malaise.

RETRANSPLANT FOR RECURRENT DISEASE

It is now recognized that recurrence can result in either fibrosing cholestatic hepatitis or cirrhosis requiring retransplant. Two major concerns regarding retransplant are as follows: What is to prevent the new liver from developing the same progressive disease? Do the results of retransplantation justify these procedures, given the organ shortage?

There are few reports about retransplantation for recurrent hepatitis C. Rosen et al.[69] found no difference in survival according to etiology of graft failure. On the other hand, Feray et al.[70] found that prognosis after re-OLT was poor in patients retransplanted for recurrent hepatitis C. At Mount Sinai, in 14 patients who underwent retransplantation for recurrent hepatitis C, we noted high perioperative mortality associated with renal failure and infectious complications.[55] More recently, we reported predictors of survival after late retransplant (>6 months after initial OLT).[71] We noted that patients retransplanted for recurrent hepatitis C had poorer survival (90-day survival, 57%; 1-year survival, 43%) compared with patients retransplanted for all other indications (90-day survival, 81%; 1-year survival, 74%). This difference in survival, however, did not reach statistical significance ($p = 0.09$), most likely due to the small number of patients. A preoperative creatinine level >2 mg/dL predicted poor survival, and the use of all intraoperative blood products (packed red blood cells, fresh frozen plasma, and platelets) correlated strongly with outcome. Previous studies have reported an increased incidence of infections in liver transplant recipients with recurrent hepatitis C.[72] In our patients who underwent re-OLT for hepatitis C compared with patients who underwent retransplantation for other disease, however, there was no significantly higher rate of infection to explain the lower survival. The difference in survival is also not explained by recurrent disease after re-OLT, as graft failure secondary to rerecurrence of hepatitis C was seen in only

9.5% of our patients retransplanted for this indication. The high mortality associated with re-OLT for recurrent hepatitis C may reflect poor patient selection and a failure to recognize predictors of poor prognosis.

SUMMARY

Hepatitis C remains a challenge for transplant surgeons and physicians. Despite our increasing understanding of the ways in which host and immune factors affect the outcome of patients transplanted for hepatitis C, we are still unable to predict the development of severe disease after transplant in individual patients. Treatment options remain poor, with major side effects and no proven long-term efficacy. Prophylaxis with combination therapy may offer some advantages over treatment, but many patients may not tolerate therapy. Retransplantation, now being increasingly performed in patients with recurrent disease, still has a high mortality rate. New more effective antiviral agents and a better understanding of the role of immunosuppression may help reduce the incidence and severity of recurrent hepatitis C after liver transplant.

ABBREVIATIONS

ALT   alanine transferase
AST   aspartate aminotransferase
HAI   hepatic activity index
HCV   hepatitis C virus
LFT   liver function test
MMF   mycophenolate mafetil
OLT   orthotopic liver transplantation
PBC   primary biliary cirrhosis
PSC   primary sclerosing cholangitis
SRR   steroid-resistant rejection

REFERENCES

1. Seaberg E, Belle H, Beringer K, Shivins J, Detre K. Liver transplantation in the US from 1987–1998: Updated results from the Pitt-UNOS Liver Transplant Registry. In: Cecka J, Terasaki P, eds. Clinical Transplants 1998. Los Angeles: UCLA Tissue Typing Laboratory, 1999
2. Wright TL, Donegan E, Hsu HH, et al. Recurrent and acquired hepatitis C viral infection in liver transplant recipients. Gastroenterology 1992;103:317–322
3. Feray C, Gigou M, Samuel D, et al. The course of hepatitis C virus infection after liver transplantation. Hepatology 1994;20:1137–1143
4. Johnson MW, Washburn K, Freeman RB, FitzMaurice SE, Dienstag J, Basgoz N, Jenkins RL, Cosimi B. Hepatitis C viral infection in liver transplantation. Arch Surg 1996;131:284–291
5. Gane EJ, Portmann BC, Naoumov NV, Smith HM, Underhill JA, Donaldson PT, Maertens G, Williams R. Long term outcome of

hepatitis C infection after liver transplantation. N Engl J Med 1996;334:815–819

6. Martin P, Munoz SJ, Di Bisceglie AM, Rubin R, Waggoner JG, Armenti VT, Moritz MJ, Jarrell BE, Maddrey WC. Recurrence of hepatitis C virus infection after orthotopic liver transplantation. Hepatology 1991;13:719–721

7. Wright TL, Donegan E, Hsu HH, et al. Recurrent and acquired hepatitis C viral infection in liver transplant recipients. Gastroenterology 1992;103:317–322

8. Chazouilleres O, Kim M, Combs C, et al. Quantitation of hepatitis C virus RNA in liver transplant recipients.Gastroenterology 1994;106:994–999

9. Greenson JK, Svoboda-Newman SM, Merion RM, Frank TS. Histologic progression of recurrent hepatitis C in liver transplant allografts. Am J Surg Pathol 1996;20:731–738

10. Schluger LK, Sheiner PA, Thung SN, et al. Severe recurrent cholestatic hepatitis C following orthotopic liver transplantation. Hepatology 1996;23:971–976

11. Shah G, Dmetris J, Gavaler J, Lewis J, Todo S, Starzl T, Van Thiel D. Incidence, prevalence, and clinical course of hepatitis C following liver transplantation. Gastoenterology 1993;103:323–329

12. DiBisceglie AM, Goodman ZD, Ishak KG, Hoofnagle JH, Melpolder JJ, Alter HJ. Long term clinical and histopathological follow-up of chronic posttransfusion hepatitis. Hepatology 1991;14:969–974

13. Sheiner PA, Schwartz M, Mor E, et al. Severe or multiple rejection episodes lead to increased early recurrence of hepatitis C after orthotopic liver transplantation. Hepatology 1995;21:30–34

14. Harrison RF, Davies MH, Goldin RD, Hubscher SG. Recurrent hepatitis B in liver allografts: A distinctive form of rapidly developing cirrhosis. Histopathology 1993;23:21–28

15. Angus PW, Locarnini SA, McCaughan GW, Jones RM, McMillan JS, Bowden DS. Hepatitis B virus precore mutant infection is associated with severe recurrent disease after liver transplantation. Hepatology 1995;21:14–18

16. Dickson RC, Caldwell SH, Ishitani MB, Lau JY, Driscoll CJ, Stevenson WC, McCullough CS, Pruett TL. Clinical and histologic patterns of early graft failure due to recurrent hepatitis C in four patients after liver transplantation. Transplantation 1996;61:701–705

17. Schoeman MN, Liddle C, Bilous M, Groerson J, Craig PI, Batey, RG, Farrell GC. Chronic nonA-nonB hepatitis: Lack of correlation between biochemical and morphological activity and effects of immunosuppressive therapy on disease progression. Aust NZ J Med 1990;20:56–62

18. Fong TL, Valinluck B, Govindarajan S, Charboneau F, Adkins RH, Redeker AG. Short-term prednisone therapy affects aminotransferase activity and hepatitis C virus RNA levels in chronic hepatitis C. Gastroenterology 1994;107:196–199

19. Magrin S, Craxi A, Fabiano C, et al. Hepatitis C viremia in chronic liver disease: Relationship to interferon-alpha or corticosteroid treatment. Hepatology 1994;19:273–279

20. Bonacini M, Govindarajan S, Blatt LM, Schmid P, Conrad A, Lindsay KL. Patients co-infected with human immunodeficiency virus and hepatitis C virus demonstrate higher levels of hepatic HCV RNA. J Virol Hepatol 1999;6:203–208

21. Rosen HR, Shackleton CR, Higa L, et al. Use of OKT3 is associated with early and severe recurrence of hepatitis C after liver transplantation. Am J Gastroenterol 1997;92:1453–1457

22. Prieto M, Berenguer M, Rayon JM, et al. High incidence of allograft cirrhosis in hepatitis C virus genotype 1b infection following transplantation: Relationship with rejection episodes. Hepatology 1999;29:250–256

23. Berenguer M, Prieto M, Cordoba J, et al. Early development of chronic active hepatitis in recurrent hepatitis C virus infection

after liver transplantation: Association with treatment of rejection. J Hepatol 1998;28:756–763

24. Charlton M, Seaberg E, for the National Institute of Diabetes and Digestive and Kidney Diseases Liver Transplantation Database. Impact of immunosuppression and acute rejection of recurrence of hepatitis C: Results of the National Institute of Diabetes and Digestive and Kidney Diseases Liver Transplantation Database. Liver Transplant Surg 1999;5:S107–S114

25. O'Grady JG, Sutherland S, Harvey F, et al. Cytomegalovirus infection and donor/recipient HLA antigens: Interdependent cofactors in the pathogenesis of vanishing bile duct syndrome after liver transplantation. Lancet 1988;2:302

26. Pouteil-Noble C, Ecochard R, Landrivon G, et al. Cytomegalovirus infection—an etiological factor for rejection? Transplantation 1993;55:851–857

27. Farges O, Saliba F, Hosseine F, et al. Incidence of rejection and infection after liver transplantation as a function of the primary disease: Possible influence of alcohol and polyclonal immunoglobulins. Hepatology 1996;23:240–248

28. Singh N, Gayowski T, Ndimbie OK, Nedjar S, Wagener MM, Yu VL. Recurrent hepatitis C virus hepatitis in liver transplant recipients receiving tacrolimus: Association with rejection and increased immunosuppression after transplantation. Surgery 1996;119:452–456

29. Loinaz C, Lumbreras C, Gonzalez-Pinto I, et al. High incidence of posttransplant hepatitis and chronic rejection associated with hepatitis C virus infection in liver transplant recipients. Transplant Proc 1995;27:1217–1218

30. Hoffmann RM, Gunther C, Diepolder HM, Zachoval R, Eissner HJ, Forst H, Anthuber M, Paumgartner G, Pape GR. Hepatitis C virus infection as a possible risk factor for ductopenic rejection (vanishing bile duct syndrome) after liver transplantation. Transplant Int 1995;8:353–359

31. Kakumu S, Takayanagi M, Iwata K, Okumura A, Aiyama T, Ishikawa T, Nadai M, Yoshioka K. Cyclosporine therapy affects aminotransferase activity but not hepatitis C virus RNA levels in chronic hepatitis C. J Gastroenterol Hepatol 1997;12:62–66

32. Sheiner PA, Boros P, Klion FM, et al. The efficacy of prophylactic interferon alfa-2b in preventing recurrent hepatitis C after liver transplantation. Hepatology 1998;28:831–838

33. Flamm SL, Marcos A, Jenkins RL, et al. Tacrolimus is associated with decreased survival in patients undergoing liver transplantation with chronic hepatitis C infection. Presented at the 15th annual meeting of the American Society of Transplant Physicians , Dallas, Texas, May 1996

34. Casavilla A, Mateo R, Rakela J, et al. Impact of hepatitis C viral infection on survival following primary liver transplantation under FK 506 (Prograf) [Abstract]. AASLD Single Topic Symposium, Reston, Virginia, March 1995

35. Casavilla FA, Rakela J, Kapur S, et al. Clinical outcome of patients infected with hepatitis C virus infection on survival after primary liver transplantation under tacrolimus. Liver Transplant Surg 1998;4:448–454

36. Lake JR for the US FK506 Multicenter Trial Investigators. Outcome of hepatitis C virus-infected primary liver transplants: 5 year follow up of the US randomized comparartive study. Abstract presented at the 16th annual meeting of the American Society of Transplant Physicians, Chicago, Illinois, May 1997

37. Zervos XA, Weppler D, Fagulidis GP, et al. Comparison of tacrolimus with micro-emulsion CyA as primary immunosuppression in hepatitis C patients after liver transplantation. Transplantation 1998;65:1044–1046

38. Ghobrial RM, Farmer DG, Baquerizo A, et al. Orthotopic liver transplantation for hepatitis C: Outcome, effect of immunosuppression, and causes of retransplantation during an 8-year single-center experience. Ann Surg 1999;229:824–831

39. Neyts J, Meerbach A, McKenna P, De Clercq E. Use of the yellow fever virus vaccine strain 17D for the study of strategies for the treatment of yellow fever virus infections. Antiviral Res 1996;30:125–132

40. Platz KP, Mueller AR, Berg T, Neuhaus R, Hopf U, Lobeck H, Neuhaus P. Searching for the optimal management of hepatitis C patients after liver transplantation. Transplant Int 1998;11(Suppl 1):S209–S211

41. Paterson DL, Singh N, Panebianco A, Wannstedt CF, Wagener MM, Gayowski T, Marino IR. Infectious complications occurring in liver transplant recipients receiving mycophenolate mofetil. Transplantation 1998;66:593–598

42. Chazouilleres O, Kim M, Ferrell L, et al. Quantitative study of hepatitis C virus in liver transplant recipients. Gastroenterology 1994;106:994–999

43. Freeman R, Tran S, Lee YM, et al. Serum hepatitis C RNA titers after liver transplantation are not correlated with immunosuppression or hepatitis. Transplantation 1996;61:542–545

44. Charlton M, Seaberg E, Wiesner R, Everhart J, Zetterman R, Lake J, Detre K, Hoofnagle J. Predictors of patient and graft survival following liver transplantation for hepatitis C. Hepatology 1998;28:823–830

45. Doughty AL, Spencer JD, Cossart YE, McCaughan GW. Cholestatic hepatitis after liver transplantation is associated with persistently high serum hepatitis C virus RNA levels. Liver Transplant Surg 1998;4:15–21

46. Gane EJ, Naoumov NV, Qian KP, et al. Longitudinal analysis of hepatitis C virus replication following liver transplantation. Gastroenterology. 1996;110:167–177

47. Berg T, Hopf U, Bechstein WO, Muller AR, Fukumoto T, Neuhaus R, Lobeck H, Neuhaus P. Pretransplant virological markers hepatitis C virus genotype and viremia level are not helpful in predicting individual outcome after orthotopic liver transplantation. Transplantation 1998;66:225–228

48. Moll C, Kahler C, Edis C, Nachbauer K, Konigsrainer A, Spechtenhauser B, Margreiter R, Vogel W. Early-level hepatitis C viremia after orthotopic liver transplantation is of prognostic significance. Transplant Proc 1998;30:698–700

49. Almasio PL, Di Marco V, Bonura C, et al. Viral and host factors in determining response of relapsers with chronic hepatitis C to retreatment with interferon. Dig Dis Sci 1999;44:1013–1019

50. Bellentani S, Pozzato G, Saccoccio G, et al. Clinical course and risk factors of hepatitis C virus related liver disease in the general population: Report from the Dionysos study. Gut 1999;44:874–880

51. Vandelli C, Renzo F, Braun HB, et al. Prediction of successful outcome in a randomised controlled trial of the long-term efficacy of interferon alpha treatment for chronic hepatitis C. J Med Virol 1999;58:26–34

52. Feray C, Gigou M, Samuel D, et al. Influence of the genotype of hepatitis C virus on the severity of recurrent liver disease after liver transplantation. Gastroenterology 1995;108:1314–1317

53. Gordon FD, Poterucha JJ, Germer J, Zein NN, Batts KP, Gross JB Jr, Wiesner R, Persing D. Relationship between hepatitis C genotype and severity of recurrent hepatitis C after liver transplantation. Transplantation 1997;63:1419–1423

54. Pageaux GP, Ducos J, Mondain AM, Costes B, Picot MC, Perrigault PF, Domergue J, Larrey D, Michel H. Hepatitis C virus genotypes and quantitation of serum hepatits C virus RNA in liver transplant recipients: Relationsip with severity of histological recurrence and implications in the pathogenesis of HCV infection. Liver Transplant Surg 1997;3:501–505

55. Sheiner PA, Kim-Schluger L, Emre S, et al. Retransplantation for recurrent hepatitis C. Liver Transplant Surg 1997;3:130–136

56. Zhou S, Terrault NA, Ferrell L, et al. Severity of liver diseas in liver transplantation recipients with hepatitis C virus infection: Relationship to genotype and level of viremia. Hepatology 1996;24:1041–1046

57. Vargas HE, Laskus T, Wang LF, et al. The influence of hepatitis C virus genotype on the outcome of liver transplantation. Liver Transplant Surg 1998;4:22–27

58. Wright HI, Gavaler JS, Van Theil DH. Preliminary experience with alpha-2b-interferon therapy of viral hepatitis in liver allograft recipients. Transplantation 1992;53:121–124

59. Wright TL, Combs C, Kim M, et al. Interferon-alpha therapy for hepatitis C virus infection after liver transplantation. Hepatology 1994;20(4 Pt 1).773–779.

60. Lau JY, Davis Gl, Kniffen J, Qian KP, Urdea MS, Chan CS, Mizokami M, Neuwald PD, Wilber JC. Significance of serum hepatitis C virus RNA levels in chronic hepatitis C. Lancet 1993;341:1501–1504

61. Yamada G, Takatani M, Kishi F, et al. Efficacy of interferon alfa therapy in chronic hepatitis C patients depends primarily on hepatitis C virus RNA level. Hepatology 1995;22:1351–1354

62. Feray C, Samuel D, Gigou M, Paradis V, David MF, Lemonnier C, Reynes M, Bismuth H. An open trial of interferon alfa recombinant for hepatitis C after liver transplantation: Antiviral effects and risk of rejection. Hepatology 1995;22(4 Pt 1):1084–1089

63. Jain A, Demetris AJ, Manez R, Tsamanadas AC, Van Thiel D, Rakela J, Starzl TE, Fung JJ. Incidence and severity of acute allograft rejection in liver transplant recipients treated with alfa interferon. Liver Transplant Surg 1998;4:197–203

64. Cattral MS, Hemming AW, Wanless IR, Al Ashgar H, Krajden M, Lilly L, Greig PD, Levy GA. Outcome of long-term ribavirin therapy for recurrent hepatitis C after liver transplantation. Transplantation 1999;67:1277–1280

65. Gane EJ, Lo SK, Riordan SM, Portmann BC, Lau JY, Naoumov NV, Williams R. A randomized study comparing ribavirin and interferon alfa monotherapy for hepatitis C recurrence after liver transplantation. Hepatology 1998;27:1403–1407

66. Bizollon T, Palazzo U, Ducerf C, Chevallier M, Elliott M, Baulieux J, Pouyet M, Trepo C. Pilot study of the combination of interferon alfa and ribavirin as therapy of recurrent hepatitis C after liver transplantation. Hepatology 1997;26:500–504

67. Singh N, Gayowski T, Wannstedt CF, Shakil AO, Wagener MM, Fung JJ, Marino IR. Interferon-alpha for prophylaxis of recurrent viral hepatitis C in liver transplant recipients: A prospective, randomized, controlled trial. Transplantation 1998;65:82–86

68. Mazzaferro V, Regalia E, Pulvirenti A, et al. Prophylaxis against HCV recurrence after liver transplantation: Effect of interferon and ribavirin combination. Transplant Proc 1997;29:519–521

69. Rosen HR, O'Reilly PM, Shackleton CR, et al. Graft loss following liver transplantation in patients with chronic hepatitis C. Transplantation 1996;62:1773–1776

70. Feray C, Habasanne A, Samuel D, Farges O, Reynes M, Bismuth H. Poor prognosis of patients retransplanted for recurrent liver disease due to hepatitis C virus. Hepatology 1995;22:135A

71. Facciuto M, Heidt D, Guarrera J, et al. Retransplantation for late liver graft failure: Predictors of mortality. Liver Transplant 2000;6:174–179

72. Singh N, Gayowski T, Wagener MM, Marino IR. Increased infections in liver transplant recipients with recurrent hepatitis C virus (HCV) hepatitis. Transplantation 1996;61:402–406

Vaccine Development for Hepatitis C

MARTIN LECHMANN, Ph.D. and T. JAKE LIANG, M.D.

ABSTRACT: *Given the global disease burden and public health impact of hepatitis C, the development of an effective vaccine is of paramount importance. However, many challenging obstacles loom ahead of this goal. The hepatitis C virus (HCV), being an RNA virus, can mutate rapidly in adaptation to the environment, thus contributing to the high sequence divergence of multiple viral isolates in the world. The highest heterogeneity has been found in the hypervariable region of the envelope glycoprotein 2, which contains a principal neutralization epitope. HCV also causes persistent infection in a high percentage of immunocompetent hosts despite active immune response. The lack of an efficient tissue culture system for propagating HCV and testing neutralizing antibodies adds further complexity to the task of vaccine development. The immunologic correlates associated with disease progression or protection are yet to be defined, but recent studies suggest that a vigorous multispecific cellular immune response is important in the resolution of infection. Induction of high-titer, long-lasting, and cross-reactive antienvelope antibodies and a vigorous multispecific cellular immune response that includes both helper and cytotoxic T lymphocytes may be necessary for an effective vaccine. Several promising approaches have been used to develop an HCV vaccine. Novel vaccine candidates based on molecular technology such as recombinant proteins, peptides, viruslike particles, naked DNA, and recombinant viruses are being explored. The final vaccine product may require multiple components that target various aspects of protective immunity. Finally, sterilizing immunity may not be necessary if a vaccine can be developed to prevent chronic infection, which is the major cause of morbidity and mortality from this disease.*

KEY WORDS: recombinant subunit vaccine, immune response, cytotoxic T cell, T helper cell, antibody, protective immunity

One of the greatest achievements in medical science can be attributed to Edward Jenner's initial description of a smallpox vaccine in 1776, when he inoculated an 8-year-old boy with cowpox (vaccinia) that protected the child against subsequent challenge with the virulent smallpox. This monumental discovery had lapsed for more than 150 years until the accomplishments of vaccine pioneers, such as Koch, von Behring,

Objectives

Upon completion of this article, the reader should be able to 1) summarize the newest approaches in HCV vaccine development and 2) list the commonly used approaches.

Accreditation

The Indiana University School of Medicine is accredited by the Accreditation Council for Continuing Medical Education to provide continuing medical education for physicians.

Credit

The Indiana University School of Medicine designates this educational activity for a maximum of 1.0 hours credit toward the AMA Physicians Recognition Award in category one. Each physician should claim only those hours of credit that he/she actually spent in the educational activity.

Disclosure

Statements have been obtained regarding the authors' relationships with financial supporters of this activity. There is no apparent conflict of interest related to the context of participation of the author of this article.

Liver Diseases Section, NIDDK, National Institutes of Health, Bethesda, Maryland

Reprint requests: T.J. Liang, M.D., Liver Diseases Section, NIDDK, National Institutes of Health, 10 Center Drive, Rm 9B16, Bethesda, MD 20892-1800. E-mail: JLiang@nih.gov

Published by Thieme Medical Publishers, Inc., 333 Seventh Avenue, New York, NY 10001, USA. Tel.: +1(212) 584-4662. 0272-8087,p;2000,20,02,211,226,ftx,en;sld00058x

Ehrlich and Pasteur, that led to successful vaccines against smallpox, rabies, typhoid fever, cholera, and plague. This concept of using benign materials derived from virulent pathogens to induce protective immunity against the same pathogens has resulted in some of the greatest human triumphs against the infectious scourges that plagued much of human history. Yet, there is still a great deal that we do not understand about how vaccines work. Such knowledge can be applied to improve on existing vaccines with respect to better efficacy and less adverse effects and to develop vaccines against viruses for which there are none today, like HIV and hepatitis C virus (HCV). In addition, the classic concept of vaccination has been extended beyond protection of infection to therapy of existing infection and cancer.

Figure 1 illustrates the various traditional and newer approaches in vaccine development. Most vaccines today are whole-organism vaccines containing inactivated whole or live attenuated bacteria or viruses. Live attenuated vaccines are rather potent in inducing a long-lasting cell-mediated and humoral immunity. These vaccines have been very successful because they resemble the natural infection closely. However, the potential risk, especially in immunocompromised hosts,

that attenuated viruses or bacteria may mutate to virulent wild-type strains exists. On the other hand, inactivated organisms or inactivated toxins are noninfectious but are less immunogenic than attenuated viruses. Therefore, adjuvants and booster injections are necessary to enhance the immunogenicity for induction of protective immunity.

The principles of the newer types of vaccines evolve around the concept that one or several genes of the pathogen are incorporated into the genome of a normally nonpathogenic organism for amplification of the immunogens. The subunit vaccine is then generated from the heterologous organism by purifying the immunogen (protein immunogen), isolating the naked DNA in the form of a plasmid carrying the gene encoding for the immunogen (DNA vaccine), or using the entire host as a live vector (recombinant viruses or bacteria). In addition, chemically synthesized peptides have also been explored as subunit vaccines. Several recombinant subunit vaccines have been successfully developed, including the yeast-derived hepatitis B vaccine. The recombinant subunit vaccines offer many advantages over the traditional approaches. First, the pathogen can be excluded from the vaccine and is therefore not in-

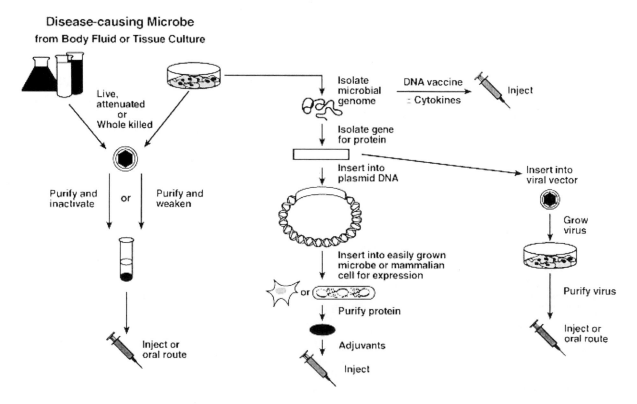

FIG. 1. Various strategies in vaccine development. The traditional vaccines, shown on the left side, are usually whole-organism vaccines containing inactivated whole or live attenuated bacteria or viruses. Because no cell culture system is available so far to propagate HCV, this strategy cannot be adapted for the development of an HCV vaccine. On the right side are illustrated the strategies of the newer types of vaccines that are being pursued for an HCV vaccine. These approaches evolve around the concept that one or several genes of the pathogen are incorporated into the genome of a normally nonpathogenic organism for amplification of the immunogens.

fectious. Second, the vaccine can be specifically designed and optimized for a particular pathogen to exclude toxins or to induce specific arms of the immune response known to be important for protection. Third, this approach can be applied for viruses like HCV that cannot be grown in cell culture. Therefore, a variety of approaches based on this concept is being investigated to improve on existing vaccines and to develop vaccines against more challenging diseases such as hepatitis C or AIDS, for which the traditional approaches have failed or cannot be adapted. However, many new approaches are limited by the poor immunogenicity of recombinant viral proteins when they are administered alone. Thus, the effort to develop new and more potent adjuvants has intensified in the past years. There is now a variety of promising novel compounds, such as lipopolysaccharide-derived monophosphoryl lipid A, saponin derivative QS21, microemulsion MF59, lipid-particle immune-stimulating complex (Iscoms), and CpG oligonucleotides (for review, see Ref. 1) that can provide substantial enhancement to the efficacy of subunit vaccines. Clinical trials are currently underway to determine their efficacy and safety in humans.

Approximately 200 million persons are chronically infected with HCV worldwide, and this large reservoir of infected persons constitutes a daunting source of potential new infections. Therefore, there is a compelling need to develop an effective vaccine. However, many obstacles to the development of a successful vaccine against hepatitis C exist. This review summarizes the current status and highlights novel promising strategies in HCV vaccine development. Because another article in this volume provides extensive coverage of the immune responses of hepatitis C, we limit our discussion of immune responses to those that are pertinent to vaccine development.

HUMORAL IMMUNITY

B cells play an important role in protection against viral infections. During primary infection, antibodies, cell-mediated immunity, or both are crucial. However, during secondary infections, antibodies are the critical mediators and are often essential for the control of viral spread. This observation is reflected by the fact that many successful antiviral vaccines are based on the induction of neutralizing antibodies. In infections with other flaviviruses such as yellow fever,[2] dengue,[3] and tickborne encephalitis virus,[4] antibodies against the envelope glycoproteins have neutralizing capacity and protect against lethal flavivirus challenge. In addition, it has been reported that antibodies against a nonstructural protein of the tickborne encephalitis virus are also able to protect against virus challenge.[5] The complete identification of neutralizing or protective epitopes in HCV

has not yet been accomplished. The envelope protein E2 of HCV has been of particular interest because it contains highly variable sequences within the N-terminal region (HVR1) that encodes neutralizing B-cell epitopes.[6] In addition, the E2 protein binds to CD81, which is thought to be a receptor for HCV,[7] although the CD81 binding region of E2 is probably not located within the HVR1 site.[8] The hypervariability of this region has been suggested as a possible mechanism through which the virus evades the immune response.[6,9,10]

Mutations within the N-terminus of HVR1 have been shown to occur rapidly in infected individuals and coincide with the disappearance of preexisting anti-HVR1 antibodies.[11] Farci et al.[9] reported in vitro neutralization of HCV with a rabbit hyperimmune serum raised against a homologous synthetic peptide derived from the HVR1 region. The anti-HVR1 serum induced protection against the homologous HCV strain in chimpanzees but not against the mutants that cannot be neutralized by the antiserum. However, the antibody response against E2 and its role in viral clearance is still controversial. Early development of anti-E2 or anti-HVR1 has been suggested to be associated with recovery from acute HCV infection in humans.[12,13] However, other studies found no correlation between anti-E2 and self-limited infection by HCV in humans and in chimpanzees.[14–17] Because protection against HCV infection did not correlate with anti-HVR1 levels in a chimpanzee immunization experiment,[18] neutralization determinants other than the HVR1 site likely exist. Finally, antibody responses to the envelope proteins develop slowly and achieve only modest titers during primary infection.[19] Therefore, neutralizing antibodies may emerge too late to prevent chronic infection. In addition, antienvelope antibodies tend to be short-lived and disappear gradually after viral clearance.[19]

CELL-MEDIATED IMMUNITY

There is accumulating evidence that failure to generate an effective immune response against HCV in the acute phase of infection is responsible for the high rate of chronicity. Most HCV proteins have been shown to be targets of helper T-cell responses and cytotoxic T lymphocyte (CTL) activities. Strong T-cell proliferative responses against HCV core,[20–24] E2,[22] NS3,[22,24,25] NS4,[21–24] and NS5[21–23] proteins have been found to be associated with self-limited infection. The identified immunodominant epitopes are highly conserved among the known HCV isolates and can be presented by different human histocompatibility leukocyte (HLA) class II molecules.[26,27] Among these epitopes, several highly conserved CD4+ T-cell immunodominant epitopes within the NS3 protein have been particularly linked to viral clearance in acute hepatitis C.[27] In addition, the ability to generate anti-HCV multispecific T-cell proliferative responses has been shown to correlate with response to interferon treatment.[28–30] Thus, broadly directed and vigorous proliferative responses against structural and nonstructural proteins seem to be important in controlling HCV infection. Analysis of the cytokine profiles of HCV-specific T cells revealed that persons displaying a T helper type I profile (antigen-dependent production of interleukin [IL]-2 and interferon-γ) that promotes cellular effector mechanisms rather than humoral immune responses are more likely to experience viral clearance.[25,28,31,32]

HLA class I-restricted CTLs can directly kill virus-infected cells and produce potent antiviral cytokines and therefore are crucial in clearing viral infections. However, CTL-mediated lysis of virus-infected host cells, if inefficient, can result in persistent infection and chronic tissue injury. In HCV-infected patients, CD8+ T-cell responses are directed against structural and nonstructural proteins in the context of different HLA molecules.[33–40] Chronic hepatitis C occurs despite a polyclonal and multispecific HCV-specific CTL activity that can be found in the peripheral blood and in the liver.[33–35,39,41–43] CTL escape mutants, including CTL antagonists, may contribute to the manifestation of chronic infection.[44,45] On the other hand, studies showed an inverse correlation between levels of HCV-specific CTL activity and viral loads, suggesting that HCV can be controlled to some extent by CTLs.[46–48] This observation is confirmed by studies in chimpanzees showing that during acute infection, CD8+ CTL activities correlated better with protection than the antibodies.[49] Additional support for this evidence comes from studies in agammaglobulinemic children in whom resolution of HCV infection can occur independently of antibodies.[50–52] Thus, the vigor and character of CTL responses in the early phase of infection are probably crucial in clearing the virus, whereas in the later phase insufficient viral-specific CTL responses may contribute to hepatocellular injury.

OBSTACLES IN DEVELOPING AN HCV VACCINE

The development of an effective vaccine against HCV faces many challenges (Table 1). First, substantial sequence diversity exists among HCV strains isolated within and between geographic areas. There are at least 6 HCV genotypes and more than 50 subtypes. This makes the development of a global HCV vaccine rather complex. Second, even within an infected person, HCV isolates with rather divergent sequences in certain region of viral genome (quasispecies) are present and mutations occur frequently during the course of infection. In particular, the N-terminus of the E2 protein contains

TABLE 1. Obstacles in Developing an HCV Vaccine

Viral factors	High sequence diversity among HCV strains within and between geographic areas
	Quasispecies are prevalent and evolve continuously during the course of infection
Host determinants	Immunologic correlates associated with disease progression or protection not well defined
Technical limitations	Lack of reliable tissue culture system for testing neutralizing antibodies and expanding or passage HCV
	Chimpanzee as the only reliable animal model for HCV infection

a hypervariable region of about 30 amino acids (HVR1), which shows extensive variation among all known isolates. The genetic variability within this region is thought to allow the virus to escape immune surveillance. Third, immunologic correlates that are associated with protection or disease progression are still being defined. The knowledge of immunogenic epitopes and their relevance to viral clearance and the existence of conserved cross-reacting epitopes are still unclear. These problems are further complicated by the lack of a reliable infectious tissue culture system for testing neutralizing antibodies or passage and expanding of the virus. The availability of such tissue culture systems has been invaluable in the successful development of other vaccines. For HCV, a surrogate assay for the determination of possible neutralizing antibodies has been developed. In this assay, antibodies are tested for their ability to neutralize the binding of highly purified recombinant E2 protein (NOB assay)[53] or antibody-captured HCV derived from high-titer sera[54] onto susceptible cells such as MOL-4 cells. This assay measures only inhibition of binding to target cells, which does not necessarily reflect neutralization of infectious virus in vivo. The only reliable model for HCV infection is the chimpanzee, which as an endangered species is not only costly but also difficult to study. Furthermore, the course of HCV infection in chimpanzee may not necessarily represent that in humans. Earlier experiments in chimpanzees in which challenge of apparently recovered chimpanzees with a homologous or heterologous strain of HCV resulted in reinfection suggest an absence of protective immunity from natural infection. In addition, HCV manages to persist in chronically infected persons despite the presence of broad antibody and T-cell responses. The viral and host factors that lead to persistence are not fully understood and remain to be elucidated in the future. Because the availability of small animal models would have greatly facilitated the development of HCV vaccine, intense effort has been under way to search for such models. Tupaia belangeri, a small primatelike animal, has been shown to be infectable by hepatitis B virus (HBV)[55] and is now being evaluated as a small animal model for HCV.[56] However, the robustness and reproducibility of this model remain to be fully confirmed. Alternatively, mouse models for HCV has been developed by either establishing HCV transgenic mice or transplanting human hepatocytes into immunodeficient mice. These models may prove to be useful in certain aspects of HCV vaccine development.

DNA VACCINE

Nucleic acid immunization is the most recent approach in vaccine development. The efficacy of DNA vaccines to protect against challenge with pathogens has been demonstrated in animal models of influenza virus,[57] malaria,[58] mycobacterium,[59] HIV,[60] and Ebola.[61] A DNA-based vaccine usually consists of purified plasmid DNA carrying sequences encoding for an antigen of interest under the control of eucaryotic promoter. After injection of the plasmid into the muscle or skin, the host cells take up the plasmid and express the antigen intracellularly. The expression of the encoded antigens by the host cells is one of the major advantages of this approach because it mimics natural infection. Furthermore, DNA immunization offers several other advantages, including the ease to generate and manipulate DNA and its potency in priming different arms of the immune response such as CTL, T helper cell, and antibody responses. Many studies have been published on the development of DNA-based vaccines against HCV. The DNA immunization approaches for HCV are summarized in Table 2.

Antibody Responses

The HCV core protein is highly conserved among various genotypes and therefore an attractive target for a DNA-based vaccine. However, studies in which mice were immunized with HCV core DNA alone showed no or only weak antibody responses.[62–64] To enhance the humoral immune responses against this nonsecreted viral protein, DNA encoding IL-4, IL-2, or granulocyte-macrophage colony-stimulating factor (GM-CSF) was coadministered along with the HCV core DNA.[62] Coimmunization with each of the cytokine genes substantially increases the seroconversion rate from 40% to 80%. Similarly, in another study, a boost with a recombinant core protein after priming with HCV DNA induced anticore antibodies, whereas core gene immunization alone could not generate IgG response in mice.[65] Other strategies for enhancing the immunogenicity of a core DNA-based vaccine included the construction of various HBV envelope-HCV chimeras designed to express secreted forms of the core protein.[64,66] In two independent studies, the chimeric expression plasmids induced anticore antibodies in all immunized mice as compared with 0%[64] and 40%[66] response rates in mice immunized with the HCV core plasmid alone. However, in only one of the two studies could the secretion of the fusion proteins be demonstrated.[64]

Because HCV is an enveloped virus and neutralizing determinants likely reside on the surface of the envelope, the major focus for developing a DNA-based HCV vaccine has been the E2 protein. Immunization studies in mice using plasmids coding for the full-

TABLE 2. DNA Immunization Approaches

Approach	HCV Antigen	Antibody	T Helper Cells	CTL	References
DNA	***Structural proteins***				
	Core, E1, E2	low	low	low	62–64, 68, 70
	Core + IL-4	↑	↓	↓	62
	Core + IL-2	↑	↑	↑	62
	Core + GM-CSF	↑	↑	→	62
	tCore-HBV	↑	↑	→	64, 66
	tE2surf*	↑	nd	nd	68
	tE2s†-GM-CSF				
	+tE1s†-GM-CSF	↑	↑	nd	70
	Core-E1-E2 under EF-1α promoter	nd	nd	↑	82
	Nonstructural proteins				
	NS3, NS4, NS5	+	+	+	74, 75
	NS3, NS4, NS5+ GM-CSF	→	↑	↑	75
DNA	Core				
+protein boost	+ recombinant core	↑	↑	→	65
DNA	tE2s†				
+ protein boost	+ recombinant E2-HSV 1 gpD	↑	nd	↑	71

+, positive response; ↑, enhanced response; →, no change in response; ↓, decreased response; nd, not done.
*C-terminus of E2 replaced by platelet-derived growth factor receptor transmembrane domain; studies in chimpanzees showed no protection.
†Signal sequence of E1 and E2 proteins replaced by the signal sequence of HSV 1 plycoprotein D.

length E1 or E2 protein showed only low antibody responses, probably because the intact E2 glycoprotein expressed alone or together with E1 is retained in the endoplasmic reticulum.[67] Therefore, various DNA constructs have been designed to enhance the expression and secretion of the envelope glycoproteins. Mice and macaques immunized with a plasmid in which the E2 protein was targeted to the cell surface by replacing the C-terminus with a transmembrane domain showed an antibody response against E2 that occurred earlier and had higher titers than animals immunized with a plasmid expressing the full-length E2.[68] Based on these results, two chimpanzees were immunized three times with this construct. Only one animal developed anti-E2 antibodies, and preliminary data from challenge studies showed no protection against viral challenge.[69] The codelivery of cytokines was also explored to enhance the immune responses against the HCV envelope proteins. Lee et al.[70] constructed various DNA vaccine vectors carrying E1 or E2 genes with or without GM-CSF. To optimize the secretion of the E1 and E2 proteins, the authors replaced the signal sequence of the E1 and the E2 proteins with the signal sequence of the herpes simplex virus type 1 (HSV 1) glycoprotein D and additionally truncated the C-terminal hydrophobic regions of the envelope proteins. The antibody responses could be greatly enhanced (4-fold higher for E1 and over 10-fold higher for E2) in buffalo rats by codelivery of a bicistronic plasmid that expressed the GM-CSF and the engineered envelope genes. A combined vaccine regimen, consistent of priming with E2 DNA and boosting with recombinant E2 protein, could also enhance antibody (immunoglobulin G2a) responses.[71] The mode of DNA delivery has also been suggested to influence the strength of antibody responses. Intradermal injection of plasmids expressing different immunogenic domains of E2 as fusion proteins with the HBV surface antigen induced up to 100-fold higher titers of antibodies compared to intramuscularly injection in mice.[72] The combination of both delivery routes may be more efficient in inducing broad antibody responses.[73]

Two studies on the DNA immunization using plasmids encoding NS3, NS4, and NS5 proteins individually or together demonstrated the successful induction of HCV-specific antibodies against NS3, NS4, and NS5 in mice and buffalo rats.[74,75] Surprisingly, the codelivery of GM-CSF did not enhance the antibody titers to HCV NS3, NS4, and NS5.[75]

Lymphoproliferative and Cytokine Responses

DNA immunization can induce lymphoproliferative responses against the structural proteins core,[62,65,66,76] E1,[77] E2,[77] and the nonstructural proteins NS3, NS4, and NS5 in mice[74] and buffalo rats.[75] However, the T-cell proliferative responses against the structural proteins are typically weak. Various approaches have been used to enhance the CD4+ T-cell responses. The codelivery of GM-CSF, IL-2, or IL-4 genes can increase significantly the lymphoproliferative responses.[62,75] Additionally, boosting with a recombinant HCV core protein after HCV core DNA immunization appears to enhance the T helper cell proliferation.[65] Spleen cells from mice immunized with an HBV envelope/HCV core chimeric construct showed higher levels of proliferative activities than those from mice immunized with the nonchimeric core construct.[66] Intramuscular DNA immunization induced predominantly interferon-γ but not IL-4 production, suggesting a Th1 response.[62,74,78] Analysis of the IgG subtypes showed an almost exclusive IgG 2a and 2b antibody production,[72,73,77] which is also consistent with a Th1-like response.

Cytotoxic T-cell Responses

Several studies have demonstrated the generation of CTL activities in mice immunized with HCV core plasmids.[65,66,76,79–81] Core-specific CTL activities were highest in mice coimmunized with an IL-2 expressing plasmid, whereas GM-CSF did not significantly augment CTL activities.[62] In addition, immunization with HBV and HCV chimeric proteins[66] or combined DNA–protein immunization[65] did not alter the generation of core-specific CTL responses. In contrast, coadministration with an IL-4 construct suppressed HCV core-specific CTL activity.[62] Furthermore, mice injected with an HCV core construct truncated at amino acid 69, which removes a known CTL epitope, showed almost no induction of CTL activities in BALB/c mice.[66]

Several studies have also addressed the CTL responses of DNA immunization against the envelope proteins E1 and E2.[71,81–83] In one of these studies, six recombinant plasmids were constructed.[81] These plasmids included the structural proteins either individually or together, E1 and E2 together, and a truncated E2 in which the N-terminal hypervariable region was deleted. In this study, CTL activities were tested against target cells infected with a recombinant vaccina virus expressing core, E1 and E2. Specific CTL responses were detected only in mice injected with plasmid constructs encoding core alone or together with E1 and E2. The authors suggested from these data that the core region might have the strongest CTL epitope in the structural region for BALB/c mice. However, studies in our laboratory (J. Satoi, personal communication) showed that in BALB/c and FBV/n mice, immunization with a plasmid expressing core alone generated core-specific cytolytic activities, whereas injection of a core/E1/E2 expressing plasmid induced CTL responses only against E2 but not against core or E1. These data suggest that the coexpression of a particular protein in the context of other proteins may generate a different CTL responses. In another study, the authors constructed plasmids encoding core, E1 and E2 individually or together, under the control of a cytomegalovirus promoter.[82] The authors compared the efficacy of these constructs with a plasmid containing coding sequences for all three structural proteins under the control of the human elongation factor 1α (EF-1a) promoter. BALB/c mice were immunized only once with these constructs, and the site of injection was given an electric pulse to enhance the efficiency of DNA uptake in cells. Spleen cells obtained from the DNA-immunized mice were assessed for their ability to lyse major histocompatibility complex (MHC)-matched target cells either pulsed with core or E1 peptide or infected with E2-expressing vaccinia virus. Only mice inoculated with the plasmid expressing core, E1, and E2 under the EF-1α promoter generated HCV-specific effector responses against all three proteins after a single immunization. Furthermore, E2 DNA immunization followed by a boost with a recombinant HSV 1 glycoprotein D HCV–E2 fusion protein enhanced the CTL responses in mice, which is closely associated with the protection of mice against challenge with a E2 expressing tumor cell line.[71] CD8+ CTL activities have also been demonstrated for the nonstructural proteins NS3 and NS5 after three intramuscular injections with NS3- and NS5-encoding plasmids.[74] In addition, a tumor model in which syngeneic cells stably transfected with an NS5 expression plasmid was used to assess CTL activity in vivo.[74] About 60% of immunized mice were protected against tumor formation, and in those who developed tumors, the tumor weight was significantly reduced as compared with the unimmunized mice.

To better approximate HCV infection in humans, a transgenic mouse model expressing the human HLA-A2.1 has been developed.[80] This transgenic mouse model can be used to study the generation of humanlike HLA-A2.1 restricted CTL responses. HLA trangsenic mice were immunized three times with a plasmid vaccine encoding the entire core protein. At 2, 6, and 14 months after the last boost, mice were challenged with recombinant vaccinia virus expressing the HCV core protein or a control vaccinia virus expressing hemagglutinin. Mice were then killed and vaccinia virus titers determined in the ovaries. DNA-immunized mice showed a reduction of vaccinia titer 6–12 logs at month 2, 7 logs at month 6, and 5 logs even at month 14 after the last immunization, as compared with the corresponding mock-immunized controls. These results suggest that the HCV core DNA vaccine generated a long-lasting protection against infection with recombinant vaccinia virus expressing HCV core in vivo, despite a weak anticore CTL response requiring at least three stimulations with peptides to detect the HCV core-specific CTL activities in the standard ^{51}Cr release assay. The authors also showed that the protection was mediated by CD8+ cells.

The nucleic acid-based vaccine studies demonstrated the potency of DNA-based vaccines to induce both humoral and cellular immune responses against various HCV proteins. However, most of these studies focused on either the humoral or cellular immune responses. Therefore, more potent vectors need to be designed to generate both strong humoral and cellular immune responses against multiple epitopes within the structural and nonstructural proteins. The codelivery of cytokines has been shown to enhance the immune responses against DNA-based HCV vaccines. Thus, the benefit of other immunomodulating molecules such as B7,[84] CD40 ligand,[85,86] or CTLA4[87] that has been shown to enhance nucleic acid immunization should be explored for HCV DNA vaccination. The delivery of DNA is also a crucial step that should be studied in more detail; factors such as the route(s) (e.g., im) and methods of delivery and the delivery systems should be optimized. Furthermore, the prime-boost combination of DNA and protein vaccines should be carefully evaluated to establish an immunization protocol that maximizes the potency of both approaches.

RECOMBINANT VIRUS

Recombinant viruses are an efficient vehicle for DNA delivery that can result in high level of recombinant protein expression in host cells. In a number of experimental models, infection of animals with recombinant viruses encoding foreign viral proteins induce protective immunity to a variety of viruses.[88–90] Several recombinant viral vectors are being evaluated for HCV vaccine development (Table 3). The defective recombinant adenovirus is an attractive candidate because of its hepatotropism, its potency to induce both humoral and cell-mediated immunities, and its ability to be administered parenterally or orally. Recombinant adenoviruses that are defective in their replication and lack the E1 and E3 regions of the genome have been used to increase the amount of foreign sequences that can be inserted. Studies in mice showed that a recombinant adenovirus containing genes for the structural proteins of HCV-induced antibody responses to each of the three structural proteins.[91] In addition, strong cytotoxic T-cell responses against core and E1 could be detected in splenocytes from mice immunized with an adenovirus carrying core and E1 genes.[92] The cytotoxic T-cell responses lasted for at least 100 days. Coadministration of a recombinant adenovirus expressing IL-12 led to a marked increase in cellular immune responses when administered at a dose of 10[7] plaque-forming units.[93] The cellular immunity

TABLE 3.   Recombinant Virus Approaches

Approach	HCV Antigen	Antibody	T Helper Cells	CTL	References
Recombinant viruses					
Adenovirus	Core-E1-E2	+	nd	nd	91
	Core-E1	nd	nd	+	92
	Core-E1 + IL-12	nd	↑	↑	93
Vaccinia	Core	nd	nd	+	94
	Core-E1-E2	nd	+	+	95*
DNA + canarypox	HCV-DNA + canarypox core-E1-E2-NS2-NS3	nd	nd	↑	†

+, positive response; ↑, enhanced response; →, no change in response; ↓, decreased response; nd, not done.
*Unpublished results from our laboratory.
†P. Pancholi et al., presented at the 6th international symposium on hepatitis C and related viruses.

was abolished when higher doses of the IL-12 expressing adenovirus were used. However, the recent tragedy of death in a gene therapy trial using adenovirus has severely dampened the enthusiasm for the use of this viral vector in humans.

Spleen cells from mice immunized with a recombinant vaccinia virus expressing the HCV core gene exhibited strong core-specific CTL activities.[94] In addition, studies in our laboratory showed that immunization with a recombinant vaccinia virus carrying sequences for the structural proteins generated strong CTL and T helper cell responses against all structural proteins in BALB/c mice. Interestingly, studies using HCV vaccinia recombinants revealed that vaccinia-specific CTL responses were greatly suppressed by vaccinia recombinants expressing the core protein, suggesting that HCV core may alter the immunogenicity of a vaccine and may play a role in the persistent of HCV infection.[95] Furthermore, a nonreplicating canarypox virus encoding polycistronic core/E1/E2/NS2/NS3 genes are being used to potentiate the immune response to HCV DNA immunization. Preliminary data suggest that a booster injection with this recombinant canarypox virus enhances the HCV-specific immune response and generates broader T-cell activity (P. Pancholi, et al., presented at the 6th international symposium on hepatitis C and related viruses).

There are some promising new studies on recombinant virus vectors approaches in the HIV field that can be also adopted for the development of an HCV vaccine. Strategies using new poxvirus vectors such as canarypox, fowlpoxvirus,[96] attenuated vaccinia strains NYVAC[96] or modified vaccinia virus strain Ankara have been developed.[97] Alphavirus vectors such as Venezuelan equine encephalitis virus[98,99] or Semiliki Forest virus[100] have also been explored as a vehicle for HIV DNA immunization. An attractive approach is the use of alphavirus replicon vector as a DNA vehicle. These replicons have the advantage that they are self-replicating, express foreign genes in infected cells, but lack the viral structural proteins and can be adminis-

tered as naked DNA vaccine. Live attenuated salmonella (*Salmonella typhimurium*) is an alternative vehicle of DNA delivery.[101] Oral or nasal immunization with this bacterial vector has been shown to induce both mucosal and systemic immune responses against DNA encoded antigens. Although all these recombinant virus approaches are very promising, safety and regulatory issues may be of concern with implementation.

PEPTIDE VACCINE

Peptide vaccines follow the basic principle that T lymphocytes recognize antigens only as peptide fragments that are generated intracellularly and bound to MHC class I or II molecules on the surface of the antigen presenting cells. Helper T cells recognize antigenic peptides that are bound to the MHC class II molecules, whereas CD8+ cytotoxic T cells are bound to the MHC class I molecules. Therefore, small peptides that are present in the extracellular milieu can bind directly to MHC class I or II molecules without undergoing the antigen processing pathway. Consequently, chemically synthesized peptides that are potent immunogenic antigens are being pursued as vaccine candidate for HCV (Table 4).

The rationale of this approach is based on the knowledge that certain T-cell epitopes on the HCV polyprotein may be important for viral clearance. Using amino acid motifs to predict the binding of peptides to MHC class I and II molecules, MHC-peptide binding assays, and CTL and T helper assays, several CTL and T helper epitopes on the HCV polyprotein that may be important for the design of a peptide vaccine have been identified.

Peptides containing epitopes from the core,[102–104] NS4,[104] and NS5[102] regions have been shown to induce strong CTL responses in BALB/c and HLA-A2.1 transgenic mice. The covalent attachment of the CTL peptide to a T helper peptide seems to be crucial for generating a strong CTL response.[102–104] In addition, enhancement of

TABLE 4. Peptide, Recombinant Subunit Protein, and HCV-LP Approaches

Approach	HCV Antigen	Antibody	T Helper Cells	CTL	Chimpanzee Study	References
Peptide						
CTL +T helper epitopes	Core, NS4, NS5	nd	nd	+		102–104
Antibody epitopes	E2 HVR1	+	nd	nd		106–108
Amino acid substitution		nd	nd	↑		105
Lipidiated		nd	nd	↑		104
Recombinant protein						
Prophylaxis	E1-E2	+	—*	—*	Prevention of chronic infection	18, 110
Therapeutic	tE1	+	nd	nd	Improvement of liver histology	111
HCV-like particles	Core-E1-E2	+	+	+		120, 121

+, positive response; —, no response; ↑, enhanced response; nd, not done.
*Michael Houghton, personal communication.

the immunogenicity of a core-specific CTL epitope has been achieved by substitution of one amino acid on the native peptide.[105] Furthermore, covalently linked T helper and CTL epitopes were more potent immunogens when delivered as lipidated peptides.[104]

Other strategies for developing peptide vaccines are using peptides to generate antibodies against linear epitopes. Because HVR1 contains a neutralizing epitope, it is an attractive target for peptide-based vaccine. A chimpanzee that was immunized with recombinant E1 and E2 glycoproteins together with HVR1 peptides derived from a different isolate was protected against inoculation of the isolate from which the peptide sequence was derived.[106] In addition, antiserum from this protected chimpanzee was shown to neutralize the homologous strain by inoculation of this mixture into another chimpanzee. Similarly, rabbits that were immunized with a series of synthetic HVR1 peptides[107] produced high titers of broadly cross-reactive antibodies to HCV that could block the binding of antibody-captured HCV to MOLT-4 cells.

The most difficult problem of choosing the HVR1 as the target for a HCV vaccine is the existence of quasispecies in this region of HCV genome. The screening of phage displayed peptide libraries has been used to identify a consensus profile from over 200 HVR1 sequences of different viral isolates. HVR1 sequences most commonly recognized by patient sera and able to bind antibodies that cross-react with a large panel of HVR1 were identified (Table 5).[108] A sequence pattern within these so-called mimotopes that was responsible for the detected cross-reactivity could be developed. Mice immunized with a mixture of the mimotopes shown in Table 5 could generate antibodies that recognized 95% of the same panel of natural HVR1 variants. This finding was confirmed by another study that among the 25 different HVR1 proteins derived from genotypes 1b, the protein that contains the sequence similar to the reported con-

sensus sequence was the most frequently recognized protein by patient's sera.[109]

The major obstacles for a peptide-based approach lie in the observation that single peptide without helper function may be a poor immunogen, and many effective vaccines are typically multivalent in generating a broad immunity against several different antigens. However, this limitation can be overcome by the coadministration of potent adjuvants or the use of multiple epitopes vaccine that contains a mixture of peptides.

RECOMBINANT PROTEIN SUBUNIT VACCINE

The initial attempt to develop an HCV vaccine was directed toward generating a recombinant protein subunit vaccine. Because it has been shown for several flaviviruses that antibodies to the envelope protein can provide protection, recombinant HCV E1 and E2 proteins were used in early vaccination studies from Chiron (Table 4).[110] However, the success was limited. In their initial effort, the E1 and E2 proteins were purified from HeLa cells infected with a recombinant vaccinia virus. The purified recombinant envelope HCV proteins were injected with an oil/water microemulsified adjuvants im 18 times into two chimpanzees and three times in additional five animals. Two to 3 weeks after the final boost, chimpanzees were challenged with a low dose of homologous HCV-1 virus. The five animals with the highest anti-E1/E2 titers did not show any signs of viral infection. The two remaining animals became infected but resolved their infection. In comparison, four similarly challenged naive chimpanzees developed chronic infection. However, rechallenge of the five protected animals with heterologous. HCV-H isolate after additional boosts with recombinant E1 and E2 proteins derived from a constitutively expressing Chinese hamster ovary cell

TABLE 5. HVR1 Mimotopes with the Highest Frequency of Reactivity

	Amino Acid Sequences	Cross-Reactivity (%)
R9	QTTVVGGSQSHTVRGLTSLFSPGASQN	60
F78	QTHTTGGQAGHQAHSLTGLFSPGAKQN	70
M122	QTTTTGGSASHAVSSLTGLFSPGSKQN	44
G31	TTHTVGGSVARQVHSLTGLFSPGPQQK	77
H1	QTHTTGGVVGHATSGLTSLFSPGPSQK	42
D6	QTTTTGGQVSHATHGLTGLFSLGPQQK	60

line led to infection in all animals, although none developed persistent infection.[18] In general, the Chinese hamster ovary cell-derived vaccine exhibited lower immunogenicity than the recombinant envelope proteins derived from vaccinia virus-infected HeLa cells and did not protect any of the vaccinated chimpanzees after challenge with the homologous virus. However, self-limited infection occurred more frequently than in nonvaccinated animals. Nonetheless, these results are encouraging in the sense that although no sterilizing immunity was achieved, chronic infection might be prevented.

Recombinant HCV proteins have also been explored for an immunotherapeutic approach. Recombinant E1 protein of genotype 1b was purified as homodimers that associated into particles of about 9 nm in diameter.[111] Two chimpanzees with chronic HCV infection received a total of nine doses of 50 μg recombinant E1 protein. One of the chimpanzees was infected with HCV genotype 1a and the other one with 1b. Vaccination resulted in improved liver histology, disappearance of viral antigens from the liver as detected by immunostaining, and decrease in alanine aminotransferase (ALT) levels in both animals. Although HCV RNA levels in the serum did not change during treatment, liver inflammation and HCV antigens reappeared and ALT levels rose after the end of treatment. An association between high levels of anti-E1 antibodies and the improvement of hepatitis C was observed.

HCV-LIKE PARTICLES

Viruslike particles are attractive as a recombinant protein vaccine, because they mimic more closely the properties of native viruses than recombinant protein subunit vaccines. Indeed, studies in various animal models have demonstrated that papillomavirus- and rotarvirus-like particles synthesized in insect cells can induce protective immunity.[112–114] In addition, several studies have shown the efficacy of viruslike particles to induce not only a strong antibody response but also a CTL response in immunized animals.[115–118] Our laboratory recently reported the synthesis of HCV-like particles (HCV-LPs) in insect cells using a recombinant bac-

ulovirus containing the cDNA of the HCV structural proteins (core, E1, and E2).[119] The HCV-LP exhibit similar morphologic, biophysical, and antigenic properties as the putative virions isolated from HCV infected humans. These noninfectious 40–50 nm HCV-LPs consist of a lipid envelope containing E1 and E2 (Fig. 2). Mice immunized with HCV-LP generated a strong humoral immune response against the structural proteins core and E2 (Table 4).[120] The antienvelope titers were detectable after the third immunization and were highest after the seventh immunization with titers ranging between 12,800 and 204,800. Antienvelope antibodies recognize E2 proteins from different genotypes and were broadly directed against various regions of the E2 protein. HCV-LPs are also capable of inducing a strong cellular immune responses in BALB/c mice.[121] Splenocytes from HCV-LP immunized mice showed T-cell proliferative responses against core and E1/E2 proteins. In addition, HCV-specific CTL activities predominantly directed against the E2 protein could be detected in HCV-LP immunized mice. Furthermore, interferon-γ but not IL-4 production produced by the HCV-specific activated T cells, suggesting a type 1-like response. Studies in which HCV-LPs were denatured before injection revealed that the immunogenicity is strongly dependent on particle formation. These studies suggest that HCV-LP may be promising as a potential vaccine candidate.

PASSIVE IMMUNIZATION

Because passive immunization has been successfully used for the prevention of hepatitis A and HBV infection, the efficacy of anti-HCV immunoglobulin to protect from hepatitis C infection has been evaluated in several studies. In one study, three chimpanzees were inoculated with HCV.[122] One hour after inoculation, one chimpanzee was treated once intravenously with hepatitis C immunoglobulin, the second with anti-HCV negative immunoglobulin, and the third animal received no treatment. Anti-HCV immunoglobulin did not prevent infection as shown by the presence of HCV RNA in serum and HCV antigen in the liver. However, liver enzyme activity was delayed in the anti-HCV immunoglobulin-treated animal and the period of acute hepatitis C was prolonged. In a more recent study, four chimpanzees received multiple infusions of anti-HCV immunoglobulins over a period of 13 weeks after inoculation with HCV.[123] In this study, HCV viremia lasted only 73 to 105 days, and there was no evidence of acute hepatitis in the treated animals. HCV RNA reoccurred in serum samples of one animal after passively transferred anti-HCV immunoglobulins disappeared. In addition, three chronically infected chimpanzees were also treated with repeated infusions of anti-HCV immuno-

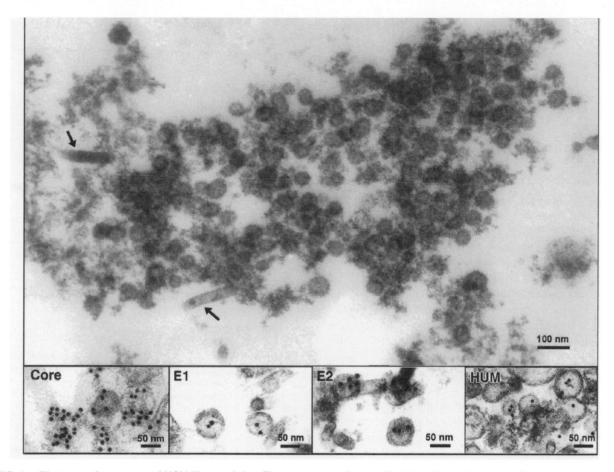

FIG. 2. Electron microscopy of HCV-like particles. The sucrose gradient purified viruslike particles were fixed and visualized by electron microscopy (arrow; bar, 40 nm). The inserts below show labeling of partially purified particles with monoclonal anticore, anti-E1, anti-E2 antibodies, and serum from an HCV-infected human (HUM) (bar, 50 nm). (Reproduced with permission from Ref. 120.)

globulins twice a week over a period of 15 weeks. In two chimpanzees, a significant decrease of HCV RNA levels in serum could be detected during treatment. After the end of treatment, HCV RNA levels decreased further. Interestingly, a substantial decrease in HCV antigen was detected in the liver. These studies suggest that antibodies alone can prevent acute HCV infection and are even beneficial when administered in the chronic phase of HCV infection. Further studies are needed to clarify which antibodies are essential for preventing acute HCV infection. The knowledge of the mechanism for antibody-mediated clearance of HCV antigens in the liver of chronically infected chimpanzees may provide further insights in preventing persistent HCV infection.

COMBINATION MODALITY

Given the lack of clearly defined correlates for a protective immunity and the relatively weak immunoge-

nicity of recombinant subunit vaccines, a successful HCV vaccine may require a multicomponent approach that stimulates various aspects of the immune response. Promising new studies on the prime-boost approaches in the HIV field could be adapted for the development of a HCV vaccine. Most encouraging approaches are priming with DNA and boosting with recombinant virus vectors or viral proteins. The efficacy of this strategy has been shown by the protection of macaque monkeys from a pathogenic challenge with simian HIV chimera (SHIV) after a prime boost regimen with DNA followed by FPV boost.[124,125] Priming with DNA followed by boosting with gp120 also generated protective responses that was far superior as either DNA or recombinant protein immunization alone.[125] Only a few studies have explored the DNA-protein prime-boost regimen for an HCV vaccine.[65,71] These studies demonstrated the potency of this strategy. Future studies, especially protection studies in chimpanzees, are needed to determine if the combination modality indeed holds the promise for the induction of broadly directed humoral and cellular immune response that is sufficient for a protective immunity against HCV.

CONCLUDING REMARKS

The development of an effective vaccine against HCV faces a variety of obstacles. The lack of a convenient experimental model system makes it very difficult to study the correlates of protective immunity and viral clearance. Studies in humans and in chimpanzees indicate thus far that an ideal vaccine should induce broad humoral, T helper, and cytotoxic T-cell responses. Therefore, the final product might be a combination of different approaches, such as a combination of DNA and recombinant subunit protein vaccines. To induce a broad cellular immune response in the general population, it is also necessary that the vaccine candidate contain epitopes that are restricted by diverse MHC alleles. In addition, given the high degree of genetic heterogenicity of HCV, this vaccine should also be able to exert cross-protective immunity against various HCV genotypes. This could be achieved by either including antigens from different genotypes or by using antigens that induce cross-protection. Mimotope sequences derived from the HVR1 that induce cross-reactivity are encouraging and may be valuable for the development of a broadly active vaccine.

Finally, because HCV-associated morbidity and mortality result from long-term sequelae of chronic infection, sterilizing immunity may not be necessary as long as vaccine-induced immunity is effective in preventing chronic infection. Following this strategy, there are encouraging reports that immunization with anti-HCV immunoglobulins or recombinant envelope proteins can alter the outcome of infection and prevent chronic infection in chimpanzees. Other promising strategies for the development of an HCV vaccine also have been evaluated in small animal models. However, their prophylactic potential would have to be determined in primate models. As we move from bench to bedside, clinical trials to test the efficacy of any vaccine candidate would have to be carefully conducted in large high-risk populations and possibly in countries where the incidence of new HCV infection remains high. Finally, the question remains as to who should receive the vaccine. High-risk populations such as health care workers, IV drug users, hemophiliacs, renal dialysis patients, infants born to infected mothers, partners of infected individuals, and highly sexually active persons should be the primary target of a vaccine program. However, universal vaccination, like the case for HBV, may be necessary to achieve the ultimate goal of global control of HCV infection.

ABBREVIATIONS

CTL	cytotoxic T lymphocyte
E	envelop
HBV	hepatitis B virus
GM-CSF	granulocyte-macrophage colony-stimulating factor
HCV	hepatitis C virus
HCV-LP	HCV-like particles
HLA	human histocompatibility leukocyte
HVR	hypervariable region
IL	interleukin
MHC	major histocompatibility complex
NS	nonstructural

REFERENCES

1. Singh M, O'Hagan D. Advances in vaccine adjuvants. Nat Biotechnol 1999;17:1075–1081
2. Brandriss MW, Schlesinger JJ, Walsh EE, Briselli M. Lethal 17D yellow fever encephalitis in mice. I. Passive protection by monoclonal antibodies to the envelope proteins of 17D yellow fever and dengue 2 viruses. J Gen Virol 1986;67:229–234
3. Bray M, Lai CJ. Dengue virus premembrane and membrane proteins elicit a protective immune response. Virology 1991;185:505–508
4. Konishi E, Pincus S, Paoletti E, Shope RE, Burrage T, Mason PW. Mice immunized with a subviral particle containing the Japanese encephalitis virus prM/M and E proteins are protected from lethal JEV infection. Virology 1992;188:714–720
5. Kreil TR, Burger I, Attakpah E, Olas K, Eibl MM. Passive immunization reduces immunity that results from simultaneous active immunization against tick-borne encephalitis virus in a mouse model. Vaccine 1998;16:955–959
6. Weiner AJ, Geysen HM, Christopherson C, et al. Evidence for immune selection of hepatitis C virus (HCV) putative envelope glycoprotein variants: Potential role in chronic HCV infections. Proc Natl Acad Sci USA 1992;89:3468–3472
7. Pileri P, Uematsu Y, Campagnoli S, et al. Binding of hepatitis C virus to CD81. Science 1998;282:938–941
8. Habersetzer F, Fournillier A, Dubuisson J, et al. Characterization of human monoclonal antibodies specific to the hepatitis C virus glycoprotein E2 with in vitro binding neutralization properties. Virology 1998;249:32–41
9. Farci P, Shimoda A, Wong D, et al. Prevention of hepatitis C virus infection in chimpanzees by hyperimmune serum against the hypervariable region 1 of the envelope 2 protein. Proc Natl Acad Sci USA 1996;93:15394–15399
10. Shimizu YK, Hijikata M, Iwamoto A, Alter HJ, Purcell RH, Yoshikura H. Neutralizing antibodies against hepatitis C virus and the emergence of neutralization escape mutant viruses. J Virol 1994;68:1494–1500
11. Kato N, Ootsuyama Y, Sekiya H, et al. Genetic drift in hypervariable region 1 of the viral genome in persistent hepatitis C virus infection. J Virol 1994;68:4776–4784
12. Allander T, Beyene A, Jacobson SH, Grillner L, Persson MA. Patients infected with the same hepatitis C virus strain display different kinetics of the isolate-specific antibody response. J Infect Dis 1997;175:26–31
13. Zibert A, Meisel H, Kraas W, Schulz A, Jung G, Roggendorf M. Early antibody response against hypervariable region 1 is asso-

ciated with acute self-limiting infections of hepatitis C virus. Hepatology 1997;25:1245–1249

14. Yuki N, Hayashi N, Kasahara A, et al. Quantitative analysis of antibody to hepatitis C virus envelope 2 glycoprotein in patients with chronic hepatitis C virus infection. Hepatology 1996;23: 947–952

15. Fournillier-Jacob A, Lunel F, Cahour A, et al. Antibody responses to hepatitis C envelope proteins in patients with acute or chronic hepatitis C. J Med Virol 1996;50:159–167

16. Grellier L, Brown D, Power J, Dusheiko G. Absence of anti-envelope antibodies and clearance of hepatitis C virus in a cohort of Irish women infected in 1977. J Viral Hepat 1997;4: 379–381

17. Prince AM, Brotman B, Lee DH, Ren L, Moore BS, Scheffel JW. Significance of the anti-E2 response in self-limited and chronic hepatitis C virus infections in chimpanzees and in humans. J Infect Dis 1999;180:987–991

18. Houghton M. Strategies and prospects for vaccination against the hepatitis C viruses. Curr Top Microbiol Immunol 2000;242: 327–329

19. Chen M, Sallberg M, Sonnerborg A, et al. Limited humoral immunity in hepatitis C virus infection. Gastroenterology 1999; 116:135–143

20. Botarelli P, Brunetto MR, Minutello MA, et al. T-lymphocyte response to hepatitis C virus in different clinical courses of infection. Gastroenterology 1993;104:580–587

21. Ferrari C, Valli A, Galati L, et al. T-cell response to structural and nonstructural hepatitis C virus antigens in persistent and self-limited hepatitis C virus infections. Hepatology 1994;19: 286–295

22. Missale G, Bertoni R, Lamonaca V, et al. Different clinical behaviors of acute hepatitis C virus infection are associated with different vigor of the anti-viral cell-mediated immune response. J Clin Invest 1996;98:706–714

23. Lechmann M, Ihlenfeldt HG, Braunschweiger I, et al. T- and B-cell responses to different hepatitis C virus antigens in patients with chronic hepatitis C infection and in healthy anti-hepatitis C virus—positive blood donors without viremia [see comments]. Hepatology 1996;24:790–795

24. Cramp ME, Carucci P, Rossol S, et al. Hepatitis C virus (HCV) specific immune responses in anti-HCV positive patients without hepatitis C viraemia. Gut 1999;44:424–429

25. Diepolder HM, Zachoval R, Hoffmann RM, et al. Possible mechanism involving T-lymphocyte response to non-structural protein 3 in viral clearance in acute hepatitis C virus infection. Lancet 1995;346:1006–1007

26. Lamonaca V, Missale G, Urbani S, et al. Conserved hepatitis C virus sequences are highly immunogenic for CD4(+) T cells: Implications for vaccine development. Hepatology 1999;30: 1088–1098

27. Diepolder HM, Gerlach JT, Zachoval R, et al. Immunodominant CD4+ T-cell epitope within nonstructural protein 3 in acute hepatitis C virus infection. J Virol 1997;71:6011–6019

28. Cramp ME, Rossol S, Chokshi S, Carucci P, Williams R, Naoumov NV. Hepatitis C virus-specific T-cell reactivity during interferon and ribavirin treatment in chronic hepatitis C. Gastroenterology 2000;118:346–355

29. Missale G, Cariani E, Lamonaca V, et al. Effects of interferon treatment on the antiviral T-cell response in hepatitis C virus genotype 1b- and genotype 2c-infected patients. Hepatology 1997;26:792–797

30. Lasarte JJ, Garcia-Granero M, Lopez A, et al. Cellular immunity to hepatitis C virus core protein and the response to interferon in patients with chronic hepatitis C [see comments]. Hepatology 1998;28:815–822

31. Woitas RP, Lechmann M, Jung G, Kaiser R, Sauerbruch T, Spengler U. CD30 induction and cytokine profiles in hepatitis C virus core-specific peripheral blood T lymphocytes. J Immunol 1997;159:1012–1018

32. Lechmann M, Woitas RP, Langhans B, et al. Decreased frequency of HCV core-specific peripheral blood mononuclear cells with type 1 cytokine secretion in chronic hepatitis C [In Process Citation]. J Hepatol 1999;31:971–978

33. Cerny A, McHutchison JG, Pasquinelli C, et al. Cytotoxic T lymphocyte response to hepatitis C virus-derived peptides containing the HLA A2.1 binding motif. J Clin Invest 1995;95: 521–530

34. Wong DK, Dudley DD, Afdhal NH, et al. Liver-derived CTL in hepatitis C virus infection: Breadth and specificity of responses in a cohort of persons with chronic infection. J Immunol 1998;160:1479–1488

35. Koziel MJ, Dudley D, Wong JT, et al. Intrahepatic cytotoxic T lymphocytes specific for hepatitis C virus in persons with chronic hepatitis. J Immunol 1992;149:3339–3344

36. Chang KM, Gruener NH, Southwood S, et al. Identification of HLA-A3 and -B7-restricted CTL response to hepatitis C virus in patients with acute and chronic hepatitis C. J Immunol 1999; 162:1156–1164

37. Koziel MJ, Dudley D, Afdhal N, et al. HLA class I-restricted cytotoxic T lymphocytes specific for hepatitis C virus. Identification of multiple epitopes and characterization of patterns of cytokine release. J Clin Invest 1995;96:2311–2321

38. Ibe M, Sakaguchi T, Tanaka K, et al. Identification and characterization of a cytotoxic T cell epitope of hepatitis C virus presented by HLA-B*3501 in acute hepatitis. J Gen Virol 1998;79:1735–1744

39. Battegay M, Fikes J, Di Bisceglie AM, et al. Patients with chronic hepatitis C have circulating cytotoxic T cells which recognize hepatitis C virus-encoded peptides binding to HLA-A2.1 molecules. J Virol 1995;69:2462–2470

40. Kaneko T, Nakamura I, Kita H, Hiroishi K, Moriyama T, Imawari M. Three new cytotoxic T cell epitopes identified within the hepatitis C virus nucleoprotein. J Gen Virol 1996; 77:1305–1309

41. Koziel MJ, Dudley D, Afdhal N, et al. Hepatitis C virus (HCV)-specific cytotoxic T lymphocytes recognize epitopes in the core and envelope proteins of HCV. J Virol 1993;67:7522–7532

42. Kita H, Hiroishi K, Moriyama T, et al. A minimal and optimal cytotoxic T cell epitope within hepatitis C virus nucleoprotein. J Gen Virol 1995;76:3189–3193

43. Chang KM, Rehermann B, McHutchison JG, et al. Immunological significance of cytotoxic T lymphocyte epitope variants in patients chronically infected by the hepatitis C virus. J Clin Invest 1997;100:2376–2385

44. Weiner A, Erickson AL, Kansopon J, et al. Persistent hepatitis C virus infection in a chimpanzee is associated with emergence of a cytotoxic T lymphocyte escape variant. Proc Natl Acad Sci USA 1995;92:2755–2759

45. Tsai SL, Chen YM, Chen MH, et al. Hepatitis C virus variants circumventing cytotoxic T lymphocyte activity as a mechanism of chronicity. Gastroenterology 1998;115:954–965

46. Hiroishi K, Kita H, Kojima M, et al. Cytotoxic T lymphocyte response and viral load in hepatitis C virus infection. Hepatology 1997;25:705–712

47. Nelson DR, Marousis CG, Davis GL, et al. The role of hepatitis C virus-specific cytotoxic T lymphocytes in chronic hepatitis C. J Immunol 1997;158:1473–1481

48. Rehermann B, Chang KM, McHutchinson J, et al. Differential cytotoxic T-lymphocyte responsiveness to the hepatitis B and C viruses in chronically infected patients. J Virol 1996;70: 7092–7102

49. Cooper S, Erickson AL, Adams EJ, et al. Analysis of a successful immune response against hepatitis C virus. Immunity 1999;10:439–449

50. Bjoro K, Froland SS, Yun Z, Samdal HH, Haaland T. Hepatitis C infection in patients with primary hypogammaglobulinemia after treatment with contaminated immune globulin. N Engl J Med 1994;331:1607–1611

51. Christie JM, Healey CJ, Watson J, et al. Clinical outcome of hypogammaglobulinaemic patients following outbreak of acute hepatitis C: 2 year follow up. Clin Exp Immunol 1997;110:4–8

52. Adams G, Kuntz S, Rabalais G, Bratcher D, Tamburro CH, Kotwal GJ. Natural recovery from acute hepatitis C virus infection by agammaglobulinemic twin children. Pediatr Infect Dis J 1997;16:533–534

53. Rosa D, Campagnoli S, Moretto C, et al. A quantitative test to estimate neutralizing antibodies to the hepatitis C virus: Cytofluorimetric assessment of envelope glycoprotein 2 binding to target cells. Proc Natl Acad Sci USA 1996;93:1759–1763

54. Esumi M, Ahmed M, Zhou YH, Takahashi H, Shikata T. Murine antibodies against E2 and hypervariable region 1 cross-reactively capture hepatitis C virus. Virology 1998;251:158–164

55. Walter E, Keist R, Niederost B, Pult I, Blum HE. Hepatitis B virus infection of tupaia hepatocytes in vitro and in vivo. Hepatology 1996;24:1–5

56. Xie ZC, Riezu-Boj JI, Lasarte JJ, et al. Transmission of hepatitis C virus infection to tree shrews. Virology 1998;244:513–520

57. Ulmer JB, Donnelly JJ, Parker SE, et al. Heterologous protection against influenza by injection of DNA encoding a viral protein [see comments]. Science 1993;259:1745–1749

58. Hoffman SL, et al. Protection against malaria by immunization with a Plasmodium yoelii circumsporozoite protein nucleic acid vaccine. Vaccine 1994;12:1529–1533

59. Huygen K, Content J, Denis O, et al. Immunogenicity and protective efficacy of a tuberculosis DNA vaccine. Nat Med 1996;2:893–898

60. Boyer JD, Ugen KE, Wang B, et al. Protection of chimpanzees from high-dose heterologous HIV-1 challenge by DNA vaccination. Nat Med 1997;3:526–532

61. Vanderzanden L, Bray M, Fuller D, et al. DNA vaccines expressing either the GP or NP genes of Ebola virus protect mice from lethal challenge. Virology 1998;246:134–144

62. Geissler M, Gesien A, Tokushige K, Wands JR. Enhancement of cellular and humoral immune responses to hepatitis C virus core protein using DNA-based vaccines augmented with cytokine-expressing plasmids. J Immunol 1997;158:1231–1237

63. Tokushige K, Wakita T, Pachuk C, et al. Expression and immune response to hepatitis C virus core DNA-based vaccine constructs. Hepatology 1996;24:14–20

64. Major ME, Vitvitski L, Mink MA, et al. DNA-based immunization with chimeric vectors for the induction of immune responses against the hepatitis C virus nucleocapsid. J Virol 1995;69:5798–5805

65. Hu GJ, Wang RY, Han DS, Alter HJ, Shih JW. Characterization of the humoral and cellular immune responses against hepatitis C virus core induced by DNA-based immunization. Vaccine 1999;17:3160–3170

66. Geissler M, Tokushige K, Wakita T, Zurawski VR Jr, Wands JR. Differential cellular and humoral immune responses to HCV core and HBV envelope proteins after genetic immunizations using chimeric constructs. Vaccine 1998;16:857–867

67. Rice CM. Flaviviridae: The viruses and their replication. In: Fields BN, Knipe DM, Howeley PM, eds. Virology. Vol. 1. 3rd ed. Philadelphia: Lippincott-Raven, 1996:931–960

68. Forns X, Emerson SU, Tobin GJ, Mushahwar IK, Purcell RH, Bukh J. DNA immunization of mice and macaques with plasmids encoding hepatitis C virus envelope E2 protein expressed intracellularly and on the cell surface. Vaccine 1999;17:1992–2002

69. Forns X, Payette PJ, Ma XY, et al. DNA immunization of macaques and chimpanzees with plasmids encoding hepatitis C virus (HCV) envelope E2 protein. Hepatology 1999;30:769

70. Lee SW, Cho JH, Sung YC. Optimal induction of hepatitis C virus envelope-specific immunity by bicistronic plasmid DNA inoculation with the granulocyte-macrophage colony-stimulating factor gene. J Virol 1998;72:8430–8436

71. Song MK, Lee SW, Suh YS, Lee KJ, Sung YC. Enhancement of immunoglobulin G2a and cytotoxic T-lymphocyte responses by a booster immunization with recombinant hepatitis C virus E2 protein in E2 DNA-primed mice. J Virol 2000;74:2920–2925

72. Nakano I, Maertens G, Major ME, et al. Immunization with plasmid DNA encoding hepatitis C virus envelope E2 antigenic domains induces antibodies whose immune reactivity is linked to the injection mode. J Virol 1997;71:7101–7109

73. Fournillier A, Nakano I, Vitvitski L, et al. Modulation of immune responses to hepatitis C virus envelope E2 protein following injection of plasmid DNA using single or combined delivery routes. Hepatology 1998;28:237–244

74. Encke J, zu Putlitz J, Geissler M, Wands JR. Genetic immunization generates cellular and humoral immune responses against the nonstructural proteins of the hepatitis C virus in a murine model. J Immunol 1998;161:4917–4923

75. Cho JH, Lee SW, Sung YC. Enhanced cellular immunity to hepatitis C virus nonstructural proteins by codelivery of granulocyte macrophage-colony stimulating factor gene in intramuscular DNA immunization. Vaccine 1999;17:1136–1144

76. Lagging LM, Meyer K, Hoft D, Houghton M, Belshe RB, Ray R. Immune responses to plasmid DNA encoding the hepatitis C virus core protein. J Virol 1995;69:5859–5863

77. Lee SW, Cho JH, Lee KJ, Sung YC. Hepatitis C virus envelope DNA-based immunization elicits humoral and cellular immune responses. Mol Cells 1998;8:444–451

78. Inchauspe G, Vitvitski L, Major ME, et al. Plasmid DNA expressing a secreted or a nonsecreted form of hepatitis C virus nucleocapsid: Comparative studies of antibody and T-helper responses following genetic immunization. DNA Cell Biol 1997;16:185–195

79. Tokushige K, Moradpour D, Wakita T, Geissler M, Hayashi N, Wands JR. Comparison between cytomegalovirus promoter and elongation factor-1 alpha promoter-driven constructs in the establishment of cell lines expressing hepatitis C virus core protein. J Virol Methods 1997;64:73–80

80. Arichi T, Saito T, Major ME, et al. Prophylactic DNA vaccine for hepatitis C virus (HCV) infection: HCV-specific cytotoxic T lymphocyte induction and protection from HCV-recombinant vaccinia infection in an HLA-A2.1 transgenic mouse model. Proc Natl Acad Sci USA 2000;97:297–302

81. Saito T, Sherman GJ, Kurokohchi K, et al. Plasmid DNA-based immunization for hepatitis C virus structural proteins: Immune responses in mice. Gastroenterology 1997;112:1321–1330

82. Nishimura Y, Kamei A, Uno-Furuta S, et al. A single immunization with a plasmid encoding hepatitis C virus (HCV) structural proteins under the elongation factor 1-alpha promoter elicits HCV-specific cytotoxic T-lymphocytes (CTL). Vaccine 1999;18:675–680

83. Gordon EJ, Bhat R, Liu Q, Wang YF, Tackney C, Prince AM. Immune responses to hepatitis C virus structural and nonstructural proteins induced by plasmid DNA immunizations [In Process Citation]. J Infect Dis 2000;181:42–50

84. Kim JJ, Bagarazzi ML, Trivedi N, et al. Engineering of in vivo immune responses to DNA immunization via codelivery of costimulatory molecule genes. Nat Biotechnol 1997;15:641–646

85. Mendoza RB, Cantwell MJ, Kipps TJ. Immunostimulatory effects of a plasmid expressing CD40 ligand (CD154) on gene immunization. J Immunol 1997;159:5777–5781

86. Ihata A, Watabe S, Sasaki S, et al. Immunomodulatory effect of a plasmid expressing CD40 ligand on DNA vaccination against human immunodeficiency virus type-1. Immunology 1999;98:436–442

87. Boyle JS, Brady JL, Lew AM. Enhanced responses to a DNA vaccine encoding a fusion antigen that is directed to sites of immune induction. Nature 1998;392:408–411

88. Jacobs SC, Stephenson JR, Wilkinson GW. High-level expression of the tick-borne encephalitis virus NS1 protein by using an adenovirus-based vector: Protection elicited in a murine model. J Virol 1992;66:2086–2095

89. Gallichan WS, Johnson DC, Graham FL, Rosenthal KL. Mucosal immunity and protection after intranasal immunization with recombinant adenovirus expressing herpes simplex virus glycoprotein B. J Infect Dis 1993;168:622–629

90. Fooks AR, Schadeck E, Liebert UG, et al. High-level expression of the measles virus nucleocapsid protein by using a replication-deficient adenovirus vector: Induction of an MHC-1-restricted CTL response and protection in a murine model. Virology 1995;210:456–465

91. Makimura M, Miyake S, Akino N, et al. Induction of antibodies against structural proteins of hepatitis C virus in mice using recombinant adenovirus. Vaccine 1996;14:28–36

92. Bruna-Romero O, Lasarte JJ, Wilkinson G, et al. Induction of cytotoxic T-cell response against hepatitis C virus structural antigens using a defective recombinant adenovirus. Hepatology 1997;25:479–477

93. Lasarte JJ, Corrales FJ, Casares N, et al. Different doses of adenoviral vector expressing IL-12 enhance or depress the immune response to a coadministered antigen: The role of nitric oxide. J Immunol 1999;162:5270–5277

94. Shirai M, Okada H, Nishioka M, et al. An epitope in hepatitis C virus core region recognized by cytotoxic T cells in mice and humans. J Virol 1994;68:3334–3342

95. Large MK, Kittlesen DJ, Hahn YS. Suppression of host immune responses by the core protein of hepatitis C virus: Possible implications for hepatitis C virus persistence. J Immunol 1999;162:931–938

96. Paoletti E, Taylor J, Meignier B, Meric C, Tartaglia J. Highly attenuated poxvirus vectors: NYVAC, ALVAC and TROVAC. Dev Biol Stand 1995;84:159–163

97. Moss B, Carroll MW, Wyatt LS, et al. Host range restricted, non-replicating vaccinia virus vectors as vaccine candidates. Adv Exp Med Biol 1996;397:7–13

98. Davis NL, Brown KW, Johnston RE. A viral vaccine vector that expresses foreign genes in lymph nodes and protects against mucosal challenge. J Virol 1996;70:3781–3787

99. Frolov I, Hoffman TA, Pragai BM, et al. Alphavirus-based expression vectors: Strategies and applications. Proc Natl Acad Sci USA 1996;93:11371–11377

100. Smerdou C, Liljestrom P. Two-helper RNA system for production of recombinant Semliki forest virus particles. J Virol 1999;73:1092–1098

101. Shata MT, Stevceva L, Agwale S, Lewis GK, Hone DM. Recent advances with recombinant bacterial vaccine vectors. Mol Med Today 2000;6:66–71

102. Shirai M, Chen M, Arichi T, et al. Use of intrinsic and extrinsic helper epitopes for in vivo induction of anti-hepatitis C virus cytotoxic T lymphocytes (CTL) with CTL epitope peptide vaccines. J Infect Dis 1996;173:24–31

103. Hiranuma K, Tamaki S, Nishimura Y, et al. Helper T cell determinant peptide contributes to induction of cellular immune responses by peptide vaccines against hepatitis C virus. J Gen Virol 1999;80:187–193

104. Oseroff C, Sette A, Wentworth P, et al. Pools of lipidated HTL-CTL constructs prime for multiple HBV and HCV CTL epitope responses. Vaccine 1998;16:823–833

105. Sarobe P, Pendleton CD, Akatsuka T, et al. Enhanced in vitro potency and in vivo immunogenicity of a CTL epitope from hepatitis C virus core protein following amino acid replacement at secondary HLA-A2.1 binding positions. J Clin Invest 1998;102:1239–1248

106. Esumi M, Rikihisa T, Nishimura S, et al. Experimental vaccine activities of recombinant E1 and E2 glycoproteins and hypervariable region 1 peptides of hepatitis C virus in chimpanzees. Arch Virol 1999;144:973–980

107. Shang D, Zhai W, Allain JP. Broadly cross-reactive, high-affinity antibody to hypervariable region 1 of the hepatitis C virus in rabbits. Virology 1999;258:396–405

108. Puntoriero G, Meola A, Lahm A, et al. Towards a solution for hepatitis C virus hypervariability: Mimotopes of the hypervariable region 1 can induce antibodies cross-reacting with a large number of viral variants. EMBO J 1998;17:3521–3533

109. Watanabe K, Yoshioka K, Ito H, et al. The hypervariable region 1 protein of hepatitis C virus broadly reactive with sera of patients with chronic hepatitis C has a similar amino acid sequence with the consensus sequence [In Process Citation]. Virology 1999;264:153–158

110. Choo QL, Kuo G, Ralston R, et al. Vaccination of chimpanzees against infection by the hepatitis C virus. Proc Natl Acad Sci USA 1994;91:1294–1298

111. Delpha E, Priem S, Verschoor E, et al. 1332therapeutic vaccination of chronically infected chimpanzees with the HCV E1 protein. Hepatology 1999;30:408A

112. Christensen ND, Reed CA, Cladel NM, Han R, Kreider JW. Immunization with viruslike particles induces long-term protection of rabbits against challenge with cottontail rabbit papillomavirus. J Virol 1996;70:960–965

113. Roy P, Bishop DH, LeBlois H, Erasmus BJ. Long-lasting protection of sheep against bluetongue challenge after vaccination with virus-like particles: Evidence for homologous and partial heterologous protection. Vaccine 1994;12:805–811

114. Laurent S, Vautherot JF, Madelaine MF, Le Gall G, Rasschaert D. Recombinant rabbit hemorrhagic disease virus capsid protein expressed in baculovirus self-assembles into viruslike particles and induces protection. J Virol 1994;68:6794–6798

115. Wagner R, Teeuwsen VJ, Deml L, et al. Cytotoxic T cells and neutralizing antibodies induced in rhesus monkeys by virus-like particle HIV vaccines in the absence of protection from SHIV infection. Virology 1998;245:65–74

116. Liu XS, Abdul-Jabbar I, Qi YM, Frazer IH, Zhou J. Mucosal immunisation with papillomavirus virus-like particles elicits systemic and mucosal immunity in mice. Virology 1998;252:39–45

117. Rudolf MP, Nieland JD, DaSilva DM, et al. Induction of HPV16 capsid protein-specific human T cell responses by virus-like particles. Biol Chem 1999;380:335–340

118. Wagner R, Deml L, Schirmbeck R, Reimann J, Wolf H. Induction of a MHC class I-restricted, CD8 positive cytolytic T-cell response by chimeric HIV-1 virus-like particles in vivo: Implications on HIV vaccine development. Behring Inst Mitt 1994;95:23–34

119. Baumert TF, Ito S, Wong DT, Liang TJ. Hepatitis C virus structural proteins assemble into viruslike particles in insect cells. J Virol 1998;72:3827–3836

120. Baumert TF, Vergalla J, Satoi J, et al. Hepatitis C Virus-like Particles Synthesized in Insect Cells as a Potential Vaccine Candidate. Gastroenterology 1999;117:1397–1407

121. Lechmann M, Vergalla J, Satoi J, Baumert TF, Vergalla J, Satoi J, Baumert TF, Liang TJ. Induction of humoral and cellular immune responses in mice by immunization with insect-cell derived HCV-like particles. Hepatology 1999;30:453A

122. Krawczynski K, Alter MJ, Tankersley DL, et al. Effect of immune globulin on the prevention of experimental hepatitis C virus infection. J Infect Dis 1996;173:822–828

123. Krawczynski K, Fattom A, Culver D, et al. Passive transfer of anti-HCV in chronic and acute HCV infection in chimpanzees—trials of experimental immune treatment. Hepatology 1999;30:423A

124. Kent SJ, Zhao A, Best SJ, Chandler JD, Boyle DB, Ramshaw IA. Enhanced T-cell immunogenicity and protective efficacy of a human immunodeficiency virus type 1 vaccine regimen consisting of consecutive priming with DNA and boosting with recombinant fowlpox virus. J Virol 1998;72:10180–10188

125. Robinson HL, Montefiori DC, Johnson RP, et al. Neutralizing antibody-independent containment of immunodeficiency virus

SEMINARS IN LIVER DISEASE—VOL. 20, NO. 2, 2000

DIAGNOSTIC PROBLEMS IN HEPATOLOGY

A 67-Year-Old Man with Hepatitis C Virus Infection and a Liver Tumor

ARIEF SURIAWINATA, M.D., KATYA IVANOV, M.D.,
MENAHEM BEN HAIM, M.D.*, and MYRON E. SCHWARTZ, M.D.*

CASE REPORT

A 67-year-old Caucasian man was found to have an incidental mass in the right lobe of the liver. He had a history of diabetes mellitus, hypertension, three operations for herniated lumbar discs, and coronary artery disease, for which he underwent three-vessel coronary artery bypass grafts 6 months prior. There was no history of liver disease, ethanol use, or occupational exposure. He had been treated with furosemide, carvedilol, transdermal nitroglycerin, and insulin.

On physical examination, the patient's blood pressure was 160/90 mmHg. Other vital signs were within normal limits. Chest auscultation was remarkable for scattered ronchi and wheezes. There were no signs of liver failure or any features of chronic liver disease.

Laboratory work-up included complete blood count, which showed mild anemia (Hgb 11.3 g/dL), a normal coagulation screen, normal chemistry and a normal liver function profile. The patient had a positive hepatitis C virus antibody (anti-HCV) by RIBA. Anti-HBs (hepatitis B surface), HBsAg (hepatitis B surface antigen) and anti-HBc (hepatitis B core) were negative. CA 19–9 was 36.2 U/mL (normal < 37.0), alpha-fetoprotein (AFP) was 2.2 ng/ml (normal < 20.0) and carcinoembryonic antigen (CEA) was 0.9 ng/mL (normal < 5.0).

Chest x-ray showed mild congestion without infiltrates or pleural effusion. Echocardiography demonstrated global hypokinesia with an ejection fraction of 45%. A sonogram of the upper abdomen demonstrated a 6-cm solid lesion in the right lobe of the liver. A CT scan showed the mass in the posterior right lobe, which was enhanced during the arterial phase (Fig. 1). A MRI confirmed a well-circumscribed lesion in the right inferior segment, which was bright on T2-weighted images. Intraoperatively, there was a 8x5 cm firm, white-gray mass involving segments VI, VII, and VIII.

Objectives

Upon completion of this article, the reader should be able to 1) summarize the newest approaches in HCV vaccine development and 2) list the commonly used approaches.

Accreditation

The Indiana University School of Medicine is accredited by the Accreditation Council for Continuing Medical Education to sponsor continuing medical education for physicians. The Indiana University School of Medicine takes responsibility for the contents, quality, and scientific integrity of this activity.

Credit

The Indiana University School of Medicine designates this educational activity for a maximum of 1.0 hours credit toward the AMA Physicians Recognition Award in category one. Each physician should claim only those hours of credit that he/she actually spent in the educational activity.

Disclosure

Statements have been obtained regarding the authors' relationships with financial supporters of this activity. There is no apparent conflict of interest related to the context of participation of the author of this article.

---

*The Lillian and Henry M. Stratton-Hans Popper Department of Pathology and *Department of Surgery of the Mount Sinai School of Medicine, New York, New York.*

Reprint requests: Dr. Suriawinata, Department of Pathology, Box 1194, Mount Sinai School of Medicine, One Gustave L. Levy Place, New York, NY 10029.

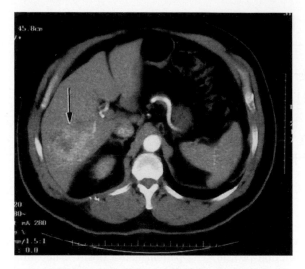

FIG. 1. Arterial phase CT scan showing 6 cm enhancing mass (arrow) in posterior right lobe of the liver.

The remaining liver parenchyma was unremarkable. The patient underwent a right hepatic lobectomy, which he tolerated well.

DIFFERENTIAL DIAGNOSIS

A 67-year-old man was found to have a 8 cm incidental tumor in the right lobe of the liver. The only other finding relevant to this condition was a positive anti-HCV. He had no known liver diseases. Serological markers for hepatitis A and B infections were all negative. His serum liver enzyme levels, AFP, CA19–9, and CEA were within normal limits.

The possibility that the mass was a malignant tumor was more than likely given the patient's age and sex, and the tumor appearance and size on imaging studies. Most common malignant tumors in the liver are metastatic tumors, with gastrointestinal tumors being one of the more common sources.[1] However, this tumor was solitary and the serum CEA level was not elevated.

Primary malignant tumor is roughly divided into hepatocellular carcinoma (HCC) arising from hepatocytes and intrahepatic cholangiocarcinoma (ICC) arising from bile duct epithelium.[2] Rarely, combined HCC and cholangiocarcinoma (CC) may develop from the bipotential precursor cells in the liver.[3–5] Nevertheless, HCC remains the more frequently encountered primary malignant tumor in patients with chronic hepatitis C virus infection.[6–10] HCV-positive HCCs generally develop on a background of cirrhosis with a male sex predominance.[11–12] Rarely, they may arise in noncirrhotic livers with chronic hepatitis C. Serum AFP level was not elevated in this patient. Normal AFP levels can be found in about 60% of patients with HCC.[13,14]

Intrahepatic cholangiocarcinoma, which is the second most common primary liver tumor, affects persons over 65 years of age, and both sexes almost equally. The degree of male predominance is much less than HCC, ranging from 1 to 2.2.[15–18] It is associated with liver fluke infestation, intrahepatic gallstones, intravenous contrast agents (Thorotrast), cystic liver diseases, primary sclerosing cholangitis, and inflammatory bowel disease.[19–24] Recently, it has been suggested that hepatitis C virus infection is involved in the pathogenesis of intrahepatic cholangiocarcinoma.[25] ICC is usually not associated with cirrhosis.[26] The tumor is often solitary, solid, firm, poorly demarcated, and gray-white in color. The levels of serum CEA and CA19–9 may be elevated in patients with ICC.[21,24,27]

More recently, several investigators have also reported an association between HCV infection and non-Hodgkin lymphoma.[28,29] Chronic antigenic stimulation in patients with chronic HCV infection was believed to play a role in the pathogenesis of lymphoma.[30] Lymphoma can also present as a solid solitary intrahepatic or hilar tumor not associated with cirrhosis.[28,31]

In our noncirrhotic patient with chronic hepatitis C, all three of these entities (i.e., HCC, ICC, lymphoma) needed be considered in the differential diagnoses. Aside from the characteristic elevated serum markers, a definitive diagnosis can be difficult to make preoperatively, because all present as solid tumors and have similar appearance on imaging studies. Biopsy of the lesion can provide a definitive diagnosis that would be important in deciding the extent of surgical resection to be carried out.

PATHOLOGIC FINDINGS

Gross Pathology

The right hepatic lobectomy specimen measured 26x17x9 cm in greatest dimension and weighed 1597 grams. The external capsule was red-brown and smooth. On sectioning, there was a well-circumscribed, firm, white-gray, nonencapsulated tumor that measured 8 × 5 × 4.5 cm (Fig. 2). The tumor had an irregular boundary and bulged through the capsule on the posterior surface. The resection margins were not involved by the tumor. Serial sectioning through the remainder of the parenchyma revealed unremarkable red-brown parenchyma. The bile ducts, hepatic arteries and hepatic veins at the resection margins were patent and unremarkable.

Histopathologic Findings

Representative sections were taken from the tumor and the nontumorous liver parenchyma. The tumor consisted of well-formed, angulated glands that varied in

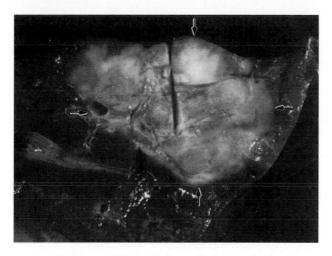

FIG. 2. Liver resection specimen showing a nonencapsulated, white-gray mass of cholangiocarcinoma (arrows).

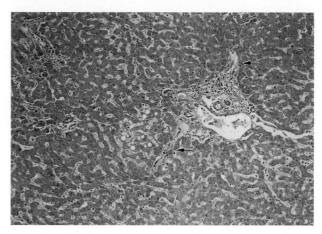

FIG. 4. Nontumorous liver showing mild lobular inflammation, mild steatosis, and a portal tract with mild lymphocytic infiltration and short septum formation (arrows) (H&E, x100).

size and were separated by dense fibrous stroma. The cells were columnar with pleomorphic nuclei and high cytoplasmic and nuclear ratio (Fig. 3). Surgical resection margins were negative for tumor. No angiolymphatic or perineural invasion was identified. The remainder of the liver parenchyma showed mild lymphocytic portal infiltration. There was mild portal fibrosis and short fibrous septum formation (Fig. 4). Rare foci of lobular inflammation were observed. There was no evidence of piecemeal necrosis or cirrhosis. The findings were consistent with chronic hepatitis C.

CLINICAL COURSE

The only postoperative complication was a small wound seroma, which was drained. Six months post surgery, the patient was doing well and his abdominal imaging studies did not show any recurrence.

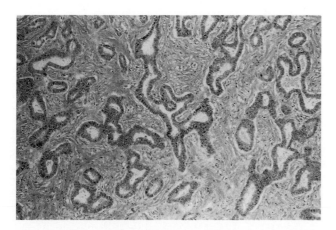

FIG. 3. Tumor cells are arranged in glandular structures separated by dense fibrous stroma (H&E, x100).

DISCUSSION

Hepatitis C virus represents one of the major causes of acute and chronic hepatitis, cirrhosis, and hepatocellular carcinoma around the world. The nature of the association between infection with HCV and hepatocarcinogenesis remains uncertain. It is not clear whether the virus acts as initiator, promoter, or both in the multistep events that result in HCC. However, most cases of HCV-associated HCC occur on the background of cirrhosis.

Recently, it been suggested that HCV infection plays a role in the pathogenesis of intrahepatic cholangiocarcinoma.[25] Yamamoto et al. found anti-HCV antibodies in 32% of patients with ICC.[32] In contrast to HCC, the development of ICC is generally unrelated to cirrhosis and has been associated with other etiologies, but not with viral hepatitis. The mechanisms of cholangiocarcinogenesis are not known. HCV has been shown to cause injury to bile duct epithelial cells.[33-35] Moreover, the presence of HCV antigens and sequences have been demonstrated in bile duct epithelium.[36-39] It has been speculated that ICC might develop in cholangioles infected with HCV or in hepatocytes, that have undergone ductal metaplasia in the areas of piecemeal necrosis.[32]

The association between HCV and ICC, in addition to the recent reports of HCV-related B cell lymphoma, reiterates the possible strong oncogenic potential of HCV not only in hepatocytes, but bile duct and lymphoid cells as well, the three cell lineages targeted by the virus.[36-39]

SUMMARY

A 67-year-old man with no known liver disease was found to have an incidental tumor in the right liver lobe.

His serum liver enzyme and alphafetoprotein were within normal limits, but he was found to be reactive for anti-HCV. The tumor was an intrahepatic cholangiocarcinoma. Since the only risk factor in this patient was hepatitis C infection, this case appears to support the recently suggested role of hepatitis C virus in the development of intrahepatic cholangiocarcinoma.

DIAGNOSES

Chronic hepatitis C virus infection
Cholangiocarcinoma

ABBREVIATIONS

AFP   alpha-fetoprotein
CEA   carcinoembryonic antigen
HBs   hepatitis B surface
HBsAg   hepatitis B surface antigen
HBc   hepatitis B core
HCC   hepatocellular carcinoma
HCV   hepatitis C virus
ICC   intrahepatic cholangiocarcinoma

REFERENCES

1. Anthony PP. Tumours and tumour-like lesions of the liver and biliary tract. In: MacSween RNW, Anthony PP, Scheuer PJ, eds. Pathology of the Liver. London: Churchill Livingstone 1994: 635–711
2. Higginson J, Steiner PE. Definition and classification of malignant epithelial neoplasms of the liver. Acta Union Internat Cancerum 1961;17:593–603
3. Theise ND, Nalesnik M, Cubukcu O, Thung SN. A stem cell tumor of the liver with differentiation to hepatocellular carcinoma and cholangiocarcinoma. Hepatology 1994;20:406A
4. Goodman ZD, Ishak KG, Langloss JM, et al. Combined hepatocellular-cholangiocarcinoma: a histologic and immunohistochemical study. Cancer 1985;55:124–135
5. Tanaka T, Imamura A, Hayashi S, et al. Minute mixed hepatoma with two components: hepatocellular and cholangiocarcinoma, which developed in liver cirrhosis with HCV. Hepatogastroenterology 1998;45:220–223
6. Colombo M. Hepatocellular carcinoma. J Hepatol 1992;15:225–236
7. Nishioka K, Watanabe J, Furuta S, et al. A high prevalence of antibody to the hepatitis C virus in patients with hepatocellular carcinoma in Japan. Cancer 1991;67:429–433
8. Liang TJ, Jeffers LJ, Reddy KR, et al. Viral pathogenesis of hepatocellular carcinoma in the United States. Hepatology 1993;18:1326–1333
9. Bruix J, Barrera JM, Calvet X, et al. Prevalence of antibodies to hepatitis C virus in Spanish patients with hepatocellular carcinoma and hepatic cirrhosis. Lancet 1989;2:1004–1006
10. Kew MC, Houghton M, Choo QL, et al. Hepatitis C virus antibodies in southern African blacks with hepatocellular carcinoma. Lancet 1990;335:873–874
11. Farinati F, Fagiuoli S, De Maria N, et al. Anti-HCV positive hepatocellular carcinoma in cirrhosis. Prevalence, risk-factors and clinical features. J Hepatol 1992;14:183–187
12. Simonetti RG, Camma C, Fiorello F, et al. Hepatitis C virus infection as a risk factor for hepatocellular carcinoma in patients with cirrhosis. A case-control study. Ann Intern Med 1992;116:97–102
13. Thung SN, Gerber MA, Sarno E, Popper H. Distribution of five antigens in hepatocellular carcinoma. Lab Invest 1979;41:101–105
14. Taketa K. Alpha-fetoprotein: reevaluation in hepatology. Hepatology 1990;12:1420–1432
15. Edmondson HA, Steiner PE. Primary carcinoma of the liver. A study of 100 cases among 48,900 necropsies. Cancer 1954;7:462–503
16. Okuda K, Kubo Y, Okazaki N, et al. Clinical aspects of intrahepatic bile duct carcinoma including hilar carcinoma. A study of 57 autopsy-proven cases. Cancer 1977:232–246
17. Mac Sween RNW. A clinicopathological review of 100 cases of primary malignant tumours of the liver. J Clin Pathol 1974;27:669–682
18. Patton RB, Horn RC. Primary liver carcinoma. Autopsy study of 60 cases. Cancer 1961;17:757–768
19. Flavel DJ. Liver-fluke infection as an aetiological feature in bile duct carcinoma of man. Trans R. Soc Trop Med Hyg 1981;75:814–824
20. Belamaric J. Intrahepatic bile duct carcinoma and C. sinensis infection in Hong Kong. Cancer 1973;31:468–473
21. Nakanuma Y, Terada T, Tanaka Y, et al. Are hepatolithiasis and cholangiocarcinoma aetiologically related? A morphological study of 12 cases of hepatolithiasis associated with cholangiocarcinoma. Virchows Arch A Pathol Anat Histopathol. 1988;406:45–58
22. Nakajima T, Kondo Y, Miyazaki M, et al. A histopathologic study of 102 cases of intrahepatic cholangiocarcinoma: histologic classification and modes of spreading. Hum Pathol 1988;19:1228–1234
23. Wee A, Ludwig J, Doffey RJ, et al. Hepatobiliary carcinoma associated with primary sclerosing cholangitis and chronic ulcerative colitis. Hum Pathol 1985;16:719–726
24. Sugihara S, Kojiro M. Pathology of cholangiocarcinoma. In: Okuda K, Ishak KG, eds. Neoplasms of the Liver. Tokyo: Springer-Verlag 1987:143–158
25. Tomimatsu M, Ishiguro N, Taniai M, et al. Hepatitis C virus antibody in patients with primary liver cancer (hepatocellular carcinoma, cholangiocarcinoma, and combined hepatocellular-cholangiocarcinoma) in Japan. Cancer 1993;72:683–688
26. Craig JR, Peters RL, Edmondson HA. Tumors of the Liver and Intrahepatic Bile Ducts. Washington, DC: Armed Forces Institute of Pathology 1989
27. Nakajima T, Kondo Y. Well-differentiated cholangiocarcinoma: diagnostic significance of morphologic and immunohistochemical parameters. Am J Surg Pathol 1989;13:569–573
28. Ascoli V, Coco F, Artini M, et al. Extranodal lymphomas associated with hepatitis C virus infection. Am J Clin Pathol. 1998;109:600–609
29. Silvestri F, Barillari G, Fanin R, et al. Hepatitis C virus infection among cryoglobulinemic and non-cryoglobulinemic B-cell non-Hodgkin's lymphomas. Haematol 1997;82:314–317
30. Lai R, Weiss LM. Hepatitis C virus and non-Hodgkin's lymphoma. Am J Clin Pathol. 1998;109:508–10
31. Suriawinata A, Ye MQ, Emre S, Strauchen J, Thung SN. Hepatocellular carcinoma and non-hodgkin lymphoma in a patient with chronic hepatitis C and cirrhosis. Arch Pathol Lab Med. (In press)
32. Yamamoto M, Takasaki K, Nakano M, Saito A . Minute nodular intrahepatic cholangiocarcinoma. Cancer 1998;82:2145–2149

33. Scheuer PJ, Ashrafzadeh P, Sherlock S, et al. The pathology of hepatitis C. Hepatology 1992;15:567–571

34. Bach N, Thung SN, Schaffner F. The histological features of chronic hepatitis C and autoimmune chronic hepatitis: a comparative analysis. Hepatology 1992;15:572–577

35. Gerber MA, Krawczynski K, Alter MJ, et al. Histopathology of community acquired chronic hepatitis C. Mod Pathol 1992;5: 483–486

36. Gerber MA. Pathobiologic effects of hepatitis C. J Hepatol 1995;22(Suppl 1):83–86

37. Krawczynski K, Beach MJ, Bradley DW, et al. Hepatitis C virus antigen in hepatocytes: immunomorphologic detection and identification. Gastroenterology 1992;103:622–629

38. Nouri-Aria KT, Sallie R, Mizokami M, et al. Intrahepatic expression of hepatitis C virus antigens in chronic liver disease. J Pathol 1995;175:77–83

39. Nouri-Aria KT, Sallie R, Sangar D. Detection of genomic and intermediate replicative strands of hepatitis C virus in liver tissue by in situ hybridization. J Clin Invest 1993;91:2226–2234

Afterword: HCV in the Decades Ahead

In the two-and-a-half decades since the discovery of non-A, non-B hepatitis, much of this affliction attributable to infection with the hepatitis C virus (HCV), a great deal has been learned. This information has permitted tremendous advances to be made in prevention, diagnosis, and treatment of HCV, but much more needs to be accomplished in the decades to come in order to fully control this virus and minimize its impact on human health. The articles contained in the first two *Seminars in Liver Disease* issues of the 21st Century not only review what is known about HCV and its disease manifestations, but offer insights into what is likely to follow. Future efforts to control HCV will divide along two lines: strategies to prevent new chronic infections, and interventions to cure or control the virus in patients who are already infected.

Before looking to the future, however, the editors wish to look back for a moment to thank the contributors. As academic life grows more hectic, it is increasingly difficult to find the time to share knowledge and ideas, yet the authors of this series went above and beyond the call of duty. They summarized vast quantities of data on topics ranging from the atomic structure of HCV proteins to the variable pattern of HCV infections around the globe, and then topped off their in-depth reviews with insightful commentaries. It was stimulating and rewarding to work with them. Their efforts benefit everyone seeking to understand and control this ubiquitous virus.

WE HAVE MET THE ENEMY AND IT IS US

Epidemiologic studies have revealed that almost all new HCV infections, with the exception of perinatal transmissions, are *theoretically* preventable, if only it were possible to change complex patterns of human behavior. In developed countries, prevention strategies in the form of blood screening programs have virtually eliminated HCV from the blood supply. Transmission continues in healthcare settings—through sticks with hollow-bore needles, and from one patient to another through exposure to contaminated supplies and equipment—but at a much lower rate than in the past. It is likely that greater vigilance on the part of the established medical community will bring this rate to even lower levels in the near future.

Unfortunately, in many parts of the world, transmission continues to occur through the use of contaminated, nondisposable needles, either in the context of "medicinal" injections or through local folk medicine and acupuncture practices. These problems need to be addressed through educational programs, by ensuring the availability of disposable equipment, and by substituting oral medications for injectable formulations whenever possible. A better handle on the world-wide prevalence and global distribution of this stealthy virus is needed in order to develop international educational and pubic health containment strategies.

At the moment, the activity most responsible for sustaining the HCV epidemic in the United States appears to be the illegal use of injection drugs. A variety of additional activities are associated with HCV prevalence, but the actual events leading to infection are not well defined. Uncertain transmission modes include cocaine "snorting," sexual intercourse, tattooing, body piercing, and the sharing of implements used for personal hygiene (toothbrushes and razors). It is suspected that some of these activities may be surrogate markers for injection drug use that is not acknowledged by the subject. Future studies are needed to distinguish true modes of viral transmission from risk factors that are associated with, but do not directly lead to, transmission. To determine the actual contribution of injection drug use, better instruments to measure stigmatized behaviors are required.

Although careful historical evaluation of the individual yields a well-known risk factor in most cases, there continues to be a definite, albeit decreasing number of instances in which the circumstances of exposure cannot be determined. Careful epidemiologic surveillance must, therefore, continue since programs to control the spread of HCV depend on knowing the routes of transmission. Finally, if HCV infection is found to occur at a high rate in certain settings, such as inside prisons, these routes of transmission also need to be identified.

PREVENTIVE INTERVENTIONS

As the success of blood screening programs and the implementation of universal precautions are bringing the number of infections associated with medical procedures to very low levels in many developed countries, new infections are increasingly concentrated in populations of individuals who inject recreational drugs, who (willingly or unwillingly) participate in activities in which the protective barrier of the skin is broken, and/or who have intimate contact with HCV-infected persons in the setting of high-risk sexual activity. One of the most effective strategies for controlling HCV in these populations may be to target the root causes of drug addiction and other high-risk behaviors. Injection drug use, high-risk sexual activity, excessive alcohol consumption—behaviors that are risk factors for HCV transmission and/or rapid disease progression—are also associated with depression, anxiety, and poverty. Access to mental health services, on the one hand, and employment opportunities, on the other, may save many individuals from a range of diseases, including, but not limited to those caused by HCV infection. Although these general strategies will not be sufficient, they can make important contributions to containment efforts.

Approaches that focus more narrowly on blocking routes of HCV transmission will also be needed. These strategies include: (1) Decreasing the illicit use of drugs; (2) reducing the risk of viral transmission during the recreational use of injection drugs (through needle exchange programs, for example); (3) reducing high-risk sexual practices; and (4) developing protective vaccines. There are formidable barriers to implementing each of these approaches.

For example, while it is of paramount importance to develop an effective vaccine for HCV, the likelihood that this will occur in the immediate future is remote. HCV is a master at frustrating the immune system during natural infections and thus it may be relatively resistant to vaccine-induced immunity. Moreover, now that screening has effectively eliminated HCV from the blood supply in many countries, and a declining minority of the population faces a significant risk of HCV infection, it will be increasingly difficult to convince government agencies that universal HCV vaccination should be required. Vaccines directed at specific high-risk groups have been difficult to deliver, as illustrated by the unsuccessful efforts to deliver the HBV vaccine to selected segments of the U.S. population. Unfortunately, many individuals at high-risk for acquiring HCV infection may be disenfranchised from the medical establishment and difficult to reach with a targeted vaccination program. Therefore, even if the technical obstacles can be overcome and a long-lasting *protective* vaccine for HCV is developed, this vaccine may be very difficult to deploy effectively in some countries. Thus,

research leading to the development of *therapeutic*, as well as *protective,* vaccines should be vigorously pursued.

In parallel, energetic and creative efforts should be made to reduce injection drug abuse, and to minimize the adverse consequences of high-risk sexual practices. Research in the fields of psychiatry, psychology, and education may lead to more effective methods of behavior modification. Through compelling public service messages, it may be possible to communicate the special dangers of injection drug use and the need to adhere to safe sex practices. Teachers can help by including age-appropriate information about HCV in course materials. Physicians, especially pediatricians, can play an essential role by making opportunities to deliver warnings and advice to their patients. To take advantage of increased awareness, drug treatment programs need to be expanded so that individuals who seek help can immediately receive support while they are still ready to accept it.

Pending the development of effective vaccines, the measures with the greatest potential to reduce the burden of hepatitis C in a cost-effective manner are the efforts of epidemiologists, public health workers, and primary care physicians, coupled to high intensity media-based campaigns of public education. Mobilizing and funding their efforts will require our unstinting support.

PINNING DOWN THE SOURCES OF VARIABILITY IN DISEASE OUTCOME

Natural History of Chronic HCV Infection

The natural history of this difficult viral infection continues to engender controversy. Accordingly, research in this area must continue, despite the fact that treatment is now widely offered in many countries, confounding the ability to conduct true natural history studies. Past studies have overcome enormous challenges. Thousands of individuals have been included and, in some cases, disease progression has been followed for decades. To realize the full benefit of these investigations, the cohorts of HCV-infected subjects and age/gender-matched control populations need to be followed for many more years.

An encouraging message has emerged from the natural history studies that have been conducted thus far. Most HCV carriers will have either: (1) a stable nonprogressive course; (2) such indolent progression that they will die from an unrelated disease before the severe sequelae of HCV become manifest; or (3) will have a sustained "curative" response to therapy. However, grim statistics from countries such as Japan and Italy, in which the incidence of HCV infection was high in the distant past, suggest that HCV eventually causes hepatocellular carcinoma in an unknown percentage of chronically-infected individuals. Even if that percentage does not turn out to be striking as an abstract number, when converted into cases based on current estimates of nearly 200 million patients with chronic HCV worldwide, it represents a great deal of human suffering. In some parts of the world, such as Egypt, the numbers of persons with chronic HCV infection are so enormous that the cost of treating everyone with interferon and ribavirin becomes prohibitive. It is, therefore, imperative to find methods to identify the individuals at greatest risk of experiencing severe, progressive liver disease and/or primary liver cancer so that medical interventions can be directed to those most likely to suffer if they are left untreated.

Efforts to identify those at greatest risk would benefit from more information about whether the circumstances of exposure (blood transfusions, accidental needlesticks, parenteral drug abuse) impact the subsequent course of disease. More information is also needed in regard to the effects of age at the time of infection, gender, and as is becoming evident, race. Recent evidence suggests that outcome may differ between African-Americans and Caucasians; this area requires further investigation. In addition, genetic analysis and family tree studies of subjects of all races may reveal inherited factors that influence disease outcome. Although children are less commonly infected than adults, and the impact of infection among them seems to be less than is the case for adults, the problem is sufficiently large that it demands more prolonged follow-up studies than have been accomplished to date. Again, special attention should be paid to the question of whether certain groups of children are more likely to have rapidly progressive liver disease than others. Research is needed to determine the impact of co-infections (HIV, HBV) and immunosuppression (drug- and disease-induced, and intrinsic) on disease progression. Outcome studies involving HCV-positive persons who are also HIV-infected, have renal disease, are on hemodialysis, or who undergo renal and hepatic transplantation, are warranted, as are studies aimed at clarifying the connection between HCV and B cell lymphoproliferative disorders, including cryoglobulinemia and lymphoma. Finally, patients who undergo liver transplantation need to be followed. Are patients transplanted in the past few years progressing to fibrosis more rapidly than earlier cohorts, as some reports suggest? What, if anything, has changed? What role should living-related organ donors play in the treatment of patients with HCV?

Studies defining the role extraneous factors play in the progression of liver disease promise to yield valuable information. There is little doubt that the likelihood of progression is greatly enhanced in the face of heavy alcohol intake, although the precise basis for this is not fully established. More information is needed concerning the impact of lesser amounts of alcohol intake and the pattern of drinking of alcohol. Smoking has also been reported to play a potentially harmful role in progression of HCV-related liver disease. Might there be additional environmental factors or contaminants that too may be harmful?

Methods for Determining Disease Progression

The essence of the problem of chronic hepatitis C is the fact of progression from the chronic inflammatory process to fibrosis, thence to cirrhosis, and ultimately hepatocellular carcinoma. Accordingly, a better understanding of the pathogenesis of chronic HCV infection is imperative. This entails not only a better understanding of the immunonologic and virologic events, but especially of the events surrounding fibrogenesis and fibrinolysis. Fibrosis has emerged as an important indicator of the severity of HCV-associated liver damage because advanced fibrosis is tied to the two most serious consequences of HCV: decompensated cirrhosis and hepatocellular carcinoma.

Better methods to diagnose and treat fibrosis, cirrhosis, and HCC are needed. The development of markers of fibrosis progression would not only identify those in special need for treatment, but would also provide information of benefit to patients concerned about future developments. At the moment, liver biopsy remains the gold standard for assessing the status of the liver. However, it carries risks and may give an incomplete picture of the processes taking place in the liver, particularly when the specimen is small and the disease is patchy. Noninvasive techniques that assess the extent of fibrosis throughout the liver are eagerly awaited. These techniques will improve safety and allow patients to be followed longitudinally without being subjected to serial biopsies.

Gene expression profiling stands out as an additional method that will advance the care of patients with HCV-associated liver disease in the years to come. This method allows the mRNA levels of thousands of genes to be measured in one assay. Gene expression profiling utilizes DNA microarrays that contain probes for thousands of cellular genes attached to solid supports. During the next five years, gene expression profiling promises to identify risk factors for disease progression, to suggest intervention strategies, and to provide sensitive and specific early markers of, *inter alia*, hepatocellular carcinoma. It is likely that the products of some genes over-expressed in the diseased liver will appear in the blood. Once these products have been identified through gene expression profiling, noninvasive serological tests can be developed to detect them. Parallel studies may help to define the immune responses associated with various outcomes—clearance of HCV vs. persistence, mild vs. aggressive disease, the role of innate immunity vs. acquired immunity, and factors leading to lymphoproliferative disorders. Collectively, these investigations will provide details about how the human body responds to the virus.

Viral Factors

Intensive collaborative efforts of molecular biologists and clinical investigators have shown the importance of viral sequences—demonstrating that HCV genotype affects the duration of interferon treatment that is needed to achieve sustained response, revealing that greater heterogeneity of viral quasispecies is associated with the establishment of chronic infection, and providing evidence that certain HCV strains appear to have a greater pathogenic potential than others. To go forward, new methods are needed to facilitate sequence analysis and to allow multiple domains of the genome to be investigated in individual patients in a timely and cost-effective manner. New methods are needed because the HCV genome contains about 9600 nucleotides, and each patient contains a mixed population of RNA sequences, a quasispecies. DNA microarrays containing probes for numerous HCV gene regions can be expected. These arrays will allow more precise analysis of HCV strains, and will help to identify clinically-important sites in the HCV genome.

Current And Future Treatment Options For Hcv Infected Patients

With current therapies (interferon alpha alone or in combination with ribavirin), HCV can be eliminated in nearly half of chronically-infected patients who are eligible for existing clinical trials. In light of this success, there is a need to develop treatment strategies for groups to whom insufficient attention has been paid—children, African-Americans, those with HIV co-infection, active drug users, HCV-infected prisoners, and patients with decompensated cirrhosis. Multicenter trials will be needed to enroll a sufficient number of patients in studies of patients with unusual conditions—such as HIV/HCV co-infected pregnant women and their babies.

An issue that has arisen recently is concern about the blanket omission from treatment of active drug users and active alcoholics. Several drug support groups have raised an alarm about this issue, suggesting that prohibition of treatment for at least a year following discontinuation of the addictive habit is inappropriate. They advocate that treatment decisions should be individualized, as is the case for treatment of HIV infection. Clearly, appropriate studies are imperative if this approach is to be recommended. Because it may be impossible to clear HCV infection in individuals who continue to inject illicit drugs, the goal of therapy, in some cases, may need to be the amelioration of liver damage, rather than the sustained elimination of the virus. Amelioration is a challenging, but critical, end point to measure. It will be valuable to have more information about how to objectively assess interventions that change the course of ongoing HCV infections, not only for studies of active drug users, but for other populations of HCV-infected individuals as well.

Although their side effects, cost, and the appreciable proportion of relapsers and nonresponders render current therapies for HCV less than optimal, their success is, nonetheless, without parallel. No anti-viral therapy for any other chronic virus clears infection in a comparable fraction of patients. Most therapies are far less effective at ridding patients of chronic viruses. Combination therapy for HIV provides an instructive example: long-term treatment reduces the level of HIV viremia but does not eliminate the virus. The investigators who helped develop curative therapies for chronic HCV infection have achieved a remarkable result.

Pharmacokinetic studies have yielded important insights into the events taking place during interferon treatment, such as the fact that HCV rebounds between doses when interferon is given three times a week. This information helped spark the development of long-acting interferons, which counter this effect. More studies of currently-approved HCV treatments are needed because it remains a mystery how either IFN or ribavirin promote HCV clearance. Given the exceptional success of IFN/ribavirin treatment for HCV, the mechanisms of action of these drugs warrant investigation. This information may instruct the development of interventions for other chronic viral diseases. Both drugs have both anti-viral and immuno-modulatory effects. If the immuno-stimulatory effects of interferon are important in HCV clearance, and if the mechanisms underlying these effects can be defined, this information may guide the development of new pharmaceuticals, more effective immune modulators, and HCV vaccines.

Clinical trials of drugs that are narrower in their mechanisms of action than ribavirin may reveal how this compound augments interferon effects and lead to new drugs. Potential ribavirin "substitutes" include new inhibitors of inosine monophosphate dehydrogenase and new immuno-modulatory drugs, such as histamines. In addition, several nonspecific medications that tend to lower the serum enzyme levels without affecting the virus itself (ursodiol, NSAIDS) have evoked interest by some in the belief that lowering of serum enzymes might enhance the efficacy of interferon. Proof for this concept is presently lacking but might be explored.

Whatever the nature of the pharmaceutical agents used for treatment, a more precise understanding of the events leading to viral eradication may permit the early discontinuation of treatment destined to fail in an individual patient. Conversely, more sensitive assays for very low levels of HCV RNA may allow patients to be stratified into those who can safely stop therapy (after 6 months, for example) and those who require extended therapy to achieve viral clearance. One simple way to enhance the sensitivity of HCV RNA detection may be to extract RNA from a larger volume of serum. It is not yet clear whether sensitivity can be enhanced by using whole blood instead of serum or plasma, but this important issue is being explored.

Future trials of new HCV treatments will need to have long follow-up periods to permit their long-term effects to be compared to those obtained with current therapies. Based on long-term follow-up of 157 patients, it appears that 90 to 95% of the individuals who have no detectable HCV RNA in serum samples drawn 6 months after the end of interferon treatment will remain free of the virus for the next 5 to 10 years. Although the number of patients is relatively small (in comparison to the number of patients who have been treated), these results are very encouraging and they set a high standard of durability that alternative treatments will need to meet or exceed.

Follow-up studies are also needed to assess the impact of interferon treatment on patients who fail to clear the virus. Some reports suggest that such patients, especially those with no markers of HBV infection, have a reduced risk of developing hepatocellular carcinoma. However, this matter is not settled, nor is it known whether interferon treatment that fails to clear HCV leads to the evolution of sequence variants with distinctive properties. Such variants might be more or less aggressive than their forebearers. Information about the biological properties of interferon-resistant variants may emerge from studies of patients who undergo liver transplantation. The grafts in these patients allow the course of the disease induced by these variants to be followed from its initial stages.

Treatment options and efficacy must improve in the decades to come. The advent of the pegylated forms of interferon and of combination therapy are promising advances. But more specific antiviral therapy targeted at interference in the life cycle of the virus must be sought. Going forward, progress on several fronts—determination of the atomic structure of HCV proteins and RNA elements, molecular modeling of such structures, advances in combinatorial chemistry, and development of rapid in vitro assays for testing inhibitors of HCV proteins—are likely to yield compounds that block HCV replication and gene expression. Development of a drug that inhibits the HCV RNA replicase could have very broad usefulness. Many viruses (e.g., poliovirus, cold viruses, rabies, influenza) use RNA replicases, but no approved drug inhibits enzymes of this class. There is an enormous financial incentive to develop anti-viral drugs active against HCV. The anticipated profits, combined with the excitement over the basic information that will emerge from the experiments needed to de-

velop HCV-specific anti-viral agents, guarantee that HCV molecular virology will be an intense and fruitful area of research in the decades ahead.

Given the state of our knowledge about the variability of HCV disease progression, it is appropriate to adopt a broad view of the interventions that may be useful: viral eradication is one clear goal, but it is also possible that some patients could benefit from therapies that minimize liver damage without clearing the virus. A broad spectrum of interventions should be considered for testing: anti-fibrotic, and anti-inflammatory drugs (IL-10, and perhaps estrogen for women), herbal preparations and nutritional supplements (including milk thistle and Sho-saiko-to, TJ-9), and programs for curbing alcohol consumption. There is a particular need for the development of therapeutic agents capable of impeding progressive fibrosis. A specific immune globulin preparation is currently under examination and may prove to be of benefit in some situations. The intense and widespread interest by the public in complementary and alternative medicines bespeaks the need to pay some attention to this issue. Many patients with HCV complain of fatigue and would benefit from interventions that ameliorate this and other symptoms that diminish the quality of life. Patients experiencing lymphoproliferative disorders and immune complex diseases may require treatment that is specifically tailored to their needs.

Because there may be little financial incentive for private industry to fund trials of interventions involving old, established drugs and inexpensive products, support from governmental agencies and private foundations will be essential. The need for this type of funding was recently emphasized in an article by Jane E. Brody in the *New York Times* (June 13, 2000). The article points out that evidence has been accumulating for the past 30 years showing that high serum levels of homocysteine are associated with cardiac disease. However, the potential value of interventions aimed at lowering homocysteine has rarely been explored because, according to Dr. Meir Stampfer of the Harvard School of Public Heath, "'there was no commercial interest in studying homocysteine,' since the way to reduce it—eating less meat and taking supplements of B vitamins—is inexpensive and not patentable."

Well-designed clinical trials can identify interventions which improve treatments and dramatically alter survival curves. Trials should be designed to test the most promising leads, and the economic potential of new interventions should not be the sole factor determining whether they are investigated. Many of the 170 million people infected with HCV live in developing countries with limited resources. The medical needs of these individuals stress the importance of affordable treatments for HCV.

Andrea D. Branch, Ph. D.
Leonard B. Seeff, M. D.

Index

Page references in *italics* indicate figures. Page references followed by "t" indicate tables.

A

Acupuncture, HCV transmission by, 8
Adolescent(s), HCV-infected
  counseling of, 40
  prevalence of, 38
Agammaglobulinemia
  HCV quasispecies in, 118
  homogeneity of HCV population in, 19, 118
Age
  at biopsy
    and grade of activity (necroinflammation), 49, *49*
    and stage of fibrosis, 49, *49*
  at diagnosis, versus age at onset, 29
  and fibrosis progression, 51
  at infection, and outcome, in children, 40
  at onset
    versus age at diagnosis, 29
    and outcomes, 29
  and outcome of HCV infection, 29, 32
  and response to antiviral therapy, 192, 194
Alanine aminotransferase, normal serum levels in HCV
    infection, management of, 191
Alcohol
  abuse, and HCV infection
    management of, 236
    outcome with, 22, 29
    prevention of, 234
    research on, advances in (future directions for), 235
  consumption
    avoidance of, by HCV-infected patients, 10, 190
    and fibrosis progression, 51, 52, 190
    and outcome of HCV infection, 29–30, *30,* 190
Alcoholism. *See* Alcohol, abuse
Aminoglycosides, mechanism of action of, 65
Aminotransferase(s), normal serum levels in HCV infection,
    management of, 191
Amplicor HCV Monitor assay (Roche), 163, 164
Amplicor test (Roche), 162–163
Animal model(s)
  of HCV-immune system interaction, 133–134
  for vaccine development, 214–215
Antigen(s), HCV, detection of, 96–97
  with human antisera, 93–94
Anti-GOR antibodies, in HCV infection, 145–146
Anti-HCV antibodies
  screening assays for, 160–161
  supplemental tests for, 161–162
Anti-idiotypic antibodies, in HCV infection, 144–145
Antinuclear autoantibody, in HCV infection, 146
Antisense drugs, for HCV infection, 65
  mechanism of action of, 65
  nonantisense effects of, 65

Antiviral drug(s), development of
  advances in (future directions for), 65–66
  bioengineered pathogens used in, 62
  nonstructural proteins of HCV and, 69–80
Antiviral therapy
  candidates for, 188
  currently licensed therapies for, 188, 188t
  HBV kinetics with, 175, *176,* 178, 178t
  HCV kinetics with, *176,* 176–178, *177,* 181
    in nonresponders, 181–182
  HCV RNA as target for, 65
  HIV kinetics with, 178, 178t
  response to
    factors affecting, 192–194, 194
    first-phase HCV decline in, 176–177, *177,* 178
    HCV genotype and, 108, 181, 188, 189t
    HCV quasispecies and, 119–120
    host factors and, 192
    immunologic factors and, 193
    predictors of, 188, 189t
    second-phase HCV clearance in, 180–181, *181*
    sustained, 166–167, *167,* 181, 188
    testing for, 166t, 166–167, *167*
    viral factors and, 193–194
  standard of care in, 188
Apoptosis, of liver-infiltrating HCV-specific T cells, 132–133
Autoimmune disease, and response to antiviral therapy, 193
Autoimmunity, in HCV infection, 144–146

B

Barbering, commercial, HCV transmission by, 8
Bayer bDNA assay, for determination of viral load, 163–164,
    164
B-cell lymphoproliferative disorders, HCV infection and,
    144, 150–154, *153,* 235
B-cell responses, in antiviral defense, 145, 150, *151*
bDNA assay, for determination of viral load, 163–164, *164*
Biopsy. *See* Liver biopsy
Blood donor(s)
  prevalence of HCV infection in, 2, 37
  screening of, 167
Blood supply, safety of, 9, 38
Blood transfusion, HCV transmission by, 4, 8, 9
  incidence of, 4
  outcomes of, 20, 22
    in children, 40–41
    long-term, 189, *189*
Body piercing, HCV transmission by, 8
Bovine viral diarrhea virus, 88
Branched DNA (bDNA) assay, for determination of viral
    load, 163–164, *164*
Breast-feeding, and maternal-infant transmission of HCV, 39

C
Cardiovascular disorder(s), interferon/ribavirin therapy
         contraindicated in, 187
CD81, HCV binding to, 128
CD5 B-cells, in autoimmunity, 145
CD4 T helper cell(s)
    in antiviral defense, 78–79, 115, 130, *131*
    and fibrosis progression, 51
    hepatic, 129
CD8 T helper cell(s)
    in antiviral defense, 78, 115, 130, *131,* 132
    hepatic, 129
Cell death
    in HCV infection, 19
    of liver-infiltrating HCV-specific T cells, 132–133
Cell-mediated immunity
    adaptive
        in acute self-limited hepatitis C, 130–131
        in chronic hepatitis C, 132
    in antiviral defense, 19, 104, 115, 129–133, 213–214
    HCV-specific, interaction with humoral immune response,
         150, *151*
Chemokine(s), 130, 132
Chemokine receptors, and T cell recruitment to liver, 132
Child(ren)
    HCV infection in
        chronic, treatment of, 42–44, 44–45
        histopathology of, 41
        liver biopsy in, 41
        natural history of, 40–42
        outcome of, 24–25, 29
            factors affecting, 235
        prevalence of, 24, 37–38
        spontaneous recovery from, 24–25, 168
        testing for, 168
    liver transplantation in, 41
    transmission of HCV in, 38–39, 168
Chimera(s), 62–63, 65
Chimpanzee, in HCV research, 133–134, 214
Cholangiosarcoma, in HCV-infected 67-year-old male,
         227–230
Circumcision, HCV transmission by, 8
Cirrhosis, HCV-associated, 18, 22–23
    in children, 41
    complications of, 47
    development of
        interval to, *25,* 25–26
        outcome after, 26, 26t
        research on, advances in (future directions for), 235
    diagnosis of, liver biopsy in, 52
    HCV genotype and, 107
    in HCV/HIV co-infection, 52
    and hepatocellular carcinoma, 20, 21, 27
    markers of, 52, *52*
    and outcome of HCV infection, 29
    prevalence of, 40
    progression to, 189–190
    and response to antiviral therapy, 192
Cocaine
    injection of, and HCV transmission, 4
    intranasal, and HCV transmission, 4
Co-infection(s)
    HCV/HBV
        management of, 191
        outcomes of, 27–28
    HCV/HIV
        in children, 38
        and cirrhosis, 52
        and fibrosis progression, 51, 52

homogeneity of HCV population in, 117–118
    management of, 191, 236
    maternal, and vertical transmission of HCV, 6, 38–39, 40
    and outcome of HCV infection, 29
    and outcome of HCV infection, 235
Colostrum, HCV RNA in, 39
Contamination, of tissue or cell population, 86
Counseling, of HCV-infected persons, 10, 39–40
C protein, 70
Cryoglobulinemia, mixed, HCV-associated, 144, 147–150
    localization of HCV antigens in, 98–99
    pathogenesis of, 147–150
    treatment of, 192
Cyclosporine, and posttransplant recurrence of HCV
         infection, 203–204
Cytokine(s), 214
    in innate immune response, 129
    response to DNA vaccine, 216
Cytotoxic T lymphocytes (CTL)
    in antiviral defense, 79–80, 104, 115, 130–131, *131,* 132,
         180, 213–214
    response to DNA vaccine, 216–217

D
Daclizumab, 204
Death(s)
    after retransplant for recurrent HCV infection, 207
    after transfusion-associated HCV infection, 189, *189*
    causes of, in HCV infection, 22, 23, 190
    HCC-related, 47
    from liver disease, in HCV-infected patients, 189–190
Dermatologic side effects, of antiviral treatment, 187
DEXH helicase family, 74
Diabetes, antiviral treatment and, 187
Diagnosis, of 67-year-old male with HCV infection and liver
         tumor, 227–230
Diagnostic testing, for HCV infection, 159–168
    in children, 168
    clinical applications of, 165–168
    costs of, 165, 165t
Diarrhea, antiviral treatment-related, 187
Dionysios study, 29
DNA, antisense, complementary to HCV
    in antiviral therapy, 65
    nonantisense effects of, 65
DNA vaccine, against HCV infection, *212,* 212–213, 215t,
         215–217
    antibody responses to, 215–216
    cytokine response to, 216
    cytotoxic T-cell responses to, 216–217
    lymphoproliferative response to, 216
Dot-blot hybridization assay, in screening for HCV genotype,
         165
dsRNA, 58, 63-64
dsRNA adenosine deaminase (dsRAD), 64–65

E
Elderly, HCV-associated liver disease in, 32
Encephalomyocarditis virus (EMCV), 64
Envelope glycoprotein(s), 70, 104
    antibody response to, 213, 215–216
Enzyme immunoassay (EIA), for anti-HCV antibodies, 160t,
         160, 160–161, *161*
    clinical applications of, 165, 167, 168
    cost of, 165t
    limitations of, 160–161, *161,* 167
Epidemiology, of HCV infection, 1–16, 37–38, 173–174, 233
    genotype analysis in, 106–107
    geographic variance in, 1–3

temporal trends in, 2–3, *3*

F

Female(s), response to antiviral therapy in, 192
Fibrosing cholestatic hepatitis, posttransplant, 202, 206–207
Fibrosis, hepatic, in HCV infection
  assessment of, indications for, 51–52
  characteristics of, 47–48
  in children, 41
  progression of, 23, 31–32, 47, 48, *49,* 235
    assessment of, methods for, 50–51
    drugs impeding, 237
    dynamic view of, *50,* 50–51
    effects of treatment on, assessment of, 53
    estimated (indirect) rate of, 50
    estimates of, 50–51
    factors affecting, 29, 51, 108
    in HCV/HIV co-infection, 52
    and interval to development of cirrhosis, *25,* 25–26
    nonquantitative assessment of, 50–51
    observed (direct) rate of, 50
  progression to, 190
  stages of, 48, *48*
    and age at biopsy, relationship of, 49, *49*
    assessment of, during or after treatment, 53
    and inflammatory grade, correlation of, 48
    and response to antiviral therapy, 194
    as time-dependent end point, 48–50
Funding, for research on HCV infection, 237

G

Gastrointestinal side effects, of antiviral treatment, 187
Gene expression profiling, in HCV infection, 235–236
Gene therapy, 65
Genetics, and outcome of HCV infection, 29
Genome, HCV, 70, 236. *See also* RNA, HCV
  alternate reading frame in, i
  genetic variability of, 104–105
  map of, 58, *58*
  mutation rates in, 104, *105*
  plasticity of, i, iii
Genotype(s), HCV, 62, 105–107
  analysis of, 164–165
    clinical applications of, 166, 166t
    cost of, 165t
    by nucleotide sequencing and phylogenetic analysis, 164
  clinical significance of, 105–108, 188, 189t
  definition of, 105–106
  and disease severity, 29
  distribution of, 106–107
  identification of, 106
  and natural history of hepatitis, 107–108
  and outcomes, 106
    after liver transplantation, 107
  and pathogenesis of HCV infection, 107–108
  and posttransplant recurrence of HCV infection, 204–205
  and response to therapy, 108, 166, 166t, 181, 188, 189t, 193t, 193–194
    in children, 44
  screening tests for, 164–165
  subtypes of, 105–106
  and vaccine development, 214
Growth factor receptor-bound protein 2 adapter protein (Grb2) signaling, NS5A and, 76

H

Hair loss, antiviral treatment-related, 187
HBV. *See* Hepatitis B/Hepatitis B virus (HBV)
HCC. *See* Hepatocellular carcinoma (HCC)

HCV. *See* Hepatitis C infection; Hepatitis C virus (HCV)
HCV-like particles, as potential HCV vaccine, 219t, 220, *221*
Healthcare-related procedures, HCV transmission in, 4–6
Healthcare worker(s)
  HCV-infected, HCV transmission from, to patients, 5–6
  occupational exposures to HCV in, 6
Helicase. *See* DEXH helicase family; Nonstructural proteins, HCV, NS3 RNA helicase
Helper T cells. *See also* CD4 T helper cell(s); CD8 T helper cell(s)
  in antiviral defense, 130–131, *131,* 213–214
Hemodialysis patient(s)
  HCV infection in
    prevalence of, 5
    transmission of, 5
  HCV testing in, 167
Hemophilia patient(s), HCV infection in, 4
  management of, 191–192
  outcome of, 29
Hepatitis A/Hepatitis A virus (HAV), iii, v
  vaccine
    candidates for, 40
    for HCV-infected patients, 10
Hepatitis B/Hepatitis B virus (HBV)
  dynamics of, mathematical modeling of, 175, *176*
  interferon therapy in, immunomodulatory effects of, 179
  kinetics of, after antiviral therapy, 175, *176*
  replication of, v, 86
  vaccine, v
    candidates for, 40
    for HCV-infected patients, 10, 40
Hepatitis C infection
  acute
    diagnosis of, 165
    liver biopsy and, 52
    long-term follow-up of, 21–22
    outcome of, HCV quasispecies and, 115–116
    recovery rate in, 30
    self-limited, adaptive cellular immune response in, 130–131
  age at onset of, and outcomes, 29
  asymptomatic, 40
  chronic, 103–104
    adaptive cellular immune response in, 132
    in children, treatment of, 42–44, 44–45
    diagnosis of, 165
    fibrosis assessment in, 51–52
    HCV quasispecies analysis in, 118
    in HIV-infected patients, diagnosis of, 168
    in immunosuppressed patients, diagnosis of, 168
    and liver tumor, in 67-year-old male, 227–230
    natural history of, 104, 234–235
    in organ transplant recipients, diagnosis of, 167–168
    with other concurrent disease, management of, 191–192
    pathogenesis of, 19, 235
    prevalence of, 37–38
    treatment of, absolute contraindications to, 186t, 186–187
  detection of, 86
  duration of
    and fibrosis progression, 51
    and grade of activity (necroinflammation), 49, *49*
    and stage of fibrosis, 49, *49*
  dynamics of, 174–175, *175*
  immune responses to, iv, v, 104
  kinetics of. *See* Kinetics, of HCV infection
  mild histologic disease, treatment of, 189–190
  nonhepatic disease caused by, management of, 192
  pathogenesis of, 62

in patients cured of childhood leukemia, 41
recurrence of, posttransplant, rate of, 202
Hepatitis C infection *(Continued)*
severity of
cofactors as determinants of, 28–30
estimates of, influence of study design on, 20–24
spontaneous recovery from, 23, 104
in children, 24–25
rates of, 30, 31t
symptoms of, 40
transfusion-associated. *See* Blood transfusion
Hepatitis C virus (HCV)
binding to cultured cells, 19
cell and tissue tropism of, 127–128
distribution throughout the body of, 85-102
diversity of, antibody and, 19
pathogenicity of, HCV quasispecies and, 117
persistence of, mechanisms of, 19, 62, 104, 111–115,
128–129, 134t, 134–136, 214
Hepatitis E/Hepatitis E virus (HEV), v
Hepatocellular carcinoma (HCC)
development of, interferon therapy and, 44, 188–189
distribution of HCV markers in, 91–92
geographic variation in, 27–28
HCV genotype and, 107
and HCV infection
association between, 18, 26–28
research on, advances in (future directions for), 235
HCV quasispecies analysis in, 118
incidence of, 22
interval to development of, in HCV infection, *25,* 25–26
pathogenesis of, 20, 21, 26–28
prevalence of, 40
prevention of, interferon and, 27, 188–189
risk for, in HCV infection, 188–189, 235
Hepatotropism, of HCV, iv
Histologic activity index (HAI), 23, 91
HIV-infected patients, chronic HCV infection in, diagnosis
of, 168
Host-virus interplay, in HCV infection, 19
Household(s), HCV transmission within, 7, 8, 8t
Human immunodeficiency virus (HIV). *See also* Co-
infection(s), HCV/HIV; HIV-infected patients
genetic variability of, 105
Humoral immunity
in antiviral defense, 19, 104, 111–115, 128–129, 213
HCV-specific, interaction with cellular immune response,
150, *151*
Hypervariable region(s)
antibody response to, 213
of HCV genome, 105, 110–111, 112–115
antibody response to, 128–129
as immunologic decoy, 116, 129
as target for HCV vaccine, 219, 220t
Hypogammaglobulinemia
homogeneity of HCV population in, 118
outcome of HCV infection in, 29

I

Illegal drug use. *See* Intravenous drug abuse, and HCV
infection
Immune escape
as mechanism of viral persistence, 111–115, 135
through HVR1 variation, 111–115
Immune response
adaptive, HCV-specific, 130–131
innate, 65, 129–130
Immune system, and HCV, interaction between, 127–136

Immunoblot, detection of HCV proteins by, 96
Immunoglobulin, anti-HCV, and prevention of HCV
infection, 220–221
Immunohistochemistry, for in situ detection of viral antigens
in liver cells, 93
Immunology, of HCV infection, iv
Immunosuppression
chronic HCV infection in, diagnosis of, 168
HCV quasispecies and, 117–118
and outcome of HCV infection, 235
and posttransplant recurrence of HCV infection, 202–203
Infectious cloned transcript(s), 62–63
Infergen. *See* Interferon therapy, alfa-con-1
Injection drug use, and HCV infection. *See* Intravenous drug
abuse, and HCV infection
Injection practice(s). *See also* Intravenous drug abuse
unsafe, HCV transmission by, 5, 9
In situ hybridization (ISH)
for detection of extrahepatic HCV replication, 98
for detection of HCV RNA, theoretic considerations in,
88–89
for detection of HCV RNA in individual liver cells, 89–91,
92–93
for detection of HCV RNA in tumor cells, 91–93
for detection of HCV-specific markers, 86, 88–91
sensitivity of, 88
specificity of, 88
Interferon
in antiviral defense, mechanism of action of, 129
immunomodulatory effects of, 179
induction of, 129
in antiviral immune response, 63
during HCV infection, 63
inhibition of HCV production, cellular mechanisms of,
179, 179–180
Interferon sensitivity determining region (ISDR), 76
Interferon therapy
alfa-2a
cost per month of, 188t
dosage and administration of, 188t
alfa-2b
cost per month of, 188t
dosage and administration of, 188t
monotherapy with, efficacy of, 188, 189t
and ribavirin, combination of. *See* Interferon therapy,
combined with ribavirin
alfa-con-1
cost per month of, 188t
dosage and administration of, 188t
combined with ribavirin, 44
absolute contraindications to, 186t, 186–187
adverse effects and side effects of, 186–187
and cryoglobulinemia, 192
effects on fibrosis progression rate, 53
effects on HCV kinetics, 182
efficacy of, 188, 189t
for naive patients, 194–195
nonresponders to
prediction of, 195
treatment of, 196
optimum duration of, determination of, 166
for posttransplant recurrence of HCV infection, 205–206
prophylaxis with, for posttransplant HCV recurrence,
206, 207
relative contraindications to, 187
response to, 166
toxicity of, monitoring, 195–196
for HCV infection, iv-v

adverse effects and side effects in children, 43, 44
in children, 42t, 42–44
contraindications to, in psychiatric patients, 186–187
effects on fibrosis progression rate, 53
factors affecting, 236
HCV kinetics with, *176,* 176–178, *177,* 178t, 180–181, *181*
HCV resistance to, NS5A in, 76
hematologic side effects of, 187
long-term benefits in adults, 44
mechanism of action of, 236
nonresponders to
    HCV kinetics with, 181–182
    prediction of, 195
pegylated forms of interferon for, 237
and prevention of HCC, 27, 44
relapse after, retreatment of, 196
response to, predictors of, 43–44
toxicity of, monitoring, 195–196
withdrawal from, rate of, 195
for posttransplant recurrence of HCV infection, 205
    prophylactic, 206–207
response to
    HCV genotype and, 108, 166, 166t, 181, 188, 189t
    HCV quasispecies and, 119–120
    predictors of, 166, 166t
    sustained, 166–167, *167,* 181, 188
    viral load and, 166, 166t
Internal ribosome entry site (IRES), of HCV genomic RNA, 59, 89
cellular proteins binding to, 61
function of, 60–61
and HCV pathogenicity, 59–60
and HCV survival, 59–60
structure of, *60,* 60–61
Intravenous drug abuse, and HCV infection, 3–4, 8, 9, 233
management of, 236
outcome of, 29
prevention of, 234
Intron-A. *See* Interferon therapy, alfa-2b
Iron content, hepatic, and response to interferon therapy, in children, 44
Irritability, antiviral treatment-related, 187

K
Kidney transplantation, and HCV infection, management of, 192
Kinetics, of HCV RNA levels in serum, 174–182
after interferon therapy, *176,* 176–178, *177,* 178t, 180–181, *181*
HCV genotype and, 181

L
La protein, 61
Leukemia, childhood, patients cured of, outcome of HCV infection in, 41
Lichen planus, 187
Line probe, in screening for HCV genotype, 165
Liver
biopsy of, 48
    adverse events and mortality with, 51, 51t
    appropriate role of, 51
    in children with HCV infection, 41
    in chronic HCV infection, 51–52
    in diagnosis of cirrhosis, 52
    in HCV infection, 235
    methods of, 51
    normal transaminase levels and, 52

in patients with several causes of liver disease, 52
in treatment decision making, 190
histopathology of, in children with HCV infection, 41
immune-mediated injury of, mechanisms of, 133
immunology of, 129
iron content of, and response to interferon therapy, in children, 44
recruitment of T cells to, 132–133
rheumatoid factor production in, 146–147
tumor of, in HCV-infected 67-year-old male, 227–230
Liver disease
HCV-related
    mode of transmission and, 20t, 28–29
    prevention of, 9–10
    progression of, 31–32
multiple causes of, liver biopsy in patients with, 52
Liver/kidney microsomal (LKM) autoantibodies, in HCV infection, 146
Liver transplantation, for HCV infection, 18–19, 201-209
in children, 41
HCV quasispecies and, 117
HCV recurrence after
    natural history of, 202
    prophylaxis for, 206–207
    rate of, 202
    retransplant for, 207
    risk factors for, 202–205
    severity of, 202
    treatment of, 192, 205–206
numbers of, 30, 202
outcome after
    HCV genotype and, 107–108
    research on, advances in (future directions for), 235
rejection of
    HCV infection as promoter of, 203
    and posttransplant recurrence of HCV, 202–203
Low-density lipoproteins (LDL), HCV binding to, 128
L-selectin, 130
Lymphocytes, hepatic, 129
Lymphoma(s). *See also* Non-Hodgkin's lymphoma
primary hepatic, distribution of HCV markers in, 92
Lymphoproliferative disorder(s), HCV-associated, 144, 150–154
Lymphoproliferative response
to DNA vaccine, 216
in HCV infection, 145

M
Male(s)
fibrosis progression in, 51
outcome of HCV infection in, 29
Maternal-infant transmission, of HCV infection, 38
and outcome, 40
rate of, 39, 45
Mathematical model(s)
of HCV response to therapy, 175–182
of viral infection, 174–175
Matrix metalloproteinase, 48
METAVIR fibrosis staging system, 48, *48*
Model(s)
animal. *See also* Chimpanzee; Mouse
    of HCV-immune system interaction, 133–134
    for vaccine development, 214–215
mathematical. *See* Mathematical model(s)
Mouse, in HCV research, 134, 215, 217
Mycophenolate mofetil, and posttransplant recurrence of HCV infection, 204

N

Natural history, of HCV infection, 18
  factors affecting, 108
Natural history, of HCV infection *(Continued)*
  genotypes and, 107–108
  HCV quasispecies and, 116–117
  in posttransplant recurrence, 202
Natural killer cells, 129, 130
  activation of, 129–130
  function of, 130
Necroinflammation, in HCV infection, grades of, 48, *48*
NK cells. *See* Natural killer cells
NKT cells. *See* Natural killer cells
NOB assay, 214
Non-A, non-B hepatitis. *See* Hepatitis C infection
Non-Hodgkin's lymphoma
  and cryoglobulinemia, in HCV infection, management of,
    192
  HCV-associated, 144, 150–154
Nonresponders
  to combination therapy
    prediction of, 195
    treatment of, 196
  HCV kinetics in, 181–182
  to interferon alfa therapy, treatment of, 196
Nonstructural proteins, HCV, 69–80, *71,* 86, 104
  CD4 T-cell response to, 78–79
  detection in infected liver, using nonhuman antibodies,
    95–96
  immunologic properties of, 78–80, 130, 132, 133, 150, 165,
    179–180, 213–214, 216
  localization in mixed cryoglobulinemia, 98–99
  NS4A (p8) protein, 70, *71*
  NS5A (p56/p58) protein, 70, *71, 179,* 179–180
    function of, 75–77
    molecular architecture of, *75,* 76
    posttranslational modification of, 75–77
  NS3/4A proteinase, 70, *72,* 72–74
  NS4B (p27) protein, 70, *71*
  NS5B (p68)/RNA-dependent RNA polymerase, 77–78
    crystal structure of, *77,* 77–78
  NS2 (p23) protein, 70, *71*
  NS3 (p70) protein, 70, *71*
  NS2/3 proteinase, 70–72
  NS3 RNA helicase, 74–75
Nontranslated region(s) (NTR), of HCV genomic RNA
  3', 58, *58,* 104–105
    structure and function of, 61–62
  5', 58, *58,* 59, 89–90, 104–105
    of different genotypes/strains, translational efficiencies
      of, 59–60
    structure of, *60,* 61, *61*

O

Occupational exposure(s), to HCV, 6
  infection rate for, 8
OKT3. *See* Tacrolimus
2',5'-Oligo(A) synthetase(s), in antiviral defense, 64, 179
Open reading frame (ORF), of HCV genomic RNA, 58, *58,*
    61, 70, 104–105
Organ donor(s), screening of, 167
Organ transplantation. *See also* Kidney transplantation; Liver
    transplantation
  HCV transmission by, 4, 9
Organ transplant recipient(s), chronic HCV infection in,
    diagnosis of, 168
Outcome(s), of HCV infection
  in acute hepatitis, 21–22
  after development of cirrhosis, 26, 26t

  in children, 24–25
    with parenteral transmission, 40–41
    with transfusion-related HCV infection, 40–41
  in cohorts studied long after defined parenteral exposure,
    20t, 22–24
  with maternal-infant transmission, 40
  measurement of, influence of study design on, 19–21
  in patients with chronic liver disease, 19–21
  in severe hepatitis, projection of, *31,* 31–33, *32*
  of transfusion-related HCV infection, 20–22, 40–41

P

Pan troglodyte. See Chimpanzee
Passive immunization, against HCV, 220–221
Pediatric population, HCV infection in, 37-40 *See also*
    Child(ren)
Peptide vaccine, against HCV infection, 218–219, 219t
Perinatal transmission, of HCV, 6, 7t
  evaluation of newborns for, 168
  outcome of infection after, 40
Peripheral blood monocytes, HCV markers in, detection of,
    97–99
Pharmacotherapy, of HCV infection, advances in (future
    directions for), 236–237
PKR (dsRNA activated protein kinase), 63–65, 76, 129, 135
  interaction with HCV genome, *179,* 179–180
  signaling, NS5A and, 76, 180
Poliovirus, 59
Polymerase chain reaction (PCR) assay. *See also* Reverse
    transcriptase polymerase chain reaction
  for determination of viral load, 163–164, *164*
    clinical applications of, 165
  for HCV genotype determination, 164–165
  in situ
    for detection of extrahepatic HCV replication, 98
    for detection of HCV RNA in individual liver cells, 91
Polyprotein processing, HCV, 70, *71*
Polypyrimidine tract binding protein (PTB), 61
p7 polypeptide, 70
Pregnancy, interferon/ribavirin therapy contraindicated in,
    186
Prevalence, of HCV infection, 18, 37–38
  age-specific, 2–3, *3*
    temporal trends in, 2–3, *3*
  in children, 24
  in dialysis patients, 5
  global, 2, *2*
  in hospital-related settings, 5
Prevention
  of HCV infection, 233
    advances in (future directions for), 234
    primary, 9
    secondary, 9–10
  of posttransplant recurrence of HCV infection, 206–207
Progression, of HCV infection, determination of, methods for,
    235–236
Prostitutes, female, prevalence of HCV infection in, 7, 7t
Protein(s), HCV. *See also* Nonstructural proteins, HCV;
    Structural proteins, HCV
  detection of, by immunoblot, 96
Psychiatric disorder(s), patients with, interferon/ribavirin
    therapy contraindicated in, 186–187

Q

Quality of life, in chronic HCV infection, treatment and,
    190–191
Quasispecies
  definition of, 19, 62, 108
  HCV, 19, 108–111

analysis of, methods for, 109–110

characterization of, 109–110

clinical implications of, 29, 111–120, 135–136

compartmentalization of, 118

composition of, 109–110, *110*

diversity of, and disease outcome, 29

evolution of, 109–110, *110*

    during acute hepatitis, 115

    in immunosuppressed patients, 117–118

genetic complexity of, 109, 110–111, *111*

genetic diversity of, 109, 110–111, *112–113,* 135

and natural history of HCV infection, 116–117, 135–136

and outcome of acute hepatitis, 115–116

and response to antiviral therapy, 119–120, 194

and vaccine development, 214

and viral transmission, 118–119

R

Race

    and outcome of HCV infection, 235

    and response to antiviral therapy, 192

Rapamycin, and posttransplant recurrence of HCV infection, 204

Rebetron. *See* Interferon therapy, combined with ribavirin

Recombinant immunoblot assay (RIBA), for anti-HCV antibodies, 161–162, *162*

    cost of, 165t

Recombinant subunit protein subunit vaccine, against HCV infection, 219t, 219–220

Recombinant viruses, in HCV vaccine development, 217–218, 218t

Relapse, after interferon alfa monotherapy, treatment of, 196

Renal failure

    chronic, HCV testing in, 167

    and HCV infection, management of, 192

    ribavirin therapy contraindicated in, 187

Replication, HCV, 59, 92

    detection of, 86

    extrahepatic, 97–99, 118, 127–128

    hepatic, 127–128

    in liver cells

        determination of, by in situ detection of viral antigens, 93–97

        evidence for, determined by ISH detection of HCV, 88–91

    markers of, detection of, 86–88

    molecular mechanisms of, 77, 86, *87*

    NS5A in, 76

    rate of, iv-v

    studies of, experimental material for, 62–63

Replication intermediates, HCV, 86, *87*

    and interferon induction, 63

Replicative intermediates. *See* Replication intermediates, HCV

Replicon(s), 62–63, 65

Research, on HCV infection

    advances in (future directions for), 234–237

    funding for, 237

Restriction fragment length polymorphism (RFLP), in screening for HCV genotype, 164

Reverse transcriptase polymerase chain reaction

    for analysis of HCV quasispecies, 109–110

    for detection of extrahepatic HCV replication, 97–98

    for detection of HCV RNA, 162–163, *163*

    for detection of HCV-specific markers, 86–88

Rheumatoid factor

    in HCV infection, 144

    in mixed cryoglobulinemia, 148–150, *149*

    production in liver, 146–147

    somatic mutations of, 150

Rh immune globulin, HCV-contaminated, outcomes after administration of, 23–24

Ribavirin therapy for HCV infection

    hemolytic effects of, 187

    mechanism of action of, 236

    "substitutes" for, 236

    teratogenicity of, 186

    and interferon, combination of. *See* Interferon therapy, combined with ribavirin

    for posttransplant recurrence of HCV infection, 205

Ribozyme

    crystal structure of, 61, *61*

    therapeutic, for HCV infection, 65

Risk factor(s), for HCV infection, 3–9, 233

    individuals with, HCV testing in, 10, 39–40

    in posttransplant recurrence, 202–205

    reduction of, advances in (future directions for), 234

RNA, HCV

    antigenomic, 58

        structural elements in, 59–62

    in contamination, 86

    detection of

        in individual liver cells, 89–91

        in tumor cells, 91–92

    double-stranded (dsRNA) replicative form, 58, 86

    genomic, 58

        landmarks of, 58–59

        structural elements in, 59–62

    and immune responses, 63–65

    input positive sense, 86, *87*

    and interferon induction, 63

    measurement of, after treatment cessation, 195–196

    negative sense, 86, *87*

        detection of, by ISH, 89

    populations of, 62

    replication of, 58

    single-strand (ssRNA), 58

    as target for antiviral drugs, 65

    tests for

        qualitative, 159, 162–163, 193

            clinical applications of, 165, 167

            cost of, 165t

        quantitative, 163–164, *164,* 193

            clinical applications of, 166, 166t

            cost of, 165t

    variants of, 62

RNA, VAI, 64

RNA, viral, double-stranded

    binding proteins, in antiviral state, 63–65

    and interferon induction, 63

    thermal denaturation of, 63, *64*

RNA-dependent RNA polymerase, 77–78

    crystal structure of, *77,* 77–78

RNA replicase, drugs active against, 237

RNase L, 64–65, 179

RNA virus(es)

    genetic variability of, 104–105

    plus strand, 59t

    positive sense, HCV as, 58

    quasispecies nature of, 108–109

Roferon-A. *See* Interferon therapy, alfa-2a

RT-PCR. *See* Reverse transcriptase polymerase chain reaction

S

Scarification, HCV transmission by, 8

Screening

    for anti-HCV antibodies, assays for, 160–161

    of blood donors, 167

    for HCV genotype, 164–165

Screening *(Continued)*
    of hemodialysis patients, 167
    of organ donors, 167
    of persons at high risk for HCV infection, 39–40
Serotyping assay(s), for HCV genotype determination, 165
Sex differences, in response to antiviral therapy in, 29, 192
Sexual activity
    HCV transmission by, prevention of, 9, 10
    high risk
        and HCV transmission, 8
        prevention of, 234
    transmission of HCV by, 6–8
Simulect, 204
Smoking, and outcome of HCV infection, research on, 235
Smooth muscle autoantibodies, in HCV infection, 146
Societal burden, of HCV infection, 18
Spastic diplegia, in children, interferon therapy and, 44
Spouse(s), HCV transmission between, 7, 8t
Stellate cell(s), 48
Steroid therapy, and posttransplant recurrence of HCV
        infection, 202–203
Structural proteins, HCV, in infected liver, detection using
        nonhuman antibodies, 94–95
Superantigens, B-cell, 145
Surveillance, epidemiologic, need for, 233

T
Tacrolimus, and posttransplant recurrence of HCV infection,
        203–204
Tattooing, HCV transmission by, 8–9
T-cell responses
    in antiviral defense, 79–80, 130–131
    HCV-specific, 80–81, 132–133
Testing, HCV, 159–168
    in blood donor screening, 167
    in children, 168
    clinical applications of, 165–168
    in diagnosis of acute hepatitis C, 165
    in diagnosis of chronic hepatitis C, 165
    in hemodialysis units, 167
    in immunosuppressed patients, 167–168
    methods for, 160–165
    in organ donor screening, 167
    in organ transplant recipients, 167–168
    in special situations, 167–168
    before treatment, 166
    during and after treatment, 166–167
Thalassemia, HCV infection in, management of, 44, 191
Thyroiditis, antiviral treatment-related, 187
Transaminase(s)
    increased levels of, anti-HIV treatments and, 52
    normal levels of, and liver biopsy, 52
Transmission, of HCV infection, iii-iv, 233. *See also*
        Maternal-infant transmission
    blocking, advances in (future directions for), 234
    in children, 38–39
    female-to-male, 7
    HCV quasispecies and, 117, 118–119
    male-to-female, 7
    male-to-male, 7t, 7–8
    mode of, and outcome, 20t, 28–29
        in children, 40–41
    nosocomial, 4–6
    parenteral, in children, 38
    patterns of, 3–9
    perinatal. *See* Perinatal transmission
    selective, 118–119
Treatment, of HCV infection. *See also* Antiviral therapy;
        Interferon therapy; Ribavirin therapy

    advances in (future directions for), 45, 236–237
    broad-spectrum approach to, 237
    in children, 42t, 42–44
    costs of, 186
    currently licensed therapies for, 188, 188t
    current status of, 236
    drug combinations for, advances in (future directions for),
        237
    effects on quality of life, in chronic HCV infection,
        190–191
    efficacy of, 186
    follow-up studies of, need for, 236–237
    in mild histologic disease, 189–190
    schedules for, in naive patients, 194–195
    standard of care in, 188
    success rate of, 186
    trials of, advances in (future directions for), 237
Tupaia belangeri, 214–215

V
Vaccine(s)
    development of
        newer approaches to, *212,* 212–213
        traditional approaches to, 212, *212*
    HAV
        candidates for, 40
        for HCV-infected patients, 10
    HBV, v
        candidates for, 40
        for HCV-infected patients, 10, 40
    HCV
        advances in (future directions for), v, 66, 222, 234
        combination modality, 221–222
        development of, 211–222
            DNA immunization approaches for, *212,* 212–213,
                215t, 215–217
            multicomponent approach to, 221–222
            obstacles to, 214t, 214–215
            recombinant viral approaches to, 217–218, 218t
        peptide, 218–219, 219t
        protective versus therapeutic, 234
    live attenuated, 212, *212*
    recombinant subunit, *212,* 212–213, 219t, 219–220
    subunit, *212,* 212–213
    whole-organism, 212, *212*
VAI RNA, 64
Vertical transmission, of HCV infection. *See* Maternal-infant
        transmission
Viral infection
    dynamics of, 174–175, *175*
    mathematical models of, 174–175
Viral load
    determination of, 163–164, *164*
    and disease outcome, 29
    and maternal-infant transmission of HCV, 38, 39
    and posttransplant recurrence of HCV infection, 204
    and response to antiviral therapy, 193–194, *194*
    and response to interferon therapy, 166, 166t
Viral titer. *See* Viral load

W
Weight loss, antiviral treatment-related, 187

Z
Zinc-dependent metalloproteinase, 70–71